M. Kaminishi, K. Takubo, K. Mafune (Eds.)

The Diversity of Gastric Carcinoma

Pathogenesis, Diagnosis, and Therapy

M. Kaminishi, K. Takubo, K. Mafune (Eds.)

The Diversity of Gastric Carcinoma

Pathogenesis, Diagnosis, and Therapy

With 172 Figures, Including 97 in Color

Springer

Michio Kaminishi, M.D., Ph.D.
Departments of Gastrointestinal Surgery, Surgical Metabolic Care and Endocrine Surgery, The University of Tokyo Graduate School of Medicine
7-3-1 Hongo, Bunkyo-ku, Tokyo 113-8655, Japan

Kaiyo Takubo, M.D., Ph.D.
Human Tissue Research Group, Tokyo Metropolitan Institute of Gerontology
35-2 Sakaecho, Itabashi-ku, Tokyo 173-0015, Japan

Ken-ichi Mafune, M.D., Ph.D., F.A.C.S.
Department of Gastrointestinal Surgery
The University of Tokyo Graduate School of Medicine
7-3-1 Hongo, Bunkyo-ku, Tokyo 113-8655, Japan

This book was financially supported by the Japan Society for the Promotion of Science (Grant-in-Aid for Publication of Scientific Research Results: Grant No. 175300).

Library of Congress Control Number: 2005921446

ISBN 4-431-21139-X Springer-Verlag Tokyo Berlin Heidelberg New York

Springer is a part of Springer Science+Business Media
springeronline.com

Typesetting: SNP Best-set Typesetter Ltd., Hong Kong
Printing and binding: Shinano, Inc., Japan

Printed on acid-free paper

Foreword

It is an honor to be asked to comment on the occasion of the publication of *The Diversity of Gastric Carcinoma: Pathogenesis, Diagnosis, and Therapy*, edited by Prof. Michio Kaminishi, Dr. Takubo, and Dr. Mafune. This book provides a very valuable, wide coverage of molecular carcinogenesis and prevention, through to diagnosis and treatment of stomach neoplasia. A particularly important aspect for gastric cancer control is the biological diversity of the tumors themselves. The stomach is a complicated organ, and the cardiac and pyloric portions have different cellular compositions and functions. The many types of cells are in a constant flux of differentiation from stem cells. Precancerous conditions such as intestinal metaplasia and atrophic gastritis are well known, and there are various factors that have already been established as promoting cancer development. They include sodium chloride intake, infection of *Helicobacter pylori*, and the host genetic background. It is therefore not surprising that stomach cancers demonstrate great diversity in their biological and clinical behavior. The practical consequence is that the clinical handling that is most suitable for each individual patient is also diverse. Each chapter of this volume is well presented by authors who are specialized in fundamental and clinical sciences and who are currently active at the forefront of their own fields. The entire book is compiled taking into account the most up-to-date knowledge, with a balanced viewpoint. This book should be widely recommended to researchers and clinicians dealing with one of most ugly and common diseases of mankind, gastric cancer.

Takashi Sugimura
President Emeritus, National Cancer Center
Chairman of Section II, The Japan Academy

Preface

Gastric cancer is still the second leading cause of cancer death worldwide, although the incidence of this disease has been gradually decreasing. Vigorous research on the mechanisms of gastric cancer development, invasion, and metastasis is required to establish prevention, early detection, and precise therapies for gastric cancer.

The diversity of gastric cancer is well known. In terms of histological classification, gastric carcinoma is divided into five types according to the general rules for gastric carcinoma of the Japanese Gastric Cancer Association. Compared with other gastroenterological carcinomas, it is characteristic in gastric cancer that respective histological types develop at a constant rate. Therefore, on the basis of clinicopathological features, gastric carcinoma is divided into two major types: diffuse and intestinal in Lauren's classification; differentiated and undifferentiated in Nakamura's classification; and gastric and intestinal phenotype by mucin immunohistochemistry. In addition, genetic and epigenetic alterations in gastric carcinogenesis have been postulated. Sex and age differences in the incidence and clinicopathological features also have been given attention. Analysis of the underlying mechanisms of the diversity of gastric carcinogenesis is likely to provide the development of not only early detection and tailor-made therapies but also prevention of gastric cancer.

In this book, the following major topics are addressed: the history of clinical and experimental gastric cancer research; undated issues of molecular and pathological research on gastric carcinogenesis; multidisciplinary methods in diagnosis, treatment and chemotherapy; and perspectives in minimally invasive surgery. We hope this book will provide a comprehensive knowledge of gastric cancer and will encourage further development of gastric cancer research and its clinical application.

We would like to express our deepest appreciation to those who have contributed their work to this book.

April 2005, Tokyo

M. Kaminishi
K. Takubo
K. Mafune

Contents

Figures in color appear at the end of each chapter in this book, regardless of the sequence of the figure numbers.

Part 4 Clinical Diagnosis

Part 5 Therapy for Gastric Carcinoma

Contributors

Aikou, Takashi (p. 329)
Department of Surgical Oncology and Digestive Surgery, Kagoshima University School of Medicine, 8-35-1 Sakuragaoka, Kagoshima 890-8520, Japan

Arai, Tomio (pp. 151, 159)
Department of Pathology, Tokyo Metropolitan Geriatric Medical Center, 35-2 Sakaecho, Itabashi-ku, Tokyo 173-0015, Japan

Arai, Yasuaki (p. 221)
Diagnostic Radiology Division, National Cancer Center Hospital, National Cancer Center, 5-1-1 Tsukiji, Chuo-ku, Tokyo 104-0045, Japan

Chong, Ja-Mun (p. 127)
Department of Human Pathology, The University of Tokyo Graduate School of Medicine, 7-3-1 Hongo, Bunkyo-ku, Tokyo 113-0033, Japan

Etoh, Tsuyoshi (p. 287)
Department of Surgery I, Oita University Faculty of Medicine, Hasama-machi, Oita 879-5593, Japan

Fujii, Hirofumi (p. 339)
Department of Radiology, Keio University School of Medicine, 35 Shinanomachi, Shinjuku-ku, Tokyo 160-8582, Japan

Fujishiro, Mitsuhiro (p. 243)
Department of Gastroenterology, The University of Tokyo Graduate School of Medicine, 7-3-1 Hongo, Bunkyo-ku, Tokyo, Japan

Fukayama, Masashi (p. 127)
Department of Human Pathology, The University of Tokyo Graduate School of Medicine, 7-3-1 Hongo, Bunkyo-ku, Tokyo 113-0033, Japan

Furukawa, Toshiharu (p. 339)
Department of Surgery, Keio University School of Medicine, 35 Shinanomachi, Shinjuku-ku, Tokyo 160-8582, Japan

Goldenring, James R. (p. 87)
Nashville VA Medical Center and the Department of Surgery, Epithelial Biology Program, Vanderbilt-Ingram Cancer Center, Vanderbilt University School of Medicine, Nashville, TN, USA

Hashimoto, Masanori (p. 203)
Department of Surgery, International Medical Center of Japan, 1-21-1 Toyama, Shinjuku-ku, Tokyo 162-8655, Japan

Hasuo, Tadateru (p. 169)
Division of Surgical Pathology, Department of Biomedical Informatics, Kobe University Graduate School of Medicine, 7-5-1 Kusunoki-cho, Chuo-ku, Kobe 650-0017, Japan

Hokita, Shuichi (p. 329)
Department of Surgical Oncology and Digestive Surgery, Kagoshima University School of Medicine, 8-35-1 Sakuragaoka, Kagoshima 890-8520, Japan

Hayashi, Yoshinori (p. 185)
Third Department of Internal Medicine, Nippon Medical School, 1-1-5 Sendagi, Bunkyo-ku, Tokyo 113-8603, Japan

Iinuma, Gen (p. 221)
Cancer Screening Division, Research Center for Cancer Prevention and Screening, National Cancer Center, 5-1-1 Tsukiji, Chuo-ku, Tokyo 104-0045, Japan

Ishigami, Sumiya (p. 329)
Department of Surgical Oncology and Digestive Surgery, Kagoshima University School of Medicine, 8-35-1 Sakuragaoka, Kagoshima 890-8520, Japan

Ishikura, Hiroshi (p. 139)
Department of Molecular Pathology, Chiba University Graduate School of Medicine, 1-8-1 Inohana, Chuo-ku, Chiba, Japan

Iwakiri, Katsuhiko (p. 185)
Third Department of Internal Medicine, Nippon Medical School, 1-1-5 Sendagi, Bunkyo-ku, Tokyo 113-8603, Japan

Kamata, Shigeyuki (p. 139)
Departments of Molecular Pathology and General Surgery, Chiba University Graduate School of Medicine, 1-8-1 Inohana, Chuo-ku, Chiba, Japan

Kameyama, Kaori (p. 339)
Department of Pathology, Keio University School of Medicine, 35 Shinanomachi, Shinjuku-ku, Tokyo 160-8582, Japan

Kaminishi, Michio (pp. 75, 87, 203, 253)
Department of Gastrointestinal Surgery, The University of Tokyo Graduate School of Medicine, 7-3-1 Hongo, Bunkyo-ku, Tokyo 113-8655, Japan

Kaneda, Atsushi (p. 97)
Carcinogenesis Division, National Cancer Center Research Institute, 5-1-1 Tsukiji, Chuo-ku, Tokyo 104-0045, Japan

Kishimoto, Takashi (p. 139)
Department of Molecular Pathology, Chiba University Graduate School of Medicine, 1-8-1 Inohana, Chuo-ku, Chiba, Japan

Kitadai, Yasuhiko (p. 51)
Department of Medicine and Molecular Science, Hiroshima University Graduate School of Biomedical Sciences, 1-2-3 Kasumi, Minami-ku, Hiroshima 734-8551, Japan

Kitagawa, Yuko (p. 339)
Department of Surgery, Keio University School of Medicine, 35 Shinanomachi, Shinjuku-ku, Tokyo 160-8582, Japan

Kitajima, Masaki (p. 339)
Department of Surgery, Keio University School of Medicine, 35 Shinanomachi, Shinjuku-ku, Tokyo 160-8582, Japan

Kitano, Seigo (p. 287)
Department of Surgery I, Oita University Faculty of Medicine, Hasama-machi, Oita 879-5593, Japan

Kobayashi, Toshiaki (p. 221)
Cancer Screening Technology Division, Research Center for Cancer Prevention and Screening, National Cancer Center, 5-1-1 Tsukiji, Chuo-ku, Tokyo 104-0045, Japan

Kojima, Kazuhiro (p. 139)
Departments of Molecular Pathology and General Surgery, Chiba University Graduate School of Medicine, 1-8-1 Inohana, Chuo-ku, Chiba, Japan

Kubo, Atsushi (p. 339)
Department of Radiology, Keio University School of Medicine, 35 Shinanomachi, Shinjuku-ku, Tokyo 160-8582, Japan

Kubota, Tetsuro (p. 339)
Department of Surgery, Keio University School of Medicine, 35 Shinanomachi, Shinjuku-ku, Tokyo 160-8582, Japan

Kumai, Koichiro (p. 339)
Center for Diagnostic and Therapeutic Endoscopy, Keio University School of Medicine, 35 Shinanomachi, Shinjuku-ku, Tokyo 160-8582, Japan

Lee, Jeffrey R. (p. 87)
Institute of Molecular Medicine and Genetics, Medical College of Georgia, Augusta, GA, USA

Li, Dong (p. 169)
Division of Surgical Pathology, Department of Biomedical Informatics, Kobe University Graduate School of Medicine, 7-5-1 Kusunoki-cho, Chuo-ku, Kobe 650-0017, Japan

Maeda, Tetsuo (p. 221)
Diagnostic Radiology Division, National Cancer Center Hospital, National Cancer Center, 5-1-1 Tsukiji, Chuo-ku, Tokyo 104-0045, Japan

Mafune, Ken-ichi (p. 271)
Department of Gastrointestinal Surgery, The University of Tokyo Graduate School of Medicine, 7-3-1 Hongo, Bunkyo-ku, Tokyo 113-8655, Japan

Matsumoto, Masataka (p. 329)
Department of Surgical Oncology and Digestive Surgery, Kagoshima University School of Medicine, 8-35-1 Sakuragaoka, Kagoshima 890-8520, Japan

Miyakawa, Kunihisa (p. 221)
Diagnostic Radiology Division, National Cancer Center Hospital, National Cancer Center, 5-1-1 Tsukiji, Chuo-ku, Tokyo 104-0045, Japan

Miyazono, Futoshi (p. 329)
Department of Surgical Oncology and Digestive Surgery, Kagoshima University School of Medicine, 8-35-1 Sakuragaoka, Kagoshima 890-8520, Japan

Mizoshita, Tsutomu (p. 3)
Division of Oncological Pathology, Aichi Cancer Center Research Institute, 1-1 Kanokoden, Chikusa-ku, Nagoya 464-8681, Japan

Moriyama, Noriyuki (p. 221)
Cancer Screening Division, Research Center for Cancer Prevention and Screening, National Cancer Center, 5-1-1 Tsukiji, Chuo-ku, Tokyo 104-0045, Japan

Mukai, Makio (p. 339)
Department of Pathology, Keio University School of Medicine, 35 Shinanomachi, Shinjuku-ku, Tokyo 160-8582, Japan

Muramatsu, Yukio (p. 221)
Cancer Screening Division, Research Center for Cancer Prevention and Screening, National Cancer Center, 5-1-1 Tsukiji, Chuo-ku, Tokyo 104-0045, Japan

Nakajima, Toshifusa (p. 29)
Cancer Institute Hospital, Japanese Foundation for Cancer Research (JFCR), Tokyo, Japan

Nakajo, Akihiro (p. 329)
Department of Surgical Oncology and Digestive Surgery, Kagoshima University School of Medicine, 8-35-1 Sakuragaoka, Kagoshima 890-8520, Japan

Nakaya, Hiroki (p. 139)
Department of Gastroenterology and Hematology, Hokkaido University Graduate School of Medicine, Sapporo, Japan

Nakayama, Hirofumi (p. 51)
Department of Molecular Pathology, Hiroshima University Graduate School of Biomedical Sciences, 1-2-3 Kasumi, Minami-ku, Hiroshima 734-8551, Japan

Natsugoe, Shoji (p. 329)
Department of Surgical Oncology and Digestive Surgery, Kagoshima University School of Medicine, 8-35-1 Sakuragaoka, Kagoshima 890-8520, Japan

Ohkura, Yasuo (p. 117)
Department of Pathology, Kyorin University School of Medicine, 6-20-2 Shinkawa, Mitaka, Tokyo 181-8611, Japan

Ohtsu, Atsushi (p. 299)
Division of Gastrointestinal Oncology/Digestive Endoscopy, National Cancer Center Hospital East, 6-5-1 Kashiwanoha, Kashiwa, Chiba 277-8577, Japan

Okumura, Hiroshi (p. 329)
Department of Surgical Oncology and Digestive Surgery, Kagoshima University School of Medicine, 8-35-1 Sakuragaoka, Kagoshima 890-8520, Japan

Omura, Kenji (p. 311)
General and Cardiovascular Surgery, Kanazawa University School of Medicine, 13-1 Takaramachi, Kanazawa 920-8641, Japan

Otani, Yoshihide (p. 339)
Department of Surgery, Keio University School of Medicine, 35 Shinanomachi, Shinjuku-ku, Tokyo 160-8582, Japan

Oue, Naohide (p. 51)
Department of Molecular Pathology, Hiroshima University Graduate School of Biomedical Sciences, 1-2-3 Kasumi, Minami-ku, Hiroshima 734-8551, Japan

Saikawa, Yoshiro (p. 339)
Department of Surgery, Keio University School of Medicine, 35 Shinanomachi, Shinjuku-ku, Tokyo 160-8582, Japan

Saito, Hiroshi (p. 221)
Cancer Screening Technology Division, Research Center for Cancer Prevention and Screening, National Cancer Center, 5-1-1 Tsukiji, Chuo-ku, Tokyo 104-0045, Japan

Sakamoto, Choitsu (p. 185)
Third Department of Internal Medicine, Nippon Medical School, 1-1-5 Sendagi, Bunkyo-ku, Tokyo 113-8603, Japan

Sasako, Mitsuru (p. 235)
Gastric Surgery Division, National Cancer Center Hospital, 5-1-1 Tsukiji, Chuo-ku, Tokyo 104-0045, Japan

Satake, Mitsuo (p. 221)
Diagnostic Radiology Division, National Cancer Center Hospital, National Cancer Center, 5-1-1 Tsukiji, Chuo-ku, Tokyo 104-0045, Japan

Semba, Shuho (p. 169)
Division of Surgical Pathology, Department of Biomedical Informatics, Kobe University Graduate School of Medicine, 7-5-1 Kusunoki-cho, Chuo-ku, Kobe 650-0017, Japan

Shimizu, Nobuyuki (p. 75)
Department of Gastrointestinal Surgery, The University of Tokyo Graduate School of Medicine, 7-3-1 Hongo, Bunkyo-ku, Tokyo 113-8655, Japan

Shimoyama, Shouji (pp. 203, 253)
Department of Gastrointestinal Surgery, The University of Tokyo Graduate School of Medicine, 7-3-1 Hongo, Bunkyo-ku, Tokyo 113-8655, Japan

Shiraishi, Norio (p. 287)
Department of Surgery I, Oita University Faculty of Medicine, Hasama-machi, Oita 879-5593, Japan

Stolte, Manfred (p. 109)
Institute of Pathology, Klinikum Bayreuth, Preuschwitzer Str. 101, 95445 Bayreuth, Germany

Supriatna, Yana (p. 139)
Department of Molecular Pathology, Chiba University Graduate School of Medicine, 1-8-1 Inohana, Chuo-ku, Chiba, Japan

Takao, Sonshin (p. 329)
Department of Surgical Oncology and Digestive Surgery, Kagoshima University School of Medicine, 8-35-1 Sakuragaoka, Kagoshima 890-8520, Japan

Takubo, Kaiyo (p. 151)
Human Tissue Research Group, Tokyo Metropolitan Institute of Gerontology, 35-2 Sakaecho, Itabashi-ku, Tokyo 173-0015, Japan

Tatematsu, Masae (pp. 3, 75)
Division of Oncological Pathology, Aichi Cancer Center Research Institute, 1-1 Kanokoden, Chikusa-ku, Nagoya 464-8681, Japan

Tokuda, Koki (p. 329)
Department of Surgical Oncology and Digestive Surgery, Kagoshima University School of Medicine, 8-35-1 Sakuragaoka, Kagoshima 890-8520, Japan

Tomimatsu, Hideto (p. 221)
Cancer Screening Division, Research Center for Cancer Prevention and Screening, National Cancer Center, 5-1-1 Tsukiji, Chuo-ku, Tokyo 104-0045, Japan

Tsukamoto, Tetsuya (p. 3)
Division of Oncological Pathology, Aichi Cancer Center Research Institute, 1-1 Kanokoden, Chikusa-ku, Nagoya 464-8681, Japan

Uozaki, Hiroshi (p. 127)
Department of Human Pathology, The University of Tokyo Graduate School of Medicine, 7-3-1 Hongo, Bunkyo-ku, Tokyo 113-0033, Japan

Vieth, Michael (p. 109)
Institute of Pathology, University of Magdeburg, Leipziger Str. 44, 39120 Magdeburg, Germany

Wakao, Fumihiko (p. 221)
Diagnostic Radiology Division, National Cancer Center Hospital, National Cancer Center, 5-1-1 Tsukiji, Chuo-ku, Tokyo 104-0045, Japan

Yamaguchi, Hirokazu (p. 87)
Department of Gastrointestinal Surgery, The University of Tokyo Graduate School of Medicine, 7-3-1 Hongo, Bunkyo-ku, Tokyo 113-8655, Japan
Institute of Molecular Medicine and Genetics, Medical College of Georgia, Augusta, GA, USA

Yasuda, Hidemitsu (p. 203)
Department of Surgery, International Medical Center of Japan, 1-21-1 Toyama, Shinjuku-ku, Tokyo 162-8655, Japan

Yasui, Wataru (p. 51)
Department of Molecular Pathology, Hiroshima University Graduate School of Biomedical Sciences, 1-2-3 Kasumi, Minami-ku, Hiroshima 734-8551, Japan

Yokozaki, Hiroshi (p. 169)
Division of Surgical Pathology, Department of Biomedical Informatics, Kobe University Graduate School of Medicine, 7-5-1 Kusunoki-cho, Chuo-ku, Kobe 650-0017, Japan

Yoshida, Masashi (p. 339)
Department of Surgery, Keio University School of Medicine, 35 Shinanomachi, Shinjuku-ku, Tokyo 160-8582, Japan

Part 1

History of Gastric Carcinoma Research

History of Gastric Carcinoma Research in Japan: Basic Aspects

Masae Tatematsu, Tetsuya Tsukamoto, and Tsutomu Mizoshita

Introduction

Human gastric cancers histologically present with various morphological structures, which is one of the most characteristic features compared with other digestive apparatus carcinomas. Great variation may even be evident within the same gastric cancerous mucosa. Many pathological and biological analyses of gastric carcinomas, including precancerous lesions, have been performed with human samples and experimental animals, and in this chapter we focus on the history of gastric carcinoma research in Japan from the point of view of basic aspects, concentrating especial attention on pathological findings.

Experimental Animals and Gastric Carcinomas

In general, spontaneous adenocarcinomas of the glandular stomach are very rare in experimental animals, although Oettle et al. reported an incidence of more than 40% in animals dying from natural causes in their *Mastomys* (*Praomys natalensis*) colony [1,2]. The tumor cells arising in the glandular stomach of old males and females were found to contain argyrophil granules when tissues fixed in formalin were colored with solutions of silver salts [3]. In short, the tumors were not gastric cancers, but rather carcinoids.

Since the 1930s, attempts to experimentally induce stomach cancers in animal have been performed by many researchers using several carcinogens such as benzo[*a*]pyrene, 3-methylcholanthrene, and 2-acethylaminofluorene [4–6]. However, the incidences of experimentally induced stomach cancer were low in all animal models, and it was only in 1967 that Sugimura et al. were able to report good yields of adenocarcinomas in the glandular stomachs of rats treated with *N*-methyl-*N*′-nitro-*N*-nitrosoguanidine (MNNG) [7]. Tumors were selectively produced with very high

Division of Oncological Pathology, Aichi Cancer Center Research Institute, 1-1 Kanokoden, Chikusa-ku, Nagoya 464-8681, Japan
e-mail: mtatemat@aichi-cc.jp

frequency when MNNG was continuously administered as a solution in drinking water [7]. In the pyloric mucosa of the rat glandular stomach thus exposed to MNNG, erosive lesions occur. Second, disordering of glandular structures and proliferation of pyloric mucosa are observed. Then, atypical glands and gastric cancer cells become detectable, and finally both differentiated and undifferentiated gastric carcinomas mimicking the histological types of human gastric cancer are induced in this model. In hamsters and dogs, MNNG also proved to be a gastric carcinogen. Oral administration of the carcinogen to hamsters at a concentration of 50–83 μg/ml in the drinking water resulted in a high incidence of tumors in the glandular stomach [8,9]. Similarly, production of stomach cancer in dogs by MNNG has been well documented [10], and with these animals it is possible to perform endoscopic observation and take stomach biopsies on a sequential basis. The presence of surfactants, such as alkylbenzenesulfonate, enhances the effect of carcinogens in the stomach of animals [11,12]. Dr. Sugimurag's group at National Cancer Center Research Institute in Tokyo has pioneered and established most of studies of experimental gastric carcinogenesis.

Stomach cancers also occur in experimental animals such as the rat, hamster, and dog given *N*-ethyl-*N'*-nitro-*N*-nitrosoguanidine (ENNG) [13,14]. Oral administration of 4-nitroquinoline 1-oxide (4-NQO) and 4-hydroxyaminoquinoline 1-oxide (4-HAQO) similarly induces carcinomas in the stomach as well as various other tissues [15,16]. However, the yields of gastric carcinomas using these chemical carcinogens are lower than with in MNNG.

The glandular stomach of mice has generally been found to be relatively resistant to carcinogen action, and administration of MNNG in the drinking water to BRSUNT/NJms mice over the life span only resulted in adenomatous hyperplasia of gastric epithelium [17]. In 1992, however, Tatematsu et al. reported induction of adenocarcinomas in the glandular stomach of BALB/c mice treated with *N*-methyl-*N*-nitrosourea (MNU) [18]. Reasonable yields were also obtained in C3H mice treated with this agent [19]. Thus, MNU in the drinking water selectively induces neoplastic lesions in the glandular stomach of mice.

Helicobacter pylori (*H. pylori*) is a major causative factor for gastric disorders, and strong epidemiological evidence has been accumulated indicating a significant relationship with active chronic gastritis, peptic ulcers, atrophic gastritis, intestinal metaplasia, and malignant lymphoma or cancer development [20–32]. Based on the epidemiological findings, *H. pylori* was defined as a "definite biological carcinogen" by WHO/IARC in 1994 [33]. Many animals have been successfully infected with human *H. pylori* to study the pathogenetic background, but none of the flat models studied proved sufficiently similar to the situation with human *H. pylori* infection and pathology [34–40]. In 1996, however, Hirayama et al. reported a Mongolian gerbil (MG) model of human *H. pylori* infection, with the bacteria detectable throughout a 12-month study period [41]. MGs can be easily infected with *H. pylori*, and the resultant chronic active gastritis, peptic ulcers, and intestinal metaplasia resemble lesions apparent in man. Then, in 1998, Tatematsu et al. described establishment of an animal model of stomach carcinogenesis using MGs with MNU and MNNG as the carcinogens [42]. *H. pylori* infection increases the incidence of both MNU- and MNNG-induced adenocarcinomas of all histological types in the MG glandular stomach [43–45]. The *H. pylori*-infected and chemical carcinogen-treated MG has thus proved very useful for the analysis of gastric carcinogenesis.

Precancerous Lesions for Gastric Carcinomas

Intestinal Metaplasia

Intestinal metaplasia (IM) has been extensively studied as a possible premalignant condition in the human stomach [46–50]. However, many questions remain regarding its pathogenesis as well as the actual relationship to gastric cancers. The present widely applied classification, into complete and incomplete types, was first proposed by Sugimura and colleagues at National Cancer Center Research Institute in Tokyo [51,52]. Classification based upon mucin secretion patterns as well as morphology has also allowed division into a small intestine type and a colonic type [53,54]. Jass and Filipe described three grades of IM (types I, II, and III) on the basis of morphology and classical mucin staining using the periodic acid-Schiff, alcian blue, and high iron diamine methods [55]. Type I corresponds to the complete and types II and III to the incomplete type with mild and severe distortion of the glandular structures. These classifications are generally accepted, but are only based on intestinal properties and do not take into account the gastric properties that are still preserved in association [56].

With recent developments in mucin histochemistry and immunohistochemistry, intestinal metaplastic cells can now be readily classified into a gastric epithelial cell type, encompassing pyloric gland cells and surface mucous cells, and an intestinal epithelial cell type, such as goblet and intestinal absorptive cells, on analysis of phenotypic expression [56]. Concerning gastric phenotypic markers, the surface mucous cell type contains galactose oxidase-Schiff (GOS) and sialidase-GOS reactive mucin, also being positive for MUC5AC and human gastric mucin (HGM). Cells of pyloric gland cell type contain class III mucin, are positive for MUC6, and show pepsinogen reactivity. Regarding intestinal epithelial markers, the goblet cell type contains mucin that is GOS negative and sialidase-GOS reactive, and exhibits sialyl-Tn antigen and MUC2 core protein. Cells of intestinal absorptive cell type demonstrate sucrase and intestinal-type alkaline phosphatase activity (I-ALP), harboring CD10 as a surface marker and the structural protein villin. Cells of Paneth cell type are reactive with antidefensin 5 antibodies [57,58].

Inada et al. have proposed a new IM classification based upon the cell differentiation status using both gastric and intestinal cell phenotypic markers [59]. Division is into two major types, a gastric and intestinal (GI) mixed type and a solely intestinal (I) type. GI-IM, which is further subdivided into six subtypes [59], predominates in the pyloric mucosa, whereas the I-IM is most frequent in the fundic region, suggesting that the pathogenesis differs between these two locations. All the subtypes of GI-IM and a subtype of I-IM without Paneth cells belong to the incomplete IM category whereas the subtype of I-IM with Paneth cells corresponds to complete IM. In many cases of GI-IM, atrophied pyloric glands are present under the intestinalized cells. To confirm this phenotypic classification, stomach mucosa was subjected to a gland isolation technique to show the characters of glands consisting of gastric and intestinal phenotypic cells through from the top to the bottom. Isolated glands were classified into gastric (G), GI mixed, and I types according to the preservation of pyloric glands and appearance of goblet cells as revealed with paradoxical concanavalin A and alcian blue staining (Fig. 1) [56]. Intestinal metaplastic glands still preserving gastric mucin can be considered as reflecting GI-IM at the cellular level, whereas others are true I-IMs, indicating more progression in the phenotypic shift from gastric toward intestinal. Thus, IM subtypes should be thought of not as independent entities, but rather as a sequence of pathological states with a gradual change from stomach to intestinal character [56,59]. Experimentally, a phenotypic shift from GI-IM to I-IM could be clearly observed on sequential observation of rat stomach treated with X-rays [60]. Heterotopic proliferative glands (HPGs) frequently develop with *H. pylori* infection in the glandular stomach of infected MGs, with a slightly dysplastic change of constituent cells [61]. Although these often resemble differentiated carcinomas, they are not malignant in character. HPGs also show a phenotypic shift from G type to GI type or I type with appearance of Paneth cells during the overall course of *H. pylori* infection [61].

With regard to direction of cell migration and differentiation of gastric and intestinal phenotypic cells in GI-IM, gastric surface mucous, intestinal absorptive, and goblet cells are found in the upper glandular portions from the proliferative zone (P-zone) and pyloric gland cells and Paneth cells are found in the lower glandular portions (Fig. 2). Hattori et al. speculated, on the basis of autoradiographic analyses, that IM might first appear in the P-zone wihin pyloric mucosa [62,63]. It is believed that stem cells (multipotent progenitor cells) are present in the P-zone in the isthmus region of the gastric glands, giving rise to all the various cell types by differentiation, so that consequently gastric glands are monoclonal in the adult stage [64,65]. In normal gastric and intestinal mucosa of C3H/HeN⇔BALB/c chimeric mice, Tatematsu et al. have previously demonstrated that each gland is composed entirely of C3H strain-specific antigen (CSA)-positive or -negative cells, with no mixed glands found, providing convincing evidence that each individual gland in the adult mouse is derived from a single progenitor cell [66,67]. Inada et al. have previously identified Paneth cells in pyloric glands in GI-IM using a specific antibody against human defensin-5 (HD-5), below the P-zone [68]. GI-IM might be the consequence of abnormal differentiation of stem cells that can produce both gastric and intestinal phenotypic cells, with the normal cell migration pattern preserved. In short, GI-IM can be considered an abnormal and unstable differentiation status between stomach and intestine [56,59] (see Fig. 2).

Homeobox genes play an important role in developing and maintaining organ differentiation. Caudal-type homeobox gene (Cdx)1 and Cdx2, mammalian members of the caudal-related homeobox gene family, are believed to be important in the early differentiation and maintenance of intestinal epithelial cells [69–72]. Cdx2 ectopic expression induces IM in the glandular stomach of transgenic mice [70,73,74], and in humans, Cdx1 and Cdx2 are widely present in the intestinal and colonic mucosa, but not in the gastric mucosa, further pointing to a contribution to the intestinal phenotype [75]. Nuclear staining of Cdx1 and Cdx2 can be detected in intestinal metaplastic cells, not in the normal gastric epithelial cells [76–78]. With regard to the gastric phenotype, cSox2 gene, a member of the transcription factor family containing an Sry-like high-mobility group (HMG) box, demonstrates localized expression in the chicken stomach [79]. Sox2 could be a key molecule for gastric differentiation in the gastrointestinal tract, also in mammals [80]. Indeed, Sox2 is found localized in the nuclei of human gastric foveolar cells [81].

In isolated glands, Sox2 has been found to gradually decrease from G, through GI, to the I type, whereas Cdx1 and Cdx2 increase through this sequence. MUC5AC and

MUC6 transcripts also decrease from G, through GI, to the I type, whereas MUC2 and villin demonstrate the inverse. Downregulation of Sox2, besides ectopic expression of Cdx genes, may thus be an important factor in the development of IM [81].

It has been suggested that "intestinal"-type carcinomas arise in intestinalized mucosa, while their "diffuse"-type counterparts develop from the gastric mucosa proper [82–85]. This hypothesis is based on morphological similarities between cancers and IM, and on the results of comparisons of carcinomas and surrounding mucosa. However, recent studies on clonality of gastric cancers and phenotypic expression of individual intestinal metaplastic or stomach cancer cells have pointed to several contradictions [60,66,78,86–96]. The details of this discrepancy are explained later in this chapter.

Pepsinogen-Altered Pyloric Glands

Pepsinogen isozymes are divided into pepsinogen isozyme (Pg) 1, Pg2, Pg3, and Pg4 in the normal rat glandular stomach. Three isozymes (Pg1, -3, -4) occur in the pyloric mucosa, and all four (Pg 1–4) in the fundic mucosa [97,98]. Of the three pepsinogen isozymes that have been separated from the pyloric mucosa by polyacrylamide gel electrophoresis [99], Pg1 disappears or preferentially decreases in areas of pyloric mucosa during the early stages of MNNG-induced rat glandular stomach carcinogenesis and before morphologically distinct preneoplastic histological changes appear [100,101]. This altered pepsinogen isozyme pattern has been also been consistently observed in gastric tumors [102]. More recent immunohistochemical studies have demonstrated individual pyloric glands low in Pg1 (thus termed Pg1-altered pyloric glands, PAPG) in otherwise normal-appearing pyloric mucosa after MNNG treatment [103] and have furthermore revealed that cells of pyloric gland cell type within gastric tumors contain little or no Pg1 [104]. In addition, induction of PAPG has been found to be dependent on the dose of MNNG administered, and numbers increase with time [103,104]. The susceptibility of different rat strains to induction of gastric carcinomas by MNNG also correlates with their susceptibility to induction of PAPG [105], and the constituent cells demonstrate a degree of independence from the surrounding pyloric glands with regard to proliferation kinetics [106]. Therefore, PAPG detected immunohistochemically are considered to be putative preneoplastic lesions in the glandular stomach of rats. An experimental protocol consisting of the following four components, (i) PAPG as the endpoint marker lesion; (ii) single dose of MNNG as the initiator; (iii) test chemical administration for 14 weeks; and (iv) administration of saturated sodium chloride solution during the test chemical exposure, has been used effectively for the detection of gastric carcinogens as well as promoters of gastric carcinogenesis in relatively short time period [107]. The altered methylation of the Pg1 gene observed in stomach cancer is acquired early in the carcinogenesis process, and progressive methylation changes occur with tumor development [108]. In mice, PAPG are also detectable immunohistochemically, suggesting possible use as a preneoplastic lesion for gastric chemical carcinogenesis in this species [109], independent of the strain [110]. Thus, PAPG can be regarded as a common change in rodents, acting as a precursor for a variety of adenocarcinoma types.

Modification of Gastric Carcinogenesis

Salt

Salt and salted foods are probable risk factors for gastric cancer, based on evidence from a large number of case-control and ecological studies [111–114]. In experimental animals, Tatematsu et al. found sodium chloride to enhance the carcinogenic effects of MNNG and 4-NQO in the rat glandular stomach [115]. It is possible that sodium chloride decreases the viscosity of the gastric mucus and so reduces the protective mucous barrier. When given alone, it has no apparent carcinogenicity in rats, but when administered with MNNG or 4-NQO it promotes gastric carcinogenesis in the rat glandular stomach [115] in a dose-dependent fashion [116]. A high concentration of sodium chloride causes initial tissue damage and consequent regenerative cell proliferation [117]. Furthermore, in 2002, Nozaki et al. demonstrated that a high-salt diet enhances the effects of *H. pylori* infection on gastric carcinogenesis, and these two factors act synergistically to promote the development of stomach cancers in the MG model, while high salt intake has a minor influence compared to *H. pylori* [118]. The available data from experimental animal models clearly support the concept that salt-preserved foods and salt increase the risk of stomach cancer in humans.

Endocrine Hormones

The frequency of gastric carcinoma is much greater in achlorhydric individuals than in those with high acid secretion [119–121], and lesions are rarely found in patients with duodenal ulcers accompanied by hypersecretion of HCl [122,123]. Indeed, gastric acid secretion may decrease during gastric cancer development in rats [124], and Tatsuta et al. have shown that prolonged administration of gastrin to rats after MNNG initiation results in a significant increase in acid production and a concomitant reduction in the incidence of stomach adenocarcinomas [125]. Histamine is similarly associated with decreased incidences of adenocarcinomas in the rat glandular stomach, but only gastrin affects the histological type [126]. Prolonged administration of gastrin to rats after MNNG exposure also suppresses development of gastric cancer precursors [127], but administration of a small dose during MNNG treatment results in the development of so-called undifferentiated adenocarcinomas [128].

A consistent sex difference is seen in areas of high and low incidence of gastric cancer; males have twice the likelihood of tumor development of females [129]. An equivalent male preponderance is also seen in the rat experimental model of gastric cancer with MNNG [130]. As Palli et al. have reported that early menopause predisposes women to gastric cancer [131], it is possible that sex steroid hormones have a role, with estrogen exerting protective effects and androgens causing enhancing effects [132]. Estrogen and progesterone receptors have been detected in adenocarcinomas of the stomach [133–138], and determination of their expression in individual tumors may facilitate understanding of their biochemical and pathophysiological behavior [139].

With regard to other hormones, Moyer et al. have demonstrated that somatostatin enhances growth of human gastric cancer cells [140]. In addition, it has been reported to enhance gastric carcinogenesis after MNNG treatment in rats [141]. However, somatostain can act as a positive regulator under certain conditions [142,143]. Iishi et al. have demonstrated that thyroxine may enhance the development of gastric cancers in rats [144] and may be related to its induction of increased proliferation of gastric epithelial cells [144,145]. Feurle et al. found that neurotensin can also act as a trophic factor on gastric antrum, leading to an increase in the thickness of the epithelium [146,147], and promotion of gastric carcinogenesis was confirmed in the MNNG rat model [148]. It also has been shown that specific binding sites for vasoactive intestinal peptide (VIP) are localized in plasma membranes of gastric glands [149] and in human gastric cell lines [150]. Iishi et al. have further demonstrated enhancement by VIP of gastric carcinogenesis induced by MNNG in rats [151], although Kobori et al. found that it exerts little or no stimulatory effects on the growth of rat stmach cancer cells [152]. Substance P, a digestive hormone, may also promote gastric carcinogenesis induced by MNNG in rats [153].

Bile

An increased risk of gastric cancer in stomach remnants long after partial gastrectomy and possibility of effects of reflux of bile and/or pancreatic juice have been reported [154–157]. Promoting effects of bile on experimental stomach tumorigenesis in the rat have also been suggested [158–162], and it has been shown that the incidence of gastric cancers induced by carcinogens is increased after partial gastrectomy, with tumor development related to the promotional effect of bile reflux [163,164]. Because gastrectomized rats not receiving any unequivocal carcinogen also frequently demonstrate cancers in the regions of anatomosis, however, not only tumor-promoting but also tumor-initiating activity is conceivable on the gastric stump [165,166]. Although the cancer incidence is very low in gastric stumps after partial stomach resection with transit reconstruction by the Billroth II technique (BII) [167], the proportion of human patients with cancer in the gastric stump after surgical procedures has been reported to range from 23% to 42% [166,168]. Such high incidences imply that strong gastric carcinogens equivalent to MNNG may be present in refluxing bile. The fact that spontaneous adenomas and carcinomas in the stomach and intestines of rodents are extremely rare makes it unlikely that unknown strong gastric carcinogens are present in their bile and/or pancreatic sections [169].

Diversion of bile secretion from the duodenum through a bypass to a distal intestinal loop, named the Roux-en-Y procedure (RY), is associated with lower incidence of neoplasms in the gastric stump [166]. Most of the proliferative lesions induced in the absence of chemical carcinogen are adenomatous hyperplasias (AHs), which are reversible after diversion of bile reflux by RY [167]. Cells of AHs can be classified phenotypically into a G type (pyloric gland and surface mucous cells) and a mixed GI or I type (intestinal absorptive and goblet cells), but most consist solely of G-type structures. All the cell types in AH show similar proportional decreases in bromodeoxyuridme (BrdU) incorporation after RY diversion, suggesting a benign nature for the lesions [170]. Thus, bile reflux is not an initiator, but rather an important promoter, in the carcinogenesis of gastric stump after partial gastrectomy.

Helicobacter pylori

From epidemiological findings, there is little room for doubt that *H. pylori* infection has a "positive correlation" with stomach cancer development [24–26,29,33,171,172]. Mongolian gerbils can be easily infected with *H. pylori*, and the resultant chronic active gastritis, peptic ulcers, and IM resemble lesions apparent in man. Thus, MGs appear to be an ideal experimental animal for detailed analysis of the roles of *H. pylori* in gastric disorders. All histological types of gastric cancer development can be observed in the glandular stomach of MGs treated with the chemical carcinogens MNU or MNNG [42], and *H. pylori* infection markedly enhances the yields of lesions [43–45]. As already noted, a high-salt diet enhances the effects of *H. pylori* infection on gastric carcinogenesis, and the two factors act synergistically to promote the development of stomach cancers in the MG model [118]. To evaluate variation in susceptibility to stomach carcinogenesis in relation to age of acquisition of *H. pylori* infection, Cao et al. designed an experiment involving inoculation of *H. pylori* followed by MNU exposure at different time points in the MG life span [173]. Early acquisition of *H. pylori* significantly increases gastric chemical carcinogenesis with MNU, as compared to the case with later infection, possibly because of differences in host gastric mucosal factors and immunological responses [173]. This finding would imply that childhood *H. pylori* infection must not be overlooked in approaches to the prevention of stomach cancer in adult life [174,175].

Several studies based on histopathology showed no carcinomas in animals treated only with *H. pylori* infection [42–45,176]. However, two reports concluded that *H. pylori* infection alone can induce well-differentiated adenocarcinomas at very high incidences in the glandular stomach of MGs [177,178], whereas another study resulted in only one poorly differentiated adenocarcinoma [179]. The incidences and histological patterns of the lesions differed greatly in these three papers. After *H. pylori* infection, glands in the stomach of MGs start to proliferate into the submucosa, disrupting the lamina muscularis mucosa. Submucosal HPGs develop in the glandular stomach of MGs with *H. pylori* infection alone, often resembling differentiated carcinomas [61]. The characteristics of the HPGs include (1) organized polarity of their component cells; (2) differentiation from G-type HPGs into I-type HPGs with mature Paneth cells; (3) formation of large cystic dilatations containing mucin, often with calcification; (4) shedding of epithelial cells and necrosis at the tips of lesions; (5) high-grade inflammation with infiltration of inflammatory cells; and (6) organized polarity of proliferating zones [61]. These characteristics are quite different from those of well-differentiated adenocarcinomas, which are characterized by obvious cellular atypia. After eradication, HPGs are obviously reduced, and gastric lesions in mucosa also disappear with few remnants of the former injury. Reversible HPGs are frequently induced solely by *H. pylori* infection in this species, and are related to severe gastritis, rather than being malignant in character. Thus, distinguishing reversible lesions from true neoplasms is necessary in investigating the relationship of *H. pylori* infection with gastric carcinogenesis in the MG model [61]. Taking into account all the available data, we conclude that *H. pylori* is a strong promoter of gastric carcinogenesis rather than an initiator. Many of these works of *H. pylori* infection and gastric carcinogenesis have been done by groups of Division of Oncological Pathology, Aichi Cancer Center Research Institute and Department of Gastrointestinal Surgery, The University of Tokyo.

Characteristics and Differentiation of Gastric Cancer Cells

Histological Classification of Gastric Carcinomas

Human gastric cancers histologically can be divided into two major groups, the "intestinal" and "diffuse" types of Lauren [82], which, respectively, correspond closely to the "differentiated" and "undifferentiated" types of Nakamura et al. [83] and Sugano et al. [180,181]. Although these classifications have been widely used, they are inadequate for studies of histogenesis of gastric carcinomas and phenotype expression at the cellular level, because of the confusion of intestinal phenotypic cancer cells with "diffuse" structure and the presence of a gastric phenotype with the "intestinal" type of Lauren [56]. It is in fact possible to analyze the phenotypic expression of each gastric cancer cell using gastric and intestinal epithelial cell markers [78,87,88,91,93,182–187]. The details of the phenotypic classification are explained later in this section.

DNA Ploidy Patterns of Gastric Cancers

The DNA ploidy pattern reflects the degree of chromosomal instability and offers a key to understanding the biological characteristics of neoplasms. There are known to be differences between differentiated and undifferentiated types of gastric cancers [188,189]. Polyploid cells appear to occur less frequently in minute than in large advanced cancers [190]. In differentiated lesions, the incidence of polyploidy is high in both early and advanced stages, whereas in undifferentiated gastric cancers it is low in early stages but significantly increases with progression. In gastric cancers, it has been shown that growth factor receptor genes such as c-erbB, c-erbB-2, c-met, and K-sam are often amplified in close relation to the histological type [192,193]. Amplifications of *c-erbB-2* and *K-sam* occur in differentiated and undifferentiated types, respectively [191–194]. Tsujimoto et al. have shown that the amplification of growth factor receptor genes is associated with polyploidy, irrespective of the DNA-ploidy mode [195]. The time course of oncogene amplification and kinds of genes amplified may also differ between differentiated and undifferentiated gastric cancers.

Monoclonal Growth of Gastric Cancers

Gastric cancer cells show heterogeneity in terms of both the histological and phenotypic types, raising the question of clonality [56]. Recently, numerous histological markers have been used for analysis of mosaicism in chimeric mice, and establishment of antibodies strictly recognizing a C3H strain-specific antigen (CSA), by Kusakabe et al., has enabled immunohistochemical discrimination of C3H cells in histological sections of C3H/HeN⇔BALB/c chimeric mice [196,197]. In normal gastric and intestinal mucosa of chimera adult mice, each individual gland is composed entirely of CSA-positive or -negative cells and no mixed glands are apparent, indicating that each is derived from a single progenitor cell [66,67]. Surface mucous cells (foveolar epithelial cells), mucous neck cells, parietal cells, and chief cells in the fundic glands thus all arise from the same cell. Similarly, surface mucous cells and pyloric gland cells in each pyloric gland are from a single progenitor cell. MNU in the drinking water selectively induces neoplastic lesions in the glandular stomach of BALB/c and C3H mice [18,19], and gastric cancers in C3H/HeN⇔BALB/c chimeric mice treated with MNU were also found to be composed of only one parental type. Thus, individual gastric cancers are derived from single cells with multipotential activitiy [66].

Phenotypic Classification and the Shift from Gastric to Intestinal Phenotype with Progression in Gastric Cancers

The phenotypic expression of malignant cells is widely thought to resemble that of the tissue of origin. Using gastric and intestinal epithelial cell markers, it is possible to analyze the phenotypic expression of each gastric cancer cell, independent of the histological type (Figs. 3, 4) [78,87,88,91,93,182,185–187,198]. MUC5AC, HGM, GOS, MUC6, and PCS class III mucin are markers of the gastric epithelial cell phenotype, whereas MUC2, sialidase-GOS, sialyl-Tn antigen, sucrase, I-ALP, CD10, and villin are typical of the intestinal epithelial cell phenotype [56,78,88,93,183–185,187,198,199]. Gastric cancers comprising epithelial elements presenting only gastric or intestinal phenotypic expression are classified as of gastric (G type) or intestinal (I type) phenotype, respectively. Those with both gastric-type cells and intestinal-type cells are classified as having a gastric and intestinal mixed phenotype (GI type), whereas the remainder exhibiting neither are grouped as unclassified (N type) [88,93,183,184,186].

In the rat glandular stomach, experimentally induced adenocarcinomas consist mainly of G-type cancer cells, with I-type cancer cells appearing later in larger tumors [89,90,199–201]. This phenotypic shift occurs in accordance with increasing depth of invasion in human signet ring cell carcinomas and with progression in human differentiated gastric cancers [91,183,185,198]. A shift from gastric to intestinal phenotypic expression is in fact observed with progression of each histological type of gastric cancer [182]. The incidence of gastric cancer cells with intestinal phenotypic expression in early differentiated cases is higher than in undifferentiated cases, suggesting that gastric cancer cells of differentiated type may be more prone to intestinalization [78,182,183]. In humans, gastric cancers at early stages, independent of the histological type, mainly consist of G-type cancer cells, and a phenotypic shift from gastric to intestinal phenotypic expression is clearly observed with progression [56].

Regarding the histogenesis of gastric cancers, it would be logical if those originating from IM should be of the I type. Even if the phenotypic expression of I-type gastric cancer cells is unstable, the incidence of I-type cancer cells in small gastric cancers should then be higher than in large gastric cancers, although expression in fact appears to be stable [90]. Sequential and quantitative analysis of the appearance of IM- and I-type gastric cancer cells during gastric carcinogenesis induced by chemical carcinogens in rats has clearly demonstrated the following points [89]. (i) Adenomatous hyperplasias consisting totally of G-type cells appear first. (ii) All adenocarcinomas consist mainly of G-type cancer cells, and in more than 50% of cases they are composed entirely of cells of G type. No tumors consisting only of I-type cells are found. (iii) The incidence of I-type cancer cells increases significantly in gastric lesions with progression from adenomatous hyperplasia through small well-differentiated adenocarcinomas to large well-differentiated adenocarcinomas. (iv) Tumor cells of G and I types may be present in the same acini in adenocarcinomas. (v) Adenocarcinomas with I-type cancer cells occasionally develop in pyloric mucosa in the absence of IM, and tumors without I-type tumor cells sometimes occur in pyloric mucosa with IM. In humans, also, there is no consistent phenotypic expression between gastric cancers and surrounding gastric mucosa between that with or without IM [93].

The phenotypes of microcarcinomas (defined as lesions less than 3.0 mm across) and their surrounding mucosa have also been found to be unrelated [78,88]. Tumors consisting mainly of G-type gastric cancer cells are commonly found within intestinal metaplastic mucosa, suggesting that IM is not a preneoplastic lesion for gastric cancers in man [182]. Differentiated gastric cancers may arise incidentally from gastric mucosa in which the carcinoma and the surrounding mucosa are becoming intestinalized independently [86,92,202]. Thus, it has been proposed that IM is important not as a precancerous lesion but as a paracancerous phenomenon [86,93,202]. Therefore, Tatematsu et al. have concluded that IM is not a preneoplastic change in gastric carcinoma, but rather that cells of the I type may appear independently in the gastric mucosa in IM or in gastric cancers (Fig. 5) [56,89–91].

Sugihara et al. and Fujimori et al. have revealed an organoid differentiation of intramucosal signet ring cell carcinomas [203,204]. The upper and lower layers of the typical intramucosal laminated structures consist of carcinoma cells containing surface mucous cell and pyloric gland cell type mucins, respectively, whereas the middle layer is occupied by immature carcinoma cells. Such a structure appears to simulate cellular differentiation occurring in normal mucosa. Similar organoid dif-

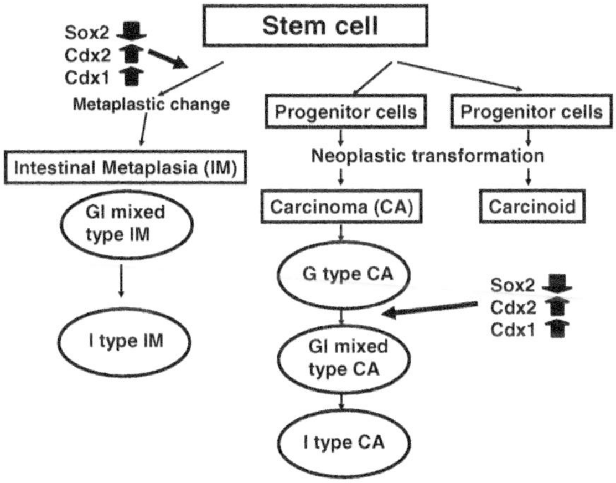

FIG. 5. Schematic illustration of the hypothesis for pathways of intestinal metaplasia and intestinalization of gastric carcinoma based on the pathological findings of human materials and experimental results with rodent models. Intestinalization progresses from GI mixed type toward I type in noncancerous (*left flow*) and cancerous (*middle flow*) tissue independently. *Sox2* has been found to gradually decrease from *G*, through *GI*, to *I* type; caudal-type homeobox gene 1 (*Cdx1*) and *Cdx2* increase through the sequence. *GI mixed type IM*, gastric and intestinal mixed-type intestinal metaplasia; *I type IM*, solely intestinal-type intestinal metaplasia; *G type CA*, gastric epithelial cell-type carcinoma; *GI mixed-type CA*, mixed gastric and intestinal epithelial cell type carcinoma; *I type CA*, intestinal epithelial cell-type carcinoma

ferentiation, mimicking pyloric gland mucosa, with GI-IM and I-IM, is often found within differentiated adenocarcinomas [183].

Expression of Homeobox Genes in Gastric Cancers

Intestinalization of gastric cancer cells differs from the non-systematic deregulation of a single gene that is often seen during carcinogenesis. Rather, orchestrated changes in the expression of various genes determining cell structures and functions are involved, as a kind of homeotic transformation. In the course of human ontogenesis, homeobox genes play key roles in developmental processes. Fetal stomach, which develops from the foregut, displays areas of "intestinal-type mucosa" with goblet cells and epithelial cells with striated borders in the antrum and cardia [205]. Intestinalization of gastric cancer cells may thus indicate a loss of ability to maintain the adult phenotype. Initiation of carcinogenesis may lead to a less-differentiated state or the capacity to differentiate in both gastric and intestinal directions, perhaps with deregulation of homeobox genes, several of which may contribute to processes leading to malignancy. Silberg et al. and Bai et al. have shown that Cdx1 is sometimes expressed in adenocarcinomas of the stomach [76,206], and Cdx2 nuclear staining has been observed in gastric carcinomas [206,207]. Almeida et al. have demonstrated a strong association between the expression of Cdx1 and Cdx2, as well as between both these and the intestinal mucin MUC2 [77]. Cdx1 and Cdx2 are indispensable for intestinal phenotypic expression even in gastric cancer cells [78,186,187], and their transcripts increase from G-, through GI-, to I-type gastric cancers [187]. There is no association with the histological type of tumor [77,78,186,187]. Cdx2 may be expressed in very early stages of gastric carcinogenesis in association with a shift from gastric to intestinal phenotypic expression [78]. The high rates for both Cdx2 and intestinal phenotypic expression in small differentiated lesions support the conclusion that the shift to intestinal phenotypic expression might occur more readily in these than in counterpart undifferentiated cancers [78].

With regard to gastric phenotypic expression, Sox2 may play an equivalent role, decreasing with the shift to I type [208].

Gene Mutations in Gastric Carcinomas

See the chapter by W. Yasui, this volume.

Prevention of Gastric Carcinomas

Polyphenols

Epidemiological studies have shown a lower risk of gastric cancer among people who consume a large amount of green tea [209], or vegetables [210]. These foods contain various polyphenols, (−)-epigallocatechin (EGCG) being a major constituent of green tea. Several experimental studies have revealed that green tea polyphenols and EGCG can inhibit chemical carcinogenesis in the duodenum [211], colon [212], skin [213–215], and lung [216,217], and in one study EGCG reduced MNNG-induced carcinogenesis of the glandular stomach in the rat [218], associated with a significant decrease in the BrdU labeling index of the mucosa. EGCG has been reported to induce apoptosis in human gastric cancer cell lines [219–221]. Tumor necrosis factor-α (TNF-α) is an endogenous tumor promoter whereas activator protein 1 (AP1) and NF-κB are directly involved in expression of the TNF-α gene. In vitro, EGCG was found to inhibit both TNF-α gene expression and TNF-α release from gastric cancer cells, mediated by inhibition of AP1 and NF-κB activation [222]. Clinical applications of EGCG without harmful effects and at low cost are conceivable.

Eradication of Helicobacter pylori

Shimizu et al. have provided direct evidence that *H. pylori* eradication may be useful as a prevention approach against gastric cancer [176]. In the *H. pylori*-infected MGs treated with MNU, the incidences of gastric cancers after curative treatment for *H. pylori* were thus significantly lower than without *H. pylori* eradication. For further evaluation, an experimental model with eradication in the early, middle, or late period was studied using *H. pylori*-infected and MNU-treated MGs [223]. *H. pylori* infection was found to strongly enhance gastric carcinogenesis initiated with the chemical carcinogen, and following eradication at an early period this effect was effectively reduced. However, after complete clearance of the bacteria, reflux esophagitis often occurs [224], and this side effect is thought to be an important risk factor for esophageal adenocarcinoma development [225]. Therefore, establishment of criteria for *H. pylori* eradication is now a top priority [176].

Restriction of Salt and Salted Food

Salt and salted foods are probable risk factors, based on evidence from a large number of case-control and ecological studies [111–114]. With regard to experimental animal models, Tatematsu et al. already reported in the 1970s that sodium chloride enhances the carcinogenic effects of MNNG and 4-NQO in the rat glandular stomach [115]. In 2002, Nozaki et al. further demonstrated that a high-salt diet acts to promote effects of *H. pylori* infection on gastric carcinogenesis, and these two factors act synergistically to drive the development of stomach cancers in the MGs model [118]. Taking into account the combination of available data, restriction of salt and salted food intake is a practical strategy for prevention of gastric cancer [226].

Conclusions

Gastric cancers develop from single cells, based on data from clonality analysis in C3H/HeN ⇔ BALB/c chimeric mice. We can conclude that IM is important not as a precancerous lesion but as a paracancerous cord from such studies of clonality of gastric cancers and of phenotypic expression of each intestinal metaplastic or stomach cancer cell. Intestinalization progresses from G, through GI, to I types in non-cancerous and cancerous tissue independently, accompanied by homeotic transformation of underlying control factors. *H. pylori* is not an initiator, but rather a strong promoter in gastric carcinogenesis, and its eradication, together with reduction in salt intake, might effectively prevent gastric cancer development.

References

1. Oettle AG (1955) Spontaneous carcinoma of the glandular stomach in a laboratory stock of *Rattus (Mastomys) natalensis*. S Afr J Med Sci 20:36
2. Oettle AG (1957) Spontaneous carcinoma of the glandular stomach in *Rattus (mastomys) natalensis*, an African rodent. Br J Cancer 11:415–433
3. Snell KC, Stewart HL (1969) Malignant argyrophilic gastric carcinoids of *Praomys (Mastomys) natalensis*. Science 163:470
4. Rusch HP, Baumann, CA, Maison GL (1940) Production of internal tumors with chemical carcinogens. Arch Pathol 29:8–19
5. Stewart HL, Snell KC (1958) Histopathogenesis of carcinoma induced in the glandular stomach of C57BL mice by the intramural injection of 20-methylcholanthrene. J Natl Cancer Inst 21:999–1035
6. Wilson RH, De Eds F, Cox AJ Jr (1941) The toxicity and carcinogenic activity of 2-acetaminofluorene. Cancer Res 1:595–608
7. Sugimura T, Fujimura S (1967) Tumour production in glandular stomach of rat by *N*-methyl-*N'*-nitro-*N*-nitrosoguanidine. Nature (Lond) 216:943–944
8. Fujimura S, Kogure K, Oboshi S, et al (1970) Production of tumors in glandular stomach of hamsters by *N*-methyl-*N'*-nitro-*N*-nitrosoguanidine. Cancer Res 30:1444–1448
9. Kogure K, Sasadaira H, Kawachi T, et al (1974) Further studies on induction of stomach cancer in hamsters by *N*-methyl-*N'*-nitro-*N*-nitrosoguanidine. Br J Cancer 29:132–142
10. Sugimura T, Tanaka N, Kawachi T, et al (1971) Production of stomach cancer in dogs by *N*-methyl-*N'*-nitro-*N*-nitrosoguanidine. Gann 62:67
11. Takahashi M, Sato H (1969) Effect of 4-nitroquinoline 1-oxide with alkylbenzenesulfonate on gastric carcinogenesis in rats. Gann Monogr 8:241–261
12. Takahashi M (1970) Effect of alkylbenzenesulfonate as a vehicle for 4-nitroquinoline 1-oxide on gastric carcinogenesis in rats. Gann 61:27–33
13. Sugimura T, Kawachi T (1976) Experimental gastric cancer (author's transl). Leber Magen Darm 6:80–90
14. Kurihara M, Shirakabe H, Murakami T, et al (1974) A new method for producing adenocarcinomas in the stomach of dogs with *N*-ethyl-*N'*-nitro-*N*-nitrosoguanidine. Gann 65:163–177
15. Mori K (1967) Carcinoma of the glandular stomach of mce by instillation of 4-nitroquinoline 1-oxide. Gann 58:389–393
16. Mori K, Ohta A (1967) Carcinoma of the glandular stomach of mice induced by 4-hydroxyaminoquinoline 1-oxide. Gann 58:551–554
17. Sugimura T, Kawachi T (1973) In: Busch H (ed) Methods in cancer research, vol VII. Academic Press. New York, pp 245–308
18. Tatematsu M, Ogawa K, Hoshiya T, et al (1992) Induction of adenocarcinomas in the glandular stomach of BALB/c mice treated with *N*-methyl-*N*-nitrosourea. Jpn J Cancer Res 83: 915–918
19. Tatematsu M, Yamamoto M, Iwata H, et al (1993) Induction of glandular stomach cancers in C3H mice treated with *N*-methyl-*N*-nitrosourea in the drinking water. Jpn J Cancer Res 84:1258–1264
20. Warren JR, Marshall B (1983) Unidentified curved bacilli on gastric epithelium in active chronic gastritis. Lancet i:1273–1275
21. Marshall BJ, Warren JR (1984) Unidentified curved bacilli in the stomach of patients with gastritis and peptic ulceration. Lancet ı:1311–1315
22. Hu PJ, Li YY, Zhou MH, et al (1995) *Helicobacter pylori* associated with a high prevalence of duodenal ulcer disease and a low prevalence of gastric cancer in a developing nation. Gut 36:198–202

23. Craanen ME, Dekker W, Blok P, et al (1992) Intestinal metaplasia and *Helicobacter pylori*: an endoscopic bioptic study of the gastric antrum. Gut 33:16–20
24. Parsonnet J, Friedman GD, Vandersteen DP, et al (1991) *Helicobacter pylori* infection and the risk of gastric carcinoma. N Engl J Med 325:1127–1131
25. Nomura A, Stemmermann GN, Chyou PH, et al (1991) *Helicobacter pylori* infection and gastric carcinoma among Japanese Americans in Hawaii. N Engl J Med 325:1132–1136
26. Forman D, Newell DG, Fullerton F, et al (1991) Association between infection with *Helicobacter pylori* and risk of gastric cancer: evidence from a prospective investigation. BMJ 302:1302–1305
27. Graham DY, Lew GM, Klein PD, et al (1992) Effect of treatment of *Helicobacter pylori* infection on the long-term recurrence of gastric or duodenal ulcer. A randomized, controlled study. Ann Intern Med 116:705–708
28. Kuipers EJ, Uyterlinde AM, Pena AS, et al (1995) Long-term sequelae of *Helicobacter pylori* gastritis. Lancet 345:1525–1528
29. Asaka M, Kato M, Kudo M, et al (1996) Atrophic changes of gastric mucosa are caused by *Helicobacter pylori* infection rather than aging: studies in asymptomatic Japanese adults. Helicobacter 1:52–56
30. Huang JQ, Sridhar S, Chen Y, et al (1998) Meta-analysis of the relationship between *Helicobacter pylori* seropositivity and gastric cancer. Gastroenterology 114:1169–1179
31. Parsonnet J, Hansen S, Rodriguez L, et al (1994) *Helicobacter pylori* infection and gastric lymphoma. N Engl J Med 330:1267–1271
32. The EUROGAST Study Group (1993) An international association between *Helicobacter pylori* infection and gastric cancer. Lancet 341:1359–1362
33. IARC Working Group on the Evaluation of Carcinogenic Risks to Humans (1994) Schistosomes, liver flukes and *Helicobacter pylori*. In: IARC Monographs on the evaluation of carcinogenic risks to humans, vol 61. IARC, Lyons, pp 1–241
34. Krakowka S, Morgan DR, Kraft WG, et al (1987) Establishment of gastric *Campylobacter pylori* infection in the neonatal gnotobiotic piglet. Infect Immun 55:2789–2796
35. Radin MJ, Eaton KA, Krakowka S, et al (1990) *Helicobacter pylori* gastric infection in gnotobiotic beagle dogs. Infect Immun 58:2606–2612
36. Lee A, Fox JG, Otto G, et al (1990) A small animal model of human *Helicobacter pylori* active chronic gastritis. Gastroenterology 99:1315–1323
37. Karita M, Kouchiyama T, Okita K, et al (1991) New small animal model for human gastric *Helicobacter pylori* infection: success in both nude and euthymic mice. Am J Gastroenterol 86:1596–1603
38. Karita M, Li Q, Cantero D, et al (1994) Establishment of a small animal model for human *Helicobacter pylori* infection using germ-free mouse. Am J Gastroenterol 89:208–213
39. Marchetti M, Arico B, Burroni D, et al (1995) Development of a mouse model of *Helicobacter pylori* infection that mimics human disease. Science 267:1655–1658
40. Fox JG, Li X, Cahill RJ, et al (1996) Hypertrophic gastropathy in *Helicobacter felis*-infected wild-type C57BL/6 mice and p53 hemizygous transgenic mice. Gastroenterology 110: 155–166
41. Hirayama F, Takagi S, Yokoyama Y, et al (1996) Establishment of gastric *Helicobacter pylori* infection in Mongolian gerbils. J Gastroenterol 31(suppl 9):24–28
42. Tatematsu M, Yamamoto M, Shimizu N, et al (1998) Induction of glandular stomach cancers in *Helicobacter pylori*-sensitive Mongolian gerbils treated with *N*-methyl-*N*-nitrosourea and *N*-methyl-*N*′-nitro-*N*-nitrosoguanidine in drinking water. Jpn J Cancer Res 89:97–104
43. Sugiyama A, Maruta F, Ikeno T, et al (1998) *Helicobacter pylori* infection enhances *N*-methyl-*N*-nitrosourea-induced stomach carcinogenesis in the Mongolian gerbil. Cancer Res 58:2067–2069
44. Shimizu N, Inada K, Nakanishi H, et al (1999) *Helicobacter pylori* infection enhances glandular stomach carcinogenesis in Mongolian gerbils treated with chemical carcinogens. Carcinogenesis (Oxf) 20:669–676

45. Shimizu N, Inada KI, Tsukamoto T, et al (1999) New animal model of glandular stomach carcinogenesis in Mongolian gerbils infected with *Helicobacter pylori* and treated with a chemical carcinogen. J Gastroenterol 34(suppl 11):61–66
46. Stemmermann GN, Hayashi T (1968) Intestinal metaplasia of the gastric mucosa: a gross and microscopic study of its distribution in various disease states. J Natl Cancer Inst 41:627–634
47. Morson BC (1955) Carcinoma arising from areas of intestinal metaplasia in the gastric mucosa. Br J Cancer 9:377–385
48. Correa P (1992) Human gastric carcinogenesis: a multistep and multifactorial process: First American Cancer Society Award Lecture on Cancer Epidemiology and Prevention. Cancer Res 52:6735–6740
49. You WC, Blot WJ, Li JY, et al (1993) Precancerous gastric lesions in a population at high risk of stomach cancer. Cancer Res 53:1317–1321
50. Yuasa Y (2003) Control of gut differentiation and intestinal-type gastric carcinogenesis. Nat Rev Cancer 3:592–600
51. Kawachi T, Kogure K, Tanaka N, et al (1974) Studies of intestinal metaplasia in the gastric mucosa by detection of disaccharidases with "Tes-Tape." J Natl Cancer Inst 53:19–30
52. Matsukura N, Suzuki K, Kawachi T, et al (1980) Distribution of marker enzymes and mucin in intestinal metaplasia in human stomach and relation to complete and incomplete types of intestinal metaplasia to minute gastric carcinomas. J Natl Cancer Inst 65:231–240
53. Teglbjaerg PS, Nielsen HO (1978) "Small intestinal type" and "colonic type" intestinal metaplasia of the human stomach, and their relationship to the histogenetic types of gastric adenocarcinoma. Acta Pathol Microbiol Scand [A] 86A:351–355
54. Segura DI, Montero C (1983) Histochemical characterization of different types of intestinal metaplasia in gastric mucosa. Cancer (Phila) 52:498–503
55. Jass JR, Filipe MI (1979) A variant of intestinal metaplasia associated with gastric carcinoma: a histochemical study. Histopathology (Oxf) 3:191–199
56. Tatematsu M, Tsukamoto T, Inada K (2003) Stem cells and gastric cancer: role of gastric and intestinal mixed intestinal metaplasia. Cancer Sci 94:135–141
57. Porter EM, van Dam E, Valore EV, et al (1997) Broad-spectrum antimicrobial activity of human intestinal defensin 5. Infect Immun 65:2396–2401
58. Porter EM, Liu L, Oren A, et al (1997) Localization of human intestinal defensin 5 in Paneth cell granules. Infect Immun 65:2389–2395
59. Inada K, Nakanishi H, Fujimitsu Y, et al (1997) Gastric and intestinal mixed and solely intestinal types of intestinal metaplasia in the human stomach. Pathol Int 47:831–841
60. Yuasa H, Inada K, Watanabe H, et al (2002) A phenotypic shift from gastric-intestinal to solely intestinal cell types in intestinal metaplasia in rat stomach following treatment with X-rays. J Toxicol Pathol 15:85–93
61. Nozaki K, Shimizu N, Tsukamoto T, et al (2002) Reversibility of heterotopic proliferative glands in glandular stomach of *Helicobacter pylori*-infected Mongolian gerbils on eradication. Jpn J Cancer Res 93:374–381
62. Hattori T, Fujita S (1979) Tritiated thymidine autoradiographic study on histogenesis and spreading of intestinal metaplasia in human stomach. Pathol Res Pract 164:224–237
63. Hattori T, Helpap B, Gedigk P (1982) The morphology and cell kinetics of pseudopyloric glands. Virchows Arch B Cell Pathol Mol Pathol 39:31–40
64. Karam SM, Leblond CP (1993) Dynamics of epithelial cells in the corpus of the mouse stomach. I. Identification of proliferative cell types and pinpointing of the stem cell. Anat Rec 236:259–279
65. Ponder BA, Schmidt GH, Wilkinson MM, et al (1985) Derivation of mouse intestinal crypts from single progenitor cells. Nature (Lond) 313:689–691
66. Tatematsu M, Fukami H, Yamamoto M, et al (1994) Clonal analysis of glandular stomach carcinogenesis in C3H/HeN↔BALB/c chimeric mice treated with *N*-methyl-*N*-nitrosourea. Cancer Lett 83:37–42

67. Tatematsu M, Masui T, Fukami H, et al (1996) Primary monoclonal and secondary polyclonal growth of colon neoplastic lesions in C3H/HeN⇔BALB/c chimeric mice treated with 1,2-dimethylhydrazine immunohistochemical detection of C3H strain-specific antigen and simple sequence length polymorphism analysis of DNA. Int J Cancer 66:234–238
68. Inada K, Tanaka H, Nakanishi H, et al (2001) Identification of Paneth cells in pyloric glands associated with gastric and intestinal mixed-type intestinal metaplasia of the human stomach. Virchows Arch 439:14–20
69. Mallo GV, Rechreche H, Frigerio JM, et al (1997) Molecular cloning, sequencing and expression of the mRNA encoding human Cdx1 and Cdx2 homeobox. Down-regulation of Cdx1 and Cdx2 mRNA expression during colorectal carcinogenesis. Int J Cancer 74:35–44
70. Silberg DG, Sullivan J, Kang E, et al (2002) Cdx2 ectopic expression induces gastric intestinal metaplasia in transgenic mice. Gastroenterology 122:689–696
71. Silberg DG, Swain GP, Suh ER, et al (2000) Cdx1 and cdx2 expression during intestinal development. Gastroenterology 119:961–971
72. Soubeyran P, Andre F, Lissitzky JC, et al (1999) Cdx1 promotes differentiation in a rat intestinal epithelial cell line. Gastroenterology 117:1326–1338
73. Eda A, Osawa H, Yanaka I, et al (2002) Expression of homeobox gene CDX2 precedes that of CDX1 during the progression of intestinal metaplasia. J Gastroenterol 37:94–100
74. Mutoh H, Hakamata Y, Sato K, et al (2002) Conversion of gastric mucosa to intestinal metaplasia in Cdx2-expressing transgenic mice. Biochem Biophys Res Commun 294:470–479
75. Mizoshita T, Inada K, Tsukamoto T, et al (2001) Expression of Cdx1 and Cdx2 mRNAs and relevance of this expression to differentiation in human gastrointestinal mucosa—with special emphasis on participation in intestinal metaplasia of the human stomach. Gastric Cancer 4:185–191
76. Silberg DG, Furth EE, Taylor JK, et al (1997) CDX1 protein expression in normal, metaplastic, and neoplastic human alimentary tract epithelium. Gastroenterology 113:478–486
77. Almeida R, Silva E, Santos-Silva F, et al (2003) Expression of intestine-specific transcription factors, CDX1 and CDX2, in intestinal metaplasia and gastric carcinomas. J Pathol 199:36–40
78. Mizoshita T, Tsukamoto T, Inada K, et al (2004) Immunohistochemically detectable Cdx2 is present in intestinal phenotypic elements in early gastric cancers of both differentiated and undifferentiated types, with no correlation to non-neoplastic surrounding mucosa. Pathol Int 54:392–400
79. Ishii Y, Rex M, Scotting PJ, et al (1998) Region-specific expression of chicken Sox2 in the developing gut and lung epithelium: regulation by epithelial-mesenchymal interactions. Dev Dyn 213:464–475
80. Yasugi S (2000) Epithelial cell differentiation during stomach development. Hum Cell 13: 177–184
81. Tsukamoto T, Inada K, Tanaka H, et al (2004) Down regulation of a gastric transcription factor, Sox2, and ectopic expression of intestinal homeobox genes, Cdx1 and Cdx2: inverse correlation during progression from gastric/intestinal-mixed to complete intestinal metaplasia. J Cancer Res Clin Oncol 130:135–145
82. Lauren P (1965) The two histological main types of gastric carcinoma: diffuse and so-called intestinal-type carcinoma: an attempt at a histo-clinical classification. Acta Pathol Microbiol Scand 64:31–49
83. Nakamura K, Sugano H, Takagi K (1968) Carcinoma of the stomach in incipient phase: its histogenesis and histological appearances. Gann 59:251–258
84. Correa P (1988) A human model of gastric carcinogenesis. Cancer Res 48:3554–3560
85. Correa P (1995) *Helicobacter pylori* and gastric carcinogenesis. Am J Surg Pathol 19(suppl 1):S37–S43
86. Egashira Y, Shimoda T, Ikegami M (1999) Mucin histochemical analysis of minute gastric differentiated adenocarcinoma. Pathol Int 49:55–61

87. Koseki K, Takizawa T, Koike M, et al (2000) Distinction of differentiated type early gastric carcinoma with gastric type mucin expression. Cancer (Phila) 89:724–732
88. Kawachi H, Takizawa T, Eishi Y, et al (2003) Absence of either gastric or intestinal phenotype in microscopic differentiated gastric carcinomas. J Pathol 199:436–446
89. Tatematsu M, Furihata C, Katsuyama T, et al (1983) Independent induction of intestinal metaplasia and gastric cancer in rats treated with *N*-methyl-*N′*-nitro-*N*-nitrosoguanidine. Cancer Res 43:1335–1341
90. Tatematsu M, Katsuyama T, Furihata C, et al (1984) Stable intestinal phenotypic expression of gastric and small intestinal tumor cells induced by *N*-methyl-*N′*-nitro-*N*-nitrosoguanidine or methylnitrosourea in rats. Gann 75:957–965
91. Tatematsu M, Furihata C, Katsuyama T, et al (1986) Gastric and intestinal phenotypic expressions of human signet ring cell carcinomas revealed by their biochemistry, mucin histochemistry, and ultrastructure. Cancer Res 46:4866–4872
92. Hattori T (1986) Development of adenocarcinomas in the stomach. Cancer (Phila) 57: 1528–1534
93. Tatematsu M, Ichinose M, Miki K, et al (1990) Gastric and intestinal phenotypic expression of human stomach cancers as revealed by pepsinogen immunohistochemistry and mucin histochemistry. Acta Pathol Jpn 40:494–504
94. Kushima R, Hattori T (1993) Histogenesis and characteristics of gastric-type adenocarcinomas in the stomach. J Cancer Res Clin Oncol 120:103–111
95. Nomura S, Kaminishi M, Sugiyama K, et al (1998) Clonal analysis of isolated intestinal metaplastic glands of stomach using X linked polymorphism. Gut 42:663–668
96. Saito A, Shimoda T, Nakanishi Y, et al (2001) Histologic heterogeneity and mucin phenotypic expression in early gastric cancer. Pathol Int 51:165–171
97. Furihata C, Iwasaki Y, Sugimura T, et al (1973) Differentiation of pepsinogen-producing cells in the fundic and pyloric mucosa of developing rats. Cell Differ 2:179–189
98. Furihata C, Saito D, Fujiki H, et al (1980) Purification and characterization of pepsinogens and a unique pepsin from rat stomach. Eur J Biochem 105:43–50
99. Furihata C, Kawachi T, Sugimura T (1972) Premature induction of pepsinogen in developing rat gastric mucosa by hormones. Biochem Biophys Res Commun 47:705–711
100. Furihata C, Sasajima K, Kazama S, et al (1975) Changes in pepsinogen isozymes in stomach carcinogenesis induced in rats by *N*-methyl-*N′*-nitro-*N*-nitrosoguanidine. J Natl Cancer Inst 55:925–930
101. Tatematsu M, Saito D, Furihata C, et al (1980) Initial DNA damage and heritable permanent change in pepsinogen isoenzyme pattern in the pyloric mucosae of rats after short-term administration of *N*-methyl-*N′*-nitro-*N*-nitrosoguanidine. J Natl Cancer Inst 64:775–781
102. Tatematsu M, Furihata C, Hirose M, et al (1977) Changes in pepsinogen isozymes in stomach cancers induced in Wistar rats by *N*-methyl-*N′*-nitro-*N*-nitrosoguanidine and in transplantable gastric carcinoma (SG2B). J Natl Cancer Inst 58:1709–1716
103. Tatematsu M, Furihata C, Mera Y, et al (1986) Immunohistochemical demonstration of induction of pyloric glands with low pepsinogen 1 (Pg 1) content in rat stomach by *N*-methyl-*N′*-nitro-*N*-nitrosoguanidine. Jpn J Cancer Res 77:238–243
104. Tatematsu M, Furihata C, Katsuyama T, et al (1987) Immunohistochemical demonstration of pyloric gland-type cells with low-pepsinogen isozyme 1 in preneoplastic and neoplastic tissues of rat stomachs treated with *N*-methyl-*N′*-nitro-*N*-nitrosoguanidine. J Natl Cancer Inst 78:771–777
105. Tatematsu M, Aoki T, Inoue T, et al (1988) Coefficient induction of pepsinogen 1-decreased pyloric glands and gastric cancers in five different strains of rats treated with *N*-methyl-*N′*-nitro-*N*-nitrosoguanidine. Carcinogenesis (Oxf) 9:495–498
106. Tatematsu M, Mutai M, Aoki T, et al (1989) Proliferation kinetics of pepsinogen altered pyloric gland cells in rats treated with *N*-methyl-*N′*-nitro-*N*-nitrosoguanidine. Carcinogenesis (Oxf) 10:907–911

107. Tatematsu M, Ozaki K, Mutai M, et al (1990) Enhancing effects of various gastric carcinogens on development of pepsinogen-altered pyloric glands in rats. Carcinogenesis (Oxf) 11:1975–1978
108. Tatematsu M, Ichinose M, Tsukada S, et al (1993) DNA methylation of the pepsinogen 1 gene during rat glandular stomach carcinogenesis induced by *N*-methyl-*N'*-nitro-*N*-nitrosoguanidine or catechol. Carcinogenesis (Oxf) 14:1415–1419
109. Yamamoto M, Furihata C, Fujimitsu Y, et al (1997) Dose-dependent induction of both pepsinogen-altered pyloric glands and adenocarcinomas in the glandular stomach of C3H mice treated with *N*-methyl-*N*-nitrosourea. Jpn J Cancer Res 88:238–244
110. Yamamoto M, Furihata C, Ogiu T, et al (2002) Independent variation in susceptibilities of six different mouse strains to induction of pepsinogen-altered pyloric glands and gastric tumor intestinalization by *N*-methyl-*N*-nitrosourea. Cancer Lett 179:121–132
111. Tajima K, Tominaga S (1985) Dietary habits and gastro-intestinal cancers: a comparative case-control study of stomach and large intestinal cancers in Nagoya, Japan. Jpn J Cancer Res 76:705–716
112. Tsugane S, Tsuda M, Gey F, et al (1992) Cross-sectional study with multiple measurements of biological markers for assessing stomach cancer risks at the population level. Environ Health Perspect 98:207–210
113. Joossens JV, Hill MJ, Elliott P, et al (1996) Dietary salt, nitrate and stomach cancer mortality in 24 countries. European Cancer Prevention (ECP) and the INTERSALT Cooperative Research Group. Int J Epidemiol 25:494–504
114. Kono S, Hirohata T (1996) Nutrition and stomach cancer. Cancer Causes Control 7:41–55
115. Tatematsu M, Takahashi M, Fukushima S, et al (1975) Effects in rats of sodium chloride on experimental gastric cancers induced by *N*-methyl-*N*-nitro-*N*-nitrosoguanidine or 4-nitroquinoline-1-oxide. J Natl Cancer Inst 55:101–106
116. Takahashi M, Nishikawa A, Furukawa F, et al (1994) Dose-dependent promoting effects of sodium chloride (NaCl) on rat glandular stomach carcinogenesis initiated with *N*-methyl-*N'*-nitro-*N*-nitrosoguanidine. Carcinogenesis (Oxf) 15:1429–1432
117. Furihata C, Ohta H, Katsuyama T (1996) Cause and effect between concentration-dependent tissue damage and temporary cell proliferation in rat stomach mucosa by NaCl, a stomach tumor promoter. Carcinogenesis (Oxf) 17:401–406
118. Nozaki K, Shimizu N, Inada K, et al (2002) Synergistic promoting effects of *Helicobacter pylori* infection and high-salt diet on gastric carcinogenesis in Mongolian gerbils. Jpn J Cancer Res 93:1083–1089
119. Comfort MW, Kelsey MP, Berkson J (1947) Gastric acidity before and after the development of carcinoma of the stomach. J Natl Cancer Inst 7:367–373
120. Gilbertsen VA, Knatterud GL (1967) Gastric analysis as a screening measure for cancer of the stomach. Cancer (Phila) 20:127–133
121. Segal HL, Samloff IM (1973) Gastric cancer—increased frequency in patients with achlorhydria. Am J Dig Dis 18:295–299
122. Fischer A, Clagett OT, McDonald JR (1947) Coexistent duodenal ulcer and gastric malignancy. Surgery (St. Louis) 21:168–174
123. Portis SA, Jaffe RH (1938) A study of peptic ulcer based on necropsy records. JAMA 110:6–13
124. Bralow SP, Gruenstein M, Meranze DR, et al (1970) Adenocarcinoma of glandular stomach and duodenum in Wistar rats ingesting *N*-methyl-*N'*-nitro-*N*-nitrosoguanidine, histopathology and associated secretory changes. Cancer Res 30:1215–1222
125. Tatsuta M, Itoh T, Okuda S, et al (1977) Effect of prolonged administration of gastrin on experimental carcinogenesis in rat stomach induced by *N*-methyl-*N'*-nitro-*N*-nitrosoguanidine. Cancer Res 37:1808–1810
126. Tatsuta M, Itoh T, Okuda S, et al (1980) Effects of gastrin and histamine on gastric carcinogenesis induced in rats by *N*-methyl-*N'*-nitro-*N*-nitrosoguanidine. Eur J Cancer 16: 631–638

127. Tatsuta M, Yamamura H, Taniguchi H, et al (1982) Gastrin protection against chemically induced gastric adenocarcinomas in Wistar rats: histopathology of the glandular stomach and incidence of gastric adenocarcinoma. J Natl Cancer Inst 69:59–66
128. Tahara E, Haizuka S (1975) Effect of gastro-entero-pancreatic endocrine hormones on the histogenesis of gastric cancer in rats induced by *N*-methyl-*N*′-nitro-*N*-nitrosoguanidine; with special reference to development of scirrhous gastric cancer. Gann 66:421–426
129. Perkin DM, Muir CS, Whelon SL, et al (1992) Cancer incidence in five continents. IARC Scientific Publication 120, vol 6. International Agency for Research on Cancer, Lyon, pp 1–1033
130. Furukawa H, Iwanaga T, Koyama H, et al (1982) Effect of sex hormones on carcinogenesis in the stomachs of rats. Cancer Res 42:5181–5182
131. Palli D, Cipriani F, Decarli A, et al (1994) Reproductive history and gastric cancer among post-menopausal women. Int J Cancer 56:812–815
132. Singh S, Poulsom R, Wright NA, et al (1997) Differential expression of oestrogen receptor and oestrogen inducible genes in gastric mucosa and cancer. Gut 40:516–520
133. Sica V, Nola E, Contieri E, et al (1984) Estradiol and progesterone receptors in malignant gastrointestinal tumors. Cancer Res 44:4670–4674
134. Tokunaga A, Nishi K, Matsukura N, et al (1986) Estrogen and progesterone receptors in gastric cancer. Cancer (Phila) 57:1376–1379
135. Wu CW, Chi CW, Chang TJ, et al (1990) Sex hormone receptors in gastric cancer. Cancer (Phila) 65:1396–1400
136. Yokozaki H, Takekura N, Takanashi A, et al (1988) Estrogen receptors in gastric adenocarcinoma: a retrospective immunohistochemical analysis. Virchows Arch A Pathol Anat Histopathol 413:297–302
137. Uehara Y, Takahashi T, Kojima O, et al (1986) Peroxidase-antiperoxidase staining for estrogen and progesterone in scirrhous type of gastric cancer: possible existence of the estrogen receptor. Jpn J Surg 16:245–249
138. Wu CW, Chang HM, Kao HL, et al (1992) The nontransformed progesterone and estrogen receptors in gastric cancer. Gastroenterology 102:1639–1646
139. Karat D, Brotherick I, Shenton BK, et al (1999) Expression of oestrogen and progesterone receptors in gastric cancer: a flow cytometric study. Br J Cancer 80:1271–1274
140. Moyer MP, Armstrong A, Aust JB, et al (1986) Effects of gastrin, glutamine, and somatostatin on the in vitro growth of normal and malignant human gastric mucosal cells. Arch Surg 121:285–288
141. Tatsuta M, Iishi H, Baba M, et al (1989) Enhancement by somatostatin of experimental gastric carcinogenesis induced by *N*-methyl-*N*′-nitro-*N*-nitrosoguanidine in Wistar rats. Cancer Res 49:5534–5536
142. Dharmsathaphorn K, Binder HJ, Dobbins JW (1980) Somatostatin stimulates sodium and chloride absorption in the rabbit ileum. Gastroenterology 78:1559–1565
143. Shapiro B, Pienta K, Heldsinger A, et al (1981) Somatostatin is an agonist and noncompetitive antagonist of gastrin in oxyntic cell function. Endocrinology 109:1117–1121
144. Iishi H, Tatsuta M, Baba M, et al (1993) Enhancement by thyroxine of gastric carcinogenesis induced by *N*-methyl-*N*′-nitro-*N*-nitrosoguanidine in Wistar rats. Br J Cancer 68: 515–518
145. Adeniyi KO, Olowookorun MO (1989) Gastric acid secretion and parietal cell mass: effects of thyroidectomy and thyroxine. Am J Physiol 256:G975–G978
146. Feurle GE, Muller B, Ohnheiser G, et al (1985) Action of neurotensin on size, composition, and growth of pancreas and stomach in the rat. Regul Pept 13:53–62
147. Feurle GE, Muller B, Rix E (1987) Neurotensin induces hyperplasia of the pancreas and growth of the gastric antrum in rats. Gut 28(suppl):19–23
148. Tatsuta M, Iishi H, Baba M, et al (1989) Promotion by neurotensin of gastric carcinogenesis induced by *N*-methyl-*N*′-nitro-*N*-nitrosoguanidine in Wistar rats. Cancer Res 49:843–846
149. Gespach C, Hui Bon Hoa D, Rosselin G (1983) Regulation by vasoactive intestinal peptide, histamine, somatostatin-14 and -28 of cyclic adenosine monophosphate levels in gastric

glands isolated from the guinea pig fundus or antrum. Endocrinology 112:1597–1606
150. Emami S, Gespach C, Forgue-Lafitte ME, et al (1983) Histamine and VIP interactions with receptor-cyclic AMP systems in the human gastric cancer cell line HGT-1. Life Sci 33: 415–423
151. Iishi H, Tatsuta M, Baba M, et al (1992) Enhancement by vaso-active intestinal peptide of gastric carcinogenesis induced by *N*-methyl-*N'*-nitro-*N*-nitrosoguanidine in rats. Int J Cancer 50:649–652
152. Kobori O, Vuillot MT, Martin F (1982) Growth responses of rat stomach cancer cells to gastro-entero-pancreatic hormones. Int J Cancer 30:65–67
153. Tatsuta M, Iishi H, Baba M, et al (1995) Promotion by substance P of gastric carcinogenesis induced by *N*-methyl-*N'*-nitro-*N*-nitrosoguanidine in Wistar rats. Cancer Lett 96: 99–103
154. Stalsberg H, Taksdal S (1971) Stomach cancer following gastric surgery for benign conditions. Lancet 2:1175–1177
155. Schrumpf E, Serck-Hanssen A, Stadaas J, et al (1977) Mucosal changes in the gastric stump 20–25 years after partial gastrectomy. Lancet 2:467–469
156. Savage A, Jones S (1979) Histological appearances of the gastric mucosa 15–27 years after partial gastrectomy. J Clin Pathol 32:179–186
157. Saegesser F, James D (1972) Cancer of the gastric stump after partial gastrectomy (Billroth II principle) for ulcer. Cancer (Phila) 29:1150–1159
158. Furihata C, Takezawa R, Matsushima T, et al (1987) Potential tumor-promoting activity of bile acids in rat glandular stomach. Jpn J Cancer Res 78:32–39
159. Kobori O, Shimizu T, Maeda M, et al (1984) Enhancing effect of bile and bile acid on stomach tumorigenesis induced by *N*-methyl-*N'*-nitro-*N*-nitrosoguanidine in Wistar rats. J Natl Cancer Inst 73:853–861
160. Kobori O, Watanabe J, Shimizu T, et al (1984) Enhancing effect of sodium taurocholate on *N*-methyl-*N'*-nitro-*N*-nitrosoguanidine-induced stomach tumorigenesis in rats. Gann 75: 651–654
161. Salmon RJ, Laurent M, Thierry JP (1984) Effect of taurocholic acid feeding on methyl-nitro-*N*-nitroso-guanidine induced gastric tumors. Cancer Lett 22:315–320
162. Yamaguchi S, Tatematsu M, Furihata C, et al (1990) Effects of bile acids on development of pepsinogen-altered pyloric glands in rats. Cancer Lett 55:129–134
163. Salmon RJ, Merle S, Zafrani B, et al (1985) Gastric carcinogenesis induced by *N*-methyl-*N'*-nitro-*N*-nitrosoguanidine: role of gastrectomy and duodenal reflux. Jpn J Cancer Res 76: 167–172
164. Sano C, Kumashiro R, Saito T, et al (1984) Promoting effect of partial gastrectomy on carcinogenesis in the remnant stomach of rats after oral administration of *N*-methyl-*N'*-nitro-*N*-nitrosoguanidine. Oncology 41:124–128
165. Kondo K, Suzuki H, Nagayo T (1984) The influence of gastro-jejunal anastomosis on gastric carcinogenesis in rats. Gann 75:362–369
166. Langhans P, Heger RA, Hohenstein J, et al (1981) Gastric stump carcinoma—new aspects deduced from experimental results. Scand J Gastroenterol Suppl 67:161–164
167. Kobayasi S, Tatematsu M, Ogawa K, et al (1991) Reversibility of adenomatous hyperplasia in the gastric stump after diversion of bile reflux in rats. Carcinogenesis (Oxf) 12: 1437–1443
168. Mason RC (1986) Duodenogastric reflux in rat gastric carcinoma. Br J Surg 73:801–803
169. Tatematsu M, Imaeda, K (1989) Tumors of the glandular stomach. In: Stinson SF, Schuller HM, Reznik GK (eds) Atlas of tumor pathology of the Fischer rat. CRC Press, Boca Raton, FL, pp 95–115
170. Imai T, Kobayasi S, Rodrigues MA, et al (1993) Reduction of cell proliferative activities of gastric stump adenomatous hyperplasias after bile reflux diversion in rats. Carcinogenesis (Oxf) 14:1765–1769

171. Asaka M, Kimura T, Kudo M, et al (1992) Relationship of *Helicobacter pylori* to serum pepsinogens in an asymptomatic Japanese population. Gastroenterology 102:760–766
172. Uemura N, Okamoto S, Yamamoto S, et al (2001) *Helicobacter pylori* infection and the development of gastric cancer. N Engl J Med 345:784–789
173. Cao X, Tsukamoto T, Nozaki K, et al (2002) Earlier *Helicobacter pylori* infection increases the risk for the *N*-methyl-*N*-nitrosourea-induced stomach carcinogenesis in Mongolian gerbils. Jpn J Cancer Res 93:1293–1298
174. Malaty HM, El-Kasabany A, Graham DY, et al (2002) Age at acquisition of *Helicobacter pylori* infection: a follow-up study from infancy to adulthood. Lancet 359:931–935
175. Correa P, Fontham ET, Bravo JC, et al (2000) Chemoprevention of gastric dysplasia: randomized trial of antioxidant supplements and anti-*Helicobacter pylori* therapy. J Natl Cancer Inst 92:1881–1888
176. Shimizu N, Ikehara Y, Inada K, et al (2000) Eradication diminishes enhancing effects of *Helicobacter pylori* infection on glandular stomach carcinogenesis in Mongolian gerbils. Cancer Res 60:1512–1514
177. Watanabe T, Tada M, Nagai H, et al (1998) *Helicobacter pylori* infection induces gastric cancer in Mongolian gerbils. Gastroenterology 115:642–648
178. Honda S, Fujioka T, Tokieda M, et al (1998) Development of *Helicobacter pylori*-induced gastric carcinoma in Mongolian gerbils. Cancer Res 58:4255–4259
179. Hirayama F, Takagi S, Iwao E, et al (1999) Development of poorly differentiated adenocarcinoma and carcinoid due to long-term *Helicobacter pylori* colonization in Mongolian gerbils. J Gastroenterol 34:450–454
180. Sugano H, Nakamura K, Kato Y (1982) Pathological studies of human gastric cancer. Acta Pathol Jpn 32(suppl 2):329–347
181. Japanese Gastric Cancer Association (1998) Japanese classification of gastric carcinoma, 2nd English edn. Gastric Cancer 1:10–24
182. Tatematsu M, Hasegawa R, Ogawa K, et al (1992) Histogenesis of human stomach cancers based on assessment of differentiation. J Clin Gastroenterol 14(suppl 1):S1–S7
183. Yoshikawa A, Inada Ki K, Yamachika T, et al (1998) Phenotypic shift in human differentiated gastric cancers from gastric to intestinal epithelial cell type during disease progression. Gastric Cancer 1:134–141
184. Tajima Y, Shimoda T, Nakanishi Y, et al (2001) Gastric and intestinal phenotypic marker expression in gastric carcinomas and its prognostic significance: immunohistochemical analysis of 136 lesions. Oncology 61:212–220
185. Bamba M, Sugihara H, Kushima R, et al (2001) Time-dependent expression of intestinal phenotype in signet ring cell carcinomas of the human stomach. Virchows Arch 438:49–56
186. Mizoshita T, Tsukamoto T, Nakanishi H, et al (2003) Expression of Cdx2 and the phenotype of advanced gastric cancers: relationship with prognosis. J Cancer Res Clin Oncol 129:727–734
187. Mizoshita T, Inada K, Tsukamoto T, et al (2004) Expression of the intestine-specific transcription factors, Cdx1 and Cdx2, correlates shift to an intestinal phenotype in gastric cancer cells. J Cancer Res Clin Oncol 130:29–36
188. Hattori T, Hosokawa Y, Fukuda M, et al (1984) Analysis of DNA ploidy patterns of gastric carcinomas of Japanese. Cancer (Phila) 54:1591–1597
189. Korenaga D, Haraguchi M, Okamura T, et al (1989) DNA ploidy and tumor invasion in human gastric cancer. Histopathologic differentiation. Arch Surg (Phila) 124:314–318
190. Hattori T, Sugihara H, Fukuda M, et al (1986) DNA ploidy patterns of minute carcinomas in the stomach. Jpn J Cancer Res 77:276–281
191. Kuniyasu H, Yasui W, Kitadai Y, et al (1992) Frequent amplification of the c-met gene in scirrhous type stomach cancer. Biochem Biophys Res Commun 189:227–232
192. Nakatani H, Sakamoto H, Yoshida T, et al (1990) Isolation of an amplified DNA sequence in stomach cancer. Jpn J Cancer Res 81:707–710

193. Yokota J, Yamamoto T, Miyajima N, et al (1988) Genetic alterations of the c-erbB-2 oncogene occur frequently in tubular adenocarcinoma of the stomach and are often accompanied by amplification of the v-erbA homologue. Oncogene 2:283–287
194. Yoshida K, Tsuda T, Matsumura T, et al (1989) Amplification of epidermal growth factor receptor (EGFR) gene and oncogenes in human gastric carcinomas. Virchows Arch B Cell Pathol Mol Pathol 57:285–290
195. Tsujimoto H, Sugihara H, Hagiwara A, et al (1997) Amplification of growth factor receptor genes and DNA ploidy pattern in the progression of gastric cancer. Virchows Arch 431: 383–389
196. Kusakabe M, Yokoyama M, Sakakura T, et al (1988) A novel methodology for analysis of cell distribution in chimeric mouse organs using a strain specific antibody. J Cell Biol 107:257–265
197. Lee GH, Nomura K, Kanda H, et al (1991) Strain specific sensitivity to diethylnitrosamine-induced carcinogenesis is maintained in hepatocytes of C3H/HeN in equilibrium with C57BL/6N chimeric mice. Cancer Res 51:3257–3260
198. Yamachika T, Inada K, Fujimitsu Y, et al (1997) Intestinalization of gastric signet ring cell carcinomas with progression. Virchows Arch 431:103–110
199. Tatematsu M, Katsuyama T, Fukushima S, et al (1980) Mucin histochemistry by paradoxical concanavalin A staining in experimental gastric cancers induced in Wistar rats by *N*-methyl-*N*-nitro-*N*-nitrosoguanidine or 4-nitroquinoline 1-oxide. J Natl Cancer Inst 64:835–843
200. Tatematsu M, Katsuyama T, Furihata C, et al (1990) Cellular differentiation and histogenesis of rat glandular stomach cancers. Jpn J Cancer Res 81:760–767
201. Yuasa H, Hirano K, Kodama H, et al (1994) Immunohistochemical demonstration of intestinal-type alkaline phosphatase in stomach tumors induced by *N*-methyl-*N′*-nitro-*N*-nitrosoguanidine in rats. Jpn J Cancer Res 85:897–903
202. Matsukuma A, Mori M, Enjoji M (1990) Sulphomucin-secreting intestinal metaplasia in the human gastric mucosa. An association with intestinal-type gastric carcinoma. Cancer (Phila) 66:689–694
203. Sugihara H, Hattori T, Fukuda M, et al (1987) Cell proliferation and differentiation in intramucosal and advanced signet ring cell carcinomas of the human stomach. Virchows Arch A Pathol Anat Histopathol 411:117–127
204. Fujimori Y, Akamatsu T, Ota H, et al (1995) Proliferative markers in gastric carcinoma and organoid differentiation. Hum Pathol 26:725–734
205. Salenius P (1962) On the ontogenesis of the human gastric epithelial cells. A histologic and histochemical study. Acta Anat (Basel) 50(suppl 46):1–76
206. Bai YQ, Yamamoto H, Akiyama Y, et al (2002) Ectopic expression of homeodomain protein CDX2 in intestinal metaplasia and carcinomas of the stomach. Cancer Lett 176:47–55
207. Seno H, Oshima M, Taniguchi MA, et al (2002) CDX2 expression in the stomach with intestinal metaplasia and intestinal-type cancer: prognostic implications. Int J Oncol 21: 769–774
208. Li XL, Eishi Y, Bai YQ, et al (2004) Expression of the SRY-related HMG box protein SOX2 in human gastric carcinoma. Int J Oncol 24:257–263
209. Kono S, Ikeda M, Tokudome S, et al (1988) A case-control study of gastric cancer and diet in northern Kyushu, Japan. Jpn J Cancer Res 79:1067–1074
210. Weisburger JH (1991) Nutritional approach to cancer prevention with emphasis on vitamins, antioxidants, and carotenoids. Am J Clin Nutr 53:226S–237S
211. Fujita Y, Yamane T, Tanaka M, et al (1989) Inhibitory effect of (–)-epigallocatechin gallate on carcinogenesis with *N*-ethyl-*N′*-nitro-*N*-nitrosoguanidine in mouse duodenum. Jpn J Cancer Res 80:503–505
212. Narisawa T, Fukaura Y (1993) A very low dose of green tea polyphenols in drinking water prevents *N*-methyl-*N*-nitrosourea-induced colon carcinogenesis in F344 rats. Jpn J Cancer Res 84:1007–1009

213. Mukhtar H, Das M, Khan WA, et al (1988) Exceptional activity of tannic acid among naturally occurring plant phenols in protecting against 7,12-dimethylbenz(*a*)anthracene-, benzo(*a*)pyrene-, 3-methylcholanthrene-, and *N*-methyl-*N*-nitrosourea-induced skin tumorigenesis in mice. Cancer Res 48:2361–2365
214. Wang ZY, Huang MT, Ferraro T, et al (1992) Inhibitory effect of green tea in the drinking water on tumorigenesis by ultraviolet light and 12-*O*-tetradecanoylphorbol-13-acetate in the skin of SKH-1 mice. Cancer Res 52:1162–1170
215. Conney AH, Wang ZY, Huang MT, et al (1992) Inhibitory effect of green tea on tumorigenesis by chemicals and ultraviolet light. Prev Med 21:361–369
216. Xu Y, Ho CT, Amin SG, et al (1992) Inhibition of tobacco-specific nitrosamine-induced lung tumorigenesis in A/J mice by green tea and its major polyphenol as antioxidants. Cancer Res 52:3875–3879
217. Katiyar SK, Agarwal R, Zaim MT, et al (1993) Protection against *N*-nitrosodiethylamine and benzo[*a*]pyrene-induced forestomach and lung tumorigenesis in A/J mice by green tea. Carcinogenesis (Oxf) 14:849–855
218. Yamane T, Takahashi T, Kuwata K, et al (1995) Inhibition of *N*-methyl-*N'*-nitro-*N*-nitrosoguanidine-induced carcinogenesis by (–)-epigallocatechin gallate in the rat glandular stomach. Cancer Res 55:2081–2084
219. Komori A, Yatsunami J, Okabe S, et al (1993) Anticarcinogenic activity of green tea polyphenols. Jpn J Clin Oncol 23:186–190
220. Hibasami H, Komiya T, Achiwa Y, et al (1998) Induction of apoptosis in human stomach cancer cells by green tea catechins. Oncol Rep 5:527–529
221. Ahmad N, Feyes DK, Nieminen AL, et al (1997) Green tea constituent epigallocatechin-3-gallate and induction of apoptosis and cell cycle arrest in human carcinoma cells. J Natl Cancer Inst 89:1881–1886
222. Okabe S, Ochiai Y, Aida M, et al (1999) Mechanistic aspects of green tea as a cancer preventive: effect of components on human stomach cancer cell lines. Jpn J Cancer Res 90: 733–739
223. Nozaki K, Shimizu N, Ikehara Y, et al (2003) Effect of early eradication on *Helicobacter pylori*-related gastric carcinogenesis in Mongolian gerbils. Cancer Sci 94:235–239
224. Labenz J, Blum AL, Bayerdorffer E, et al (1997) Curing *Helicobacter pylori* infection in patients with duodenal ulcer may provoke reflux esophagitis. Gastroenterology 112: 1442–1447
225. Naef AP, Savary M, Ozzello L (1975) Columnar-lined lower esophagus: an acquired lesion with malignant predisposition. Report on 140 cases of Barrett's esophagus with 12 adenocarcinomas. J Thorac Cardiovasc Surg 70:826–835
226. Tsugane S, Sasazuki S, Kobayashi M, et al (2004) Salt and salted food intake and subsequent risk of gastric cancer among middle-aged Japanese men and women. Br J Cancer 90: 128–134

Color Plates

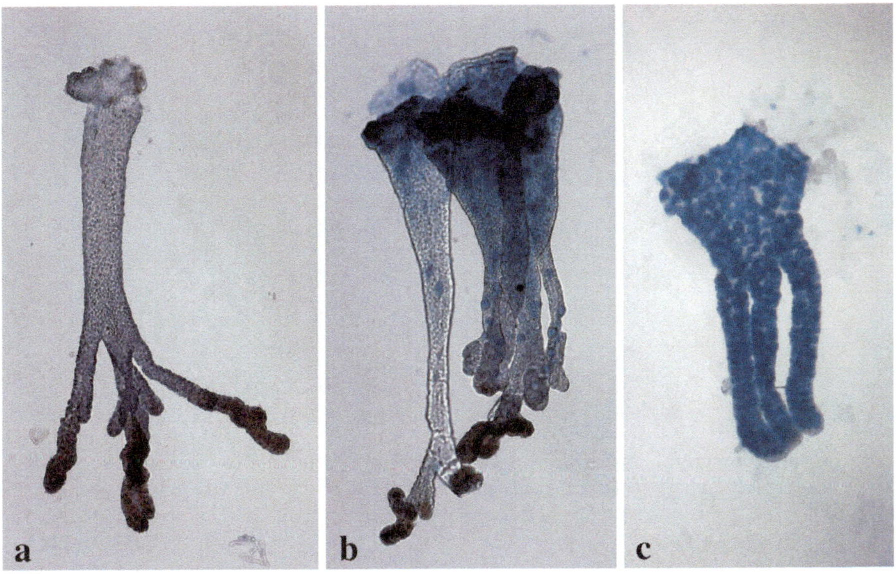

Fig. 1. Isolated stomach glands from pyloric mucosa. **a** Gastric (G) type; **b** gastric and intestinal (GI) mixed type; **c** intestinal (I) type. Alcian blue-paradoxical concanavalin A (AB-PCA) stain. ×200

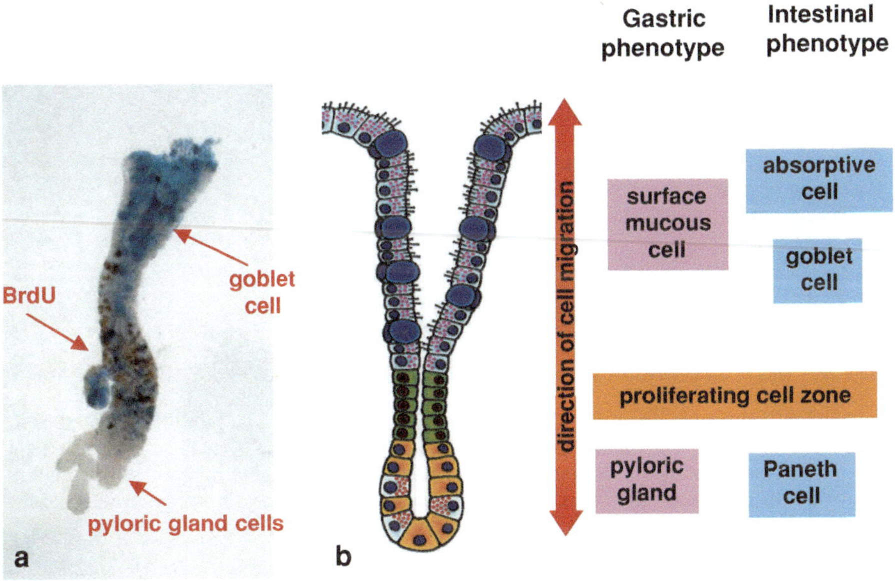

Fig. 2. Direction of cell migration and differentiation of gastric and intestinal phenotypic cells in GI mixed intestinal metaplasia (IM). **a** Isolated GI mixed intestinal metaplastic glands incubated in the presence of 10 mg/ml bromodeoxyuridine (*BrdU*) for 2 h. Proliferating cells are visualized with BrdU immunohistochemistry and goblet cells with alcian blue. ×100. **b** Schematic view of cell differentiation (*left panel*) and direction of cell migration in GI mixed intestinal metaplastic glands consisting of both gastric (*highlighted red*) and intestinal (*highlighted blue*) phenotypic cells (*right panel*)

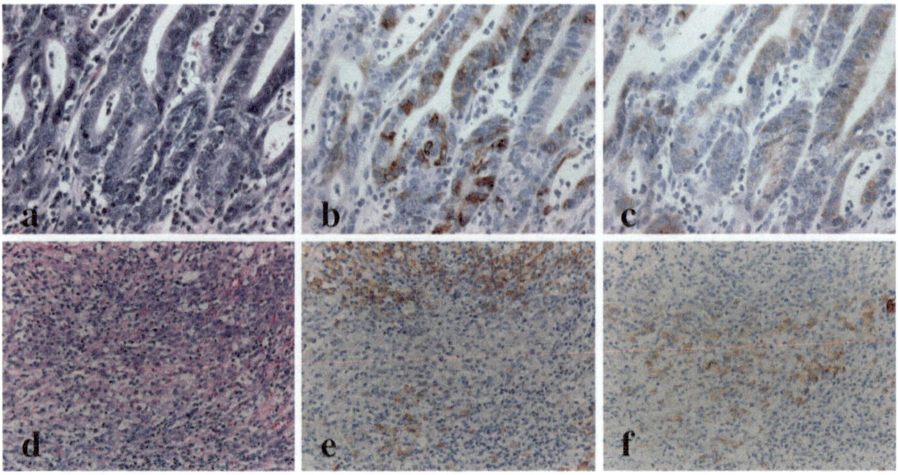

Fig. 3. Gastric phenotypic expression in both differentiated (**a–c**) and undifferentiated (**d–f**) type gastric carcinomas. **a, d** Hematoxyln and eosm (H&E) stain; **b, e** MUC5AC is detected in the cytoplasm of cancer cells; **c, f** MUC6 is apparent in the cytoplasm of tumor cells. ×320

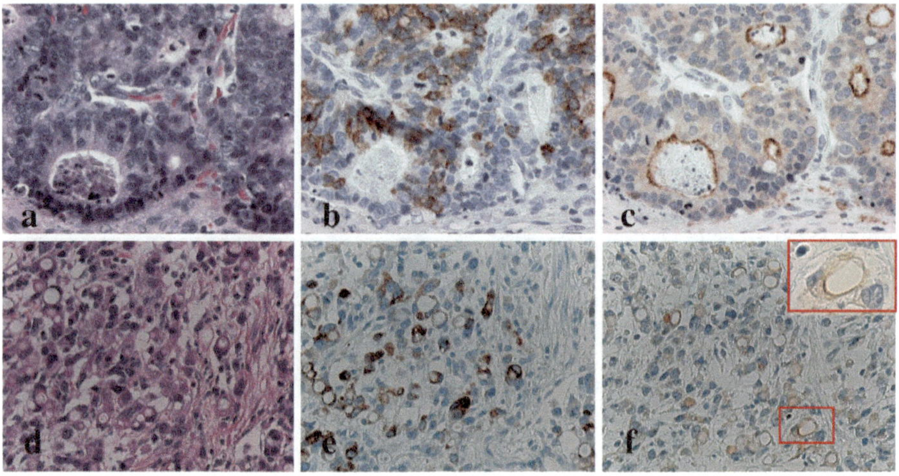

Fig. 4. Intestinal phenotypic expression in both differentiated (**a–c**) and undifferentiated (**d–f**) type gastric carcinomas. **a, d** H&E stain; **b, e** MUC2 is evident in the cytoplasm of cancer cells; **c, f** villin is apparent at the luminal surfaces of cancer cells. *Inset*, higher magnification of villin-positive tumor cells in a signet ring cell carcinoma **a–c** ×400; **d–f** ×320; *red squares* indicate a element ×640

Historical Review of Research and Treatment of Gastric Cancer in Japan: Clinical Aspect

Toshifusa Nakajima

Introduction

Gastric cancer has been decreasing in incidence in Western countries, but it still remains a leading cause of death in the world. Recent Japanese statistics (http://homepage3.nifty.com/mickeym/simin/140toukei-sibou.html) show that mortality due to gastric cancer is the second highest among males and the highest among females. However, in the past two decades, the death rate itself has been gradually decreasing in Japan as well as in Western countries, and this change is regarded as the result of the development of diagnosis, surgical techniques, effective chemotherapeutic agents, and patient care. Figure 1 shows the chronological changes in 5-year survival rate of gastric cancer patients treated in the Cancer Institute Hospital (1946–1999) by clinical stage, which clearly demonstrates the gradual increase decade by decade in all stages, especially remarkable in moderately advanced stage II and III diseases, and also shows concurrent decrease in morbidity and mortality. These improvements in treatment results are not prominent in other countries. The historical review of gastric cancer research in Japan may give some encouragement to clinicians who still struggle with the high morbidity and mortality rate of gastric cancer.

Diagnosis of Gastric Cancer

Development in the morphological diagnosis of gastric cancer in early days originated from the invention of the X-ray fluoroscopy apparatus, which Holzknecht [1,2] applied for the diagnosis of gastric disease in 1906 (Table 1). It has become one of the routine procedures in the diagnosis of gastric cancer. Conventional fluoroscopy and direct radiography were useful to detect advanced gastric cancer by a deformity, or filling defect using barium meal but were not sufficient for detection of early-stage cancer that could be cured by surgery.

Poor treatment results drove physicians to develop an effective mass-survey system with the aim of detecting early-stage cancer. Hauser employed X-ray fluoroscopy as a

Cancer Institute Hospital, Japanese Foundation for Cancer Research (JFCR), Tokyo, Japan
e-mail: nakajima@jfcr.or.jp

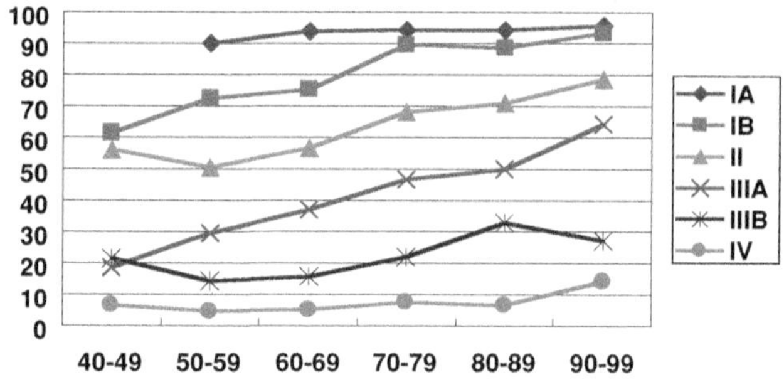

FIG. 1. Chronological changes in 5-year survival rates by clinical stage for 10688 patients who underwent surgery at Cancer Institute Hospital from 1946 to 1998

TABLE 1. Historical events in diagnosis

Year	Reporter	Events
1906	Holzknecht	Gastrofluoroscopy for gastric cancer
1911	Elsner	Hard gastroscope
1929	Porges	Gastrocamera
1932	Schindler	Soft gastroscope
1934	Kirihara	Soft gastroscope in Japan
1934	Hauser	Mass surgery with gastrofluoroscopy
1944	Castro	Indirect gastrofluoroscopy
1950	Uji, Sugiura	Gastrocamera
1953	Irie	Mass surgery with indirect gastrofluoroscopy
1957	Hiroschowitz	Fiberscope
1958	Shirakabe	Double-contrast method for early cancer
1958	Ariga, Kurokawa	Systematic mass survey in regional district

tool of mass survey of this disease in 1934, and Castro invented indirect radiography of the stomach in 1944, which facilitated later development in the mass-survey system [3]. In Japan, where gastric cancer had been prevalent, Irie initiated the mass-survey system with indirect radiography in 1953 [3], and this system was later incorporated into one of the important national health policies, which owed greatly to the endeavor of Ariga [4] and Kurokawa. Fluoroscopy was further developed as a tool of early detection of gastric cancer by incorporation of the double-contrast method by Shirakabe [5] in 1958. He found a mixture of barium meal and air in the stomach gives a clear contrast shadow of early cancer in the gastric mucosa. The curative resection rate was relatively low until this novel technique had been incorporated into clinical routines and the mass-survey system in Japan.

Endoscopy is another important tool for finding gastric cancer. Elsner [6] invented a metal gastroscopy in 1911, followed by a soft gastroscopy by Schinder in 1932, and in Japan, improved by Kirihara in 1934. The gastrocamera was invented by Uji [7] and Sugiura in 1950, which allowed color photography of the gastric lumen. The gastrocamera attracted the enthusiastic attention of physicians and drove them to detect mucosal, or early-stage, cancer. Hiroschowitz [8] demonstrated the principle of light transmission through glass fibers in 1957, and Japanese researchers and industries succeeded in the practical use of fiberscopy. Thus, the 1950s was a memorable era of the beginning of the early detection of gastric cancer in Japan. Tasaka [9] reported the nation-wide registry of early gastric cancer in 1962, and the incidence of early gastric cancer was 6.2% of resected cases. Recent statistics show that early-stage cancer is seen in more than half of the resected specimens among major cancer centers in Japan, which owes greatly to the recent development of diagnostic modalities.

Pathology and Biology

Pathology and biology are important for clinicians, not only to confirm the diagnosis but also to make an individual treatment plan for a given patient. Borrmann [10] reported macroscopic classification of tumor types in 1926, and his study has given most important information to clinicians as to how to proceed with treatment plans. He classified gastric cancer into four types according to the gross appearance of tumors, namely (1) localized, protruded, (2) localized, ulcerated, (3) infiltrating, ulcerated, and (4) diffuse, infiltrating types. This classification is the prototype of the later Japanese classification of macroscopic tumor types, and later studies reported a close correlation between the types of tumors and pattern of metastasis. In contrast to the macroscopic classification of advanced gastric cancer by Borrmann, that of early gastric cancer was defined in 1962 in Japan based on the proposal by Murakami et al. [11]. They defined three basic types (I, II, III) and four subbasic types (IIa, IIb, IIc, IIc + III) according to the macroscopic appearance of early gastric cancer.

Lymph node metastasis is the most frequent pattern of metastasis of gastric cancer. Inoue [12] reported close observation of the regional lymph node system in the upper abdomen of cadavers, and completed the map of lymphatic nodes and channels around the stomach in 1936. This map is also the prototype of lymph node station in the Japanese Classification of Gastric Carcinoma in 1961, and provided the basis for the theoretical concept of radical lymphadenectomy in Japan.

Associated with the diagnostic development of gastric cancer, relatively early-stage cancer increased in number among the resected cases. Although Borrmann already described incidental mucosa cancer in his text, Ayabe [13] reported the first two cases of mucosal cancer that were diagnosed preoperatively in 1949, and triggered enthusiasm for early diagnosis of gastric cancer in the 1950s. He introduced in his text that Bertrand and Konjetzny had separately reported a case of early gastric cancer with regional node metastasis, despite no infiltrative changes of atypical cells in the submucosal layer. He insisted that atypical cells in the mucosal epithelium that had hyperstained, various-sized nuclei, and the disappearance of normal glandular structures even with no metastasis, were enough to suggest malignancy. His idea is consistent with those of Bertrand, Konjetzny, and current Japanese pathologists. Western pathologists were reluctant to admit it as malignant when there were abnormal changes in epithelial cells without invasion into submucosal layer or lymph nodes, and instead defined such changes as dysplasia [14,15]. Thus, such discrepancy in the diagnosis of cancer or dysplasia in the mucosa between Japan and Western countries has continued for more than 50 years. Referring to the reports by Bertrand and Konjetzney might give some hints to solve this discrepancy between Japan and Western countries.

Although Hauser discussed the pathogenesis of gastric cancer arising from the scar of chronic gastric ulcer in 1883, in Japan, Takizawa, Ohta, Murakami, and many other researchers devoted their efforts to such issues as histological classification, macroscopic classification of early cancer, pathogenesis, morphological aspects of early cancer, malignant cycles of early cancer, and the process of developing from early to advanced cancer [16].

The current of early cancer detection resulted in founding the Japan Anti-Cancer Association (chaired by Shioda, Sugimura) in 1958, the Japanese Research Society for Gastric Cancer Study (chaired by Kajitanl, Niski) in 1962, and several research societies for early gastric cancer or mass-screening in 1962. Recently *Helicobacter pylori* has attracted the attention of etiologists and physicians because of its potential to cause gastric cancer, but it is still controversial as to its definite evidence for carcinogenesis [17].

Surgery

Dawn of Gastric Cancer Treatment [1,18,19]

No one is likely to disagree with the idea that surgery still remains the first choice of treatment modalities for gastric cancer, even at the beginning of the 21st century. The first gastrectomy was attempted by Pean in 1879, and successfully followed by Billroth in 1881 (Table 2). Mikulicz also succeeded in making the precise diagnosis of gastric cancer with gastroscopy and performed successful distal gastrectomy in 1883. Schlatter succeeded in total gastrectomy in 1897. In the same year, in Japan, Kondo [20] reported his first success in distal gastrectomy, followed by Itoh who succeeded in the first case of total gastrectomy in 1906. He placed a proximal cut line in the cardia, and true total gastrectomy was owing to Miyake in 1918, who placed the proximal cut line in the esophagus. Successful cardiectomy was reported by Mikulicz in 1896. Miyake [21] reported in 1914 his 10 years experience, in which resectability was 42.9% (167/389), postoperative mortality was 14.6%, and 3-year survival rate was 19.2% (19/39). Mutou [22] compared the mortality rate between Japan and Western countries in 1965: (1) decreased tendency of mortality rate in Japan and Western countries was observed associated with decades; (2) Japanese mortality rate ranged from 13.8% to 21.1% before World War II and fell below 10% after the war, whereas, in Western countries it ranged from 11.0% to 38.8% in the former period and from 6.0% to 18.6% in the latter period; and (3) these results suggested that Japanese surgery was superior to that in Western countries in terms of number of operated cases and treatment results.

Standard Gastrectomy

From the point of view of radicality, eradication of malignant lesions as complete as possible might allow us to expect longer survival of patients with gastric cancer. Radical gastrectomy aims to eradicate both the primary lesion and lymphatic spread regional to the stomach. Based on meticulous examination of the surgical stump of resected specimens, Tomoda [23] advocated wide indication of total gastrectomy in 1950. This idea coincides with total gastrectomy *de principe* in the later period [24]. As is discussed in the next paragraph, systematic radical lymph node dissection was advocated by Kuru [25], Kajitani [26], and Jinnai [27]. To avoid the suture insufficiency of gastroduodenostomy, Nakayama fixed the posterior wall of the remnant stomach

TABLE 2. Historical events in surgery

Year	Reporter	Events
1879	Pean	First attempt of distal gastrectomy
1881	Billroth	First success in distal gastrectomy
1883	Mikulicz	Diagnosis with gastroscopy and successful gastrectomy
1896	Mikulicz	First success in cardiectomy
1897	Schlatter	First success in total gastrectomy
1897	Kondo	First success in distal gastrectomy in Japan
1908	Voelcker	Success in cardiectomy
1918	Miyake	First success in total gastrectomy in Japan
1940	Seo	Jejunal interposition after total gastrectomy
1940	Morton	Total gastrectomy *de principe*
1942	Kajitani	Wide dissection of lymph nodes
1947	Brunshwig	Pancreaticoduodenectomy (PD) for distal gastric cancer involving pancreas head
1949	Yoshioka, Kajitani	PD for distal gastric cancer in Japan
1950	Tomoda	Total gastrectomy de principe
1950	Weinberg	Vital staining of lymph nodes during surgery
1952	Kajitani	Extended radical dissection
1953	Appleby	Appleby surgery
1955	Kajitani, Yamada	Vital lymph node staining with sky blue
1961	Jinnai	Extended radical gastrectomy
1969	Wada	Introduction of Appleby surgery into Japan
1969	Hauser	Lymph node scanning with isotope
1980	Takekoshi	Endoscopic mucosal resection (EMR) with endoscopic double snare polypectomy (EDSP)
	Hirao	EMR with endoscopic resection with hypertonic saline-epinephrine (ERHSE)
1984	Tada	EMR with strip biopsy
1984	Kajitani, Ohashi	Left upper abdominal evisceration
1984	Aiko	Lymph node scanning with isotope in Japan
1987	Takahashi	Lymph node staining with active carbon particles
1992	Goh	Laparoscopic Billroth II gastrectomy (ulcer)
1994	Kitano Uyama	Laparotomy-assisted gastrectomy (LAG) with abdominal wall elevating method
1999	Bonenkamp	Randomized controlled trial (RCT) of D1 vs. D2 dissection in radical gastrectomy

to the pancreas head [28]. Before this report, most surgeons preferred Billroth II type anastomosis after Miyagi [29], or the Shioda method because of its safety. General consensuses on safe and radical gastrectomy were reflected in the statement of radical gastrectomy in the General Rules for the Gastric Cancer Study issued by the Japanese Research Society for Gastric Cancer Study in 1961 in Japan. Instead of total gastrectomy *de principe*, the resection line has been recommended to be placed properly according to the tumor type, namely, 3 cm in localized cancer, and 5 cm in diffused cancer apart from the tumor margin. There is no comparative study related to total versus subtotal gastrectomy in our country, but two randomized controlled trials (RCTs) [30,31] are available in Europe. There were no differences in stump recurrence at resection margin and survival benefit between the two methods.

Since 1961, D2 dissection (eradication of all nodes in N1–N2 stations) has been the Japanese standard procedure of radical gastrectomy for locally advanced gastric cancer. The General Rules define the degree of lymph node dissection as R0–R3 (later D0–D3) according to the anatomic stations of lymph nodes. Radicality of surgery is defined as curative (D-number ≧ N-number with M0) or noncurative (D-number < N-number, or M1) in relation to the extent of surgery and spread of disease based on the meticulous postoperative dissection of the resected specimen. All documents of operative findings are described and recorded in relation to the extent of disease (T, N, and M categories) and extent of surgery (type of surgery and radicality) based on the General Rules. It has provided the common basis of documentation to facilitate the Nationwide Registry of Gastric Cancer since 1969 [32].

Lymph Node Dissection

As stated previously, metastasis to the lymph nodes is the most frequent type of cancer spread, which could only be controlled by surgeons with meticulous lymphadenectomy. Kajitani [26] stressed the importance of wide dissection of regional lymph nodes to eradicate lymphatic spread in 1944, and Jinnai [27] also advocated a systematic radical gastrectomy in 1961. Use of intraoperative vital dye staining of lymph nodes with pontamine sky blue was reported by Weinberg and Greaney [33] in 1950 to facilitate the identification of regional lymph nodes to perform radical dissection. Intraoperative or preoperative lymph node staining was studied by many investigators with sky blue [34] or iodine contrast medium [35], radioisotopes [35–37], or activated carbon particles [38]. Approach to the regional lymphatic channels with radioisotopes paved the way to later development of sentinel node navigation surgery, although its significance is still controversial in gastric cancer surgery.

D2 dissection is supported in Japan and in some Asian and Western countries [39–42] as a standard surgery for locally advanced gastric cancer. D2 dissection has been advocated from the theoretical and anatomic point of view to minimize the residual tumor after surgery. There is no critical evaluation on the comparison between D1 and D2 in Japan. However, in Europe, a large-scale phase III trial was performed in Holland, reporting that higher incidences of postoperative morbidity and mortality were observed in D2 than in D1 [43], and in 1999, later results of two prospective randomized controlled trials (RCT) in Europe [44,45] reported that no survival advantage of D2 was observed over D1. These reports seemed to be a challenge to D2 supporters and led to heated arguments among surgeons [46–48]. Up to date, the results seem to be accepted as true in most Western countries, but are subject to criticism by D2 supporters because very high postoperative morbidity and mortality are thought to have spoiled the survival benefit of radical dissection, mainly due to low hospital and surgeon volumes. The benefit of D2 surgery should be established by further RCT to determine whether to adopt it as a standard surgery.

Extended Surgery

As part of the combined multiorgan resection of involved organs that are adjacent to the stomach, pancreatoduodenectomy (PD) for distal gastric cancer involving the head of the pancreas was reported by Brunshwig in 1947 [19]. In Japan, Yoshioka [49] and Kajitani [50] also paved the way to extended radical surgery with PD in 1949.

Appleby [51], in 1953, advocated an approach to the celiac axis for the radical eradication of the whole stomach, distal pancreas, spleen, and regional lymph nodes. This procedure was introduced to Japan by Wada [52] in 1969. Extended lymph node dissection was advocated by Jinnai [27] in 1961. Prophylactic combined resection, including pancreatosplenectomy or splenectomy, has been justified as the standard procedure to perform complete D2 dissection of lymph nodes along the lienal artery and those at the splenic hilum in upper or middle gastric cancer in Japan. However, these prophylactic combined resections involving the pancreas are subject to argument in Western countries because of the high incidence of postoperative complications. Dissection of lymph nodes along the abdominal aorta, which was initiated in the Cancer Institute Hospital in the 1950s, attracted the attention of surgeons to these terminal nodes in 1976 by yielding long-term survivors who had nodal involvement in the terminal stations [53]. Indications for paraaortic nodes were discussed positively [54–56] and negatively [57]. Left upper abdominal evisceration (LUAE) was proposed by Kajitani for the eradication of proximal advanced gastric cancer in 1984 [58]. LUAE includes total gastrectomy, pancreatosplenectomy, transverse colectomy, and sometimes left hepatectomy if necessary. These methods of extended radical gastrectomy have been proposed from the theoretical and anatomic points of view, and somewhat improved treatment results of moderately advanced gastric cancer, namely, stage II and III disease [59]. However, the survival benefit is not yet confirmed by prospective RCTs.

Less-Invasive Surgery

In contrast to extended gastrectomy, modified minimized gastrectomy has attracted the attention of surgeons in accordance with the increased number of occurrences of relatively early-stage cancer. Modified gastrectomy includes reduction of the resected area, reduced extent of lymphadenectomy (D1 or less), and some function-preserving procedures such as pylorus ring or vagal nerve preservation [60]. Mucosal cancer supposedly without lymphatic spread is safely subjected to endoscopic mucosal resection (EMR) in Japan since 1980 [61–64].

Endoscopic intervention later developed into the laparoscopic approach to gastrectomy. In 1992, Goh et al. [65] reported success in laparoscopic Billroth II gastrectomy for gastric ulcer, and Kitano et al. [66] and Uyama et al. [67] succeeded in laparoscopic gastrectomy for early cancer in 1994. These minimal invasive approaches clearly have contributed to improvements in the postoperative quality of life of treated patients, but still remained to be evaluated in terms of radicality and technical skill.

Common Podium for Research and Practice

Associated with developments in treatment modality, clinicians have had a variety of treatment options according to disease extent, and some confusion was raised concerning the proper indication. The Japanese Gastric Cancer Association (JGCA) issued gastric cancer treatment guidelines for doctors [60] and patients [68] in 2001 to provide a standard indication to the complexity of various disease extents. The Japanese Classification of Gastric Carcinoma [69] and Treatment Guidelines now consist of two columns that provide a common podium for research and practice of gastric cancer.

Chemotherapy

Short History of Chemotherapy for Advanced Gastric Cancer in Japan [70,71]

Modern anticancer chemotherapy is well known to have its origin from a chemical weapon in World War II, nitrogen mustard. One of the various derivatives, nitromin, developed by Ishidate et al. [72], was incorporated into clinical practice in the early 1950s in our country. A rush of clinical reports appeared in medical journals on its marginal anticancer effect associated with serious side effects. Nitromin was succeeded in the late 1950s by mitomycin C (MMC) and 5-fluorouracil (5-FU), a stem combination regimen in later studies for advanced gastric cancer. Tegafur and adriamycin (ADM) were introduced to clinical practice in the late 1960s, and used as a single agent or a part of combination regimens for advanced gastric cancer. Their response rates (RR) were around or less than 20% with minimum survival benefit. FAM therapy [73], a combination of 5-FU, ADM, and MMC, was widely used as a standard regimen in Western countries, and primarily produced a 50% RR, although such high response was not proved in the following trials (Table 3).

Incorporation of cisplatin (CDDP) to clinical trials in the late 1970s was an epoch-making event in terms of its contribution to improving RR of CDDP-containing regimens. Recent effective regimens include a combination of 5-FU and CDDP, which is followed by S-1, taxanes, and CPT-11 in current chemotherapy. Phase I and II studies of S-1-based regimens [74–76], or a combination of taxanes and CDDP [77], or CPT-11 and CDDP [78,79] showed RR higher than 50% with potential survival benefit, although phase III trials do not yet include the standard chemotherapy to date.

Oral Chemotherapy

Principles of traditional Western chemotherapy had been based on the total cell kill theory in the treatment of leukemia [80], and systemic dose-intensive regimens have been employed until recently. Therefore, Western oncologists did not favor the oral administration of anticancer drugs.

However, the efficacy of oral chemotherapy has been established in breast [81] and lung cancer [82], but not in gastrointestinal (GI) cancer [83–85], in Western countries. Negative results of previous trials of GI tract cancers in Western countries could be attributed to the use of active-type drugs. In contrast, oral administration of masked compounds has been a popular and characteristic drug delivery route in Japan. This delivery route is reported to have an advantage of keeping a constant drug concentration in the peripheral blood for a relatively long time because of gradual conversion from masked to active type in the liver. It is also convenient for treating patients at home. Oral tegafur, 5-FU, 5′-DFUR (doxifluridine), and HCFU (carmofur) were used in Japan in the 1980s, and UFT (tegafur, uracil) and S-1 (TS-1) were applied in the 1990s to this delivery route. Reviewing recent literature shows that beneficial evidence of oral chemotherapy has been accumulated not only in our country but also in Western countries. One RCT showed that a combination of UFT and leucovorin (both oral) showed a comparable effect with less toxicity than intravenous 5-FU and leucovorin (LV) in colorectal cancer [86,87]. A comparative UFT/LV study between Japan and the United

TABLE 3. Historical events in cancer chemotherapy

Year	Reporter	Event
1952	Tasaka, Ohtsuki, Katsunuma	Chemotherapy with nitromin
1956	Yamamoto	Chemosensitivity test with CAP (cylinder agar plate method)
1957	Ishibashi Nishioka	Sensitivity test with I.N.K. (Institute for Infectious Diseases, National Institute for Health, Kimoto Clinic) method
1957	Heidelberger	5-Fluorouracil
1959	Tasaki, Taguchi, Tasaka, Kimura	Chemotherapy for gastric cancer with mitomycin C (MMC)
1962	Moore, Longmire	Adjuvant chemotherapy with Thio-TEPA Multicenter randomized controlled study
1962	Shiba	Adjuvant chemotherapy with MMC
1962	Inokuchi	Intraceliac artery chemotherapy
1964	Skipper	Total cell kill theory
1964	Watkins	Continuous intraarterial (ia) chemotherapy pump
1964	Kondo	Succinic dehydrogenase inhibition (SDI) test
1967	Karnofsky	Performance status and outcome
1967	Yamagata	Chemotherapy response criteria by Japanese Society for Clinical Oncology
1972	Folkman	Tumor dormancy concept
1976	Ohsawa	Introduction of in vivo chemosensitivity test with nude mouse
1979	WHO	Chemotherapy Response Criteria
1982	Miura	Introduction of infusaid (implantable continuous infusion pump)
1993, 1994	Hermans	Meta-analysis of adjuvant chemotherapy
1995	Holmgren	Angiogenesis suppression
	Takahashi	Long NC for new endpoint of chemotherapy, and tumor dormancy therapy
1998	Sakata	49% response rate (RR) with S-1 alone
2000	Therasse	RECIST
2001	Macdonald	Survival benefit with adjuvant chemoradiotherapy

States showed similar effects and mild toxicities in advanced colorectal cancer [88]. A combination of VP-16, UFT, and leucovorin was also proved to be effective in advanced gastric cancer [89]. 5′-DFUR–based chemotherapy was also active in advanced gastric cancer [90,91]. S-1, as a single agent, was proved to have an outstanding RR, up to 50%, with marginal survival benefit [74,92], and S-1-based combination chemotherapy seems to be useful regarding both safety and higher local response [75,76,93]. These results seems to crush persistent adherence to i.v. chemotherapy in Western countries [94], and oral chemotherapy should properly be evaluated to be one of the useful delivery routes in GI tract cancers.

Regional Chemotherapy

Chemotherapy outcome may partly depend on the local concentration of drugs at the tumor site. To increase drug concentration, regional chemotherapy has been attempted in various delivery routes such as intraarterial or intraabdominal. One-shot intraarterial (ia) chemotherapy was used in the early days with the introduction of a catheter into the artery. Inokuchi et al. reported a method of ia chemotherapy into the celiac artery with an artificial artery and plastic catheter [95]. Invention of portable, and later implantable, infusion pumps [96–98] and implantable portal devices facilitated continuous ia chemotherapy. Good local response and some survival benefit were reported by many clinicians [99–101], but the survival benefit of ia chemotherapy is not established compared with systemic chemotherapy. Survival benefit would be obtained by curative resection after achieving tumor reduction with regional chemotherapy. Nakajima et al. [102] reported long-term survivors, more than 5 years, who had extensive paraaortic lymph node metastasis treated with systemic and ia chemotherapy followed by radical surgery.

Reevaluation of Endpoints and Evaluation Criteria in Chemotherapy

Response rate (RR) has been adopted as the primary endpoint in almost all cancer clinical trials. However, it should essentially be a surrogate endpoint for survival benefit. Survival benefit is usually evaluated by median survival time (MST), survival rate at a certain time, or median time to progression (TTP). Recent trials often employ both RR and MST for their endpoints. RR sometimes correlates with survival time, but does not correlate with other time measures. It is an important issue to solve the conflict in evaluation when there is a discrepancy between local response and survival endpoints. 5′-DFUR is reported to yield a low, not encouraging, RR with a very long stable state so long as the drug is administered [103]. If RR is employed as the only endpoint, this kind of drug might not be evaluated as being effective. Takahashi and Nishioka [104] employed the concept of tumor dormancy to make a reasonable explanation of these observations, and recommended median TTP as an endpoint superior to RR in this case. TTP may be better than MST because the former endpoint could eliminate the effect of secondary survival benefit, which might be actually attributed to second- or third-line chemotherapy with recent new drugs. Quality of life (QOL) and cost–benefit efficiency may serve as a complimentary endpoint when survival benefit is equal in a comparative study. As mentioned previously, comparative study of oral UFT/leucovorin and i.v. 5-FU/leucovorin is a good example of this endpoint. There are several QOL evaluation criteria available in Japan and in Europe.

Common evaluation criteria for treatment response are mandatory to make a fair evaluation of effect and to compare the results from different groups. For this purpose, WHO issued common response criteria of chemotherapy in 1979, followed by the Japanese Society of Clinical Oncology [105] in 1986. Recent RECIST criteria [106] are widely accepted for available response evaluation. NCI-CTC [107] is also commonly used in many recent trials for evaluation of toxicity. Japanese clinical trials employ JSCO or JGCA response criteria combined with these for gastric cancer chemotherapy.

Adjuvant and Neoadjuvant Chemotherapy

Prophylactic use of anticancer drugs after curative gastrectomy aims at suppressing cancer relapse from minimum residual foci after curative surgery. Clinical trial of adjuvant chemotherapy for gastric cancer in Japan was initiated in the late 1950s. According to reviews [108–110] on adjuvant chemotherapy trials in Japan, two groups, namely the National Hospital Group (chaired by Dr. Y. Koyama) and University Hospital Group (Dr. H. Imanaga), took leadership in conducting multicenter trials in phase III type with MMC alone, or MMC and 5-FU-based combination chemotherapy such as MFC (combination of MMC, 5-FU, and cytosine arabinoside) [111–113]. The Japanese Research Foundation for Multi-disciplinary Therapy (formerly chaired by Inokuchi, succeeded by Saji) carried out a series of clinical trials of nonspecific immunotherapy with PSK (Krestine: a polysaccaride), or OK-432 in the late 1970s [114,115], and also oral chemotherapy with tegafur was incorporated into clinical trials in the late 1970s [116–120]. The Japan Clinical Oncology Group (JCOG), supported by the Ministry of Welfare and Labor, is also active in clinical trials in this field [119,121]. These studies suggested no overall survival benefit, but some marginal benefit in certain subsets, namely moderately advanced stage II or III disease. Meta-analysis in Western countries and ours [122–127] revealed significant survival benefit from adjuvant chemotherapy in gastric cancer, and further studies are warranted for yielding solid evidence for survival benefit by single (namely not combined) trial. In response to this need, a large-scale adjuvant chemotherapy trial is now comparing curative gastrectomy followed by adjuvant S-1 with surgery alone (ACTS-GC trial).

Encouraged by good response to recent chemotherapy for advanced cancer, neoadjuvant chemotherapy has become an alternate approach for locally advanced gastric cancer. The concept of neoadjuvant chemotherapy was introduced by Frei et al. [128], who claimed that preoperative chemotherapy could minimize the viability of residual microfoci left behind after surgery. However, in Japan, neoadjuvant chemotherapy has been used in inoperable advanced gastric cancer, with the aim of downstaging the disease enough to be operable. Table 4 shows a series of novel neoadjuvant chemotherapy trials in our country and abroad, which sometimes yielded more than 50% RR and long-term survivors. Most Japanese neoadjuvant chemotherapies include a combination of 5-FU or its derivatives and CDDP as an essential part of the regimens [102,129,130]. Protracted continuous infusion of 5-FU associated with low-dose CDDP is a favorite regimen for neoadjuvant therapy among surgical oncologists [131–134] because of its relatively high response rate with mild toxicities, although

TABLE 4. Neoadjuvant chemo (radio) therapy with excellent results

Year	Reporter	Event
1993	Yonemura	Good local response (66%) and survival benefit (MST 17 months) in stage IV patients with PMUE
1996	Kondo	Low-dose cisplaton (CDDP) + protracted 5-fluorouracil (5-FU) produced good local response (55%) and increased resectability (71%)
1996	Suga	UFT + CDDP yielded good local response in scirrhous cancer
1997	Nakajima	FLEP yielded good local response (50%) and long survivors in unresectable cancer (5-year survival rate, 17.7%)
2001	Lowy	Continuous 5-FU and pre- and intraoperative radiotherapy produced good local response (RR, 74%)

MST, median survival time; PMUE, CDDP + MMC + etoposide + UFT; FLEP, 5-FU + leucovorin + etposide + CDDP; RR, response rate

the late survival outcome is not yet available in most trials. Comparative study is necessary between the standard and low-dose regimen of FP therapy.

It is difficult to carry out phase III trials of neoadjuvant chemotherapy in inoperable disease to determine survival benefit, and no trials are available in our country. However, some trials were done abroad in operable disease. These trials showed that neoadjuvant chemotherapy failed to suggest either survival benefit [135] or improvement in curability [136]. However, this approach is mandatory in Japan to clarify the survival benefit of neoadjuvant chemotherapy.

Chemosensitivity Test

As an in vitro chemosensitivity test for gastric cancer in Japan, CAP (cylinder agar plate) method [137] and INK method (Institute for Infectious Diseases, National Institute for Health, and Kimoto Clinic [138]) were used in early days. Ishibashi et al. [139] reported with the INK method that 33% (6/18) of gastric cancers responded to nitromin, 40% (8/26) to sarkomycin, and 29% (5/17) to TESPA. In 1964, Kondo et al. [140] reported with the succinic dehydrogenase inhibition (SDI) test that the response rate was 62% to nitromin, 24% to mitomycin C, and 34% to toyomycin. Ohsawa [141] introduced to Japan the in vivo sensitivity test with xenograft transplanted in the nude mouse in 1975. Since then, various in vitro and in vivo sensitivity tests have been developed in Japan. According to Tanigawa [142], the most popular test currently is CD-DST (collagen gel droplet embedded drug sensitivity test), followed by the MTT assay, HDRA (histoculture drug response assay), and SDI test. These sensitivity tests seem to produce a favorable outcome in clinical trials [143], but the clinical significance still remains to be elucidated.

Summary

The history of basic and clinical research in gastric cancer originated from the 19th century in Europe, but surprisingly rapid response to this flow abroad occurred in Japan in every aspect of research and treatment of this disease. Researchers in early days devoted their best efforts to conquer the most frequent cancer in Japan. Diagnosis of gastric cancer has been highly elaborated with the aid of the double-contrast method of X-ray fluoroscopy and meticulous endoscopic apparatus, which facilitated both minimum and extended surgery according to the extent of disease. Effective anticancer drugs are available now, some of which were developed originally in our country. Daily use of gene diagnosis and treatment could be expected in the near future. Now we can enjoy a high level of treatment results in the fields of surgery and chemotherapy and should try to establish a global standard of diagnosis and treatment of gastric cancer. International corroboration is mandatory to achieve these goals, and we could expect the International and Japanese Gastric Cancer Associations and the WHO Collaborating Center for Primary Prevention, Diagnosis and Treatment of Gastric Cancer (chaired by Suemasu, Maruyama, Sasako) will take a leading role in this field. Gastric cancer still remains one of the prevailing cancers in our country, and our next goal should be based in prophylaxis to reduce the incidence of gastric cancer.

References

1. Ishikawa K, Sakai S (1996) Historical review. In: Gastric cancer in Japan (in Japanese). Kanehara Shuppan, Tokyo, pp 1–19
2. Shirakabe H, Nishizawa M (1996) X-ray and nuclear diagnosis. In: Gastric cancer in Japan (in Japanese). Kanehara Shuppan, Tokyo, pp 191–217
3. Shirakabe H, Nishizawa N (1996) Mass-screening system. In: Gastric cancer in Japan (in Japanese). Kanehara Shuppan, Tokyo, pp 349–360
4. Ariga K, Takahashi A (1965) Mass screening of gastric cancer (in Japanese). Nanzando, Tokyo, pp 4–5
5. Shirakabe H (1963) Merit and demerit of double contrast method in upper gastrointestinal tract series (in Japanese). Rinshou Kenkyu 40:768–770
6. Sakita T, Takasu Y (1996) Endoscopy, cytology and biopsy diagnosis of gastric cancer. In: Gastric cancer in Japan (in Japanese). Kanehara Shuppan, Tokyo, pp 241–305
7. Uji T (1953) Study on the photography of gastric mucosa and its clinical application (in Japanese). Tokyo Igaku Zasshi 61:135–142
8. Hirschowitz B, Curtiss LE, Peters CW, Pollard HM (1958) Demonstration of new gastroscope, the "fiberscope." Gastroenterology 35:50–53
9. Tasaka S (1962) Nation-wide registry of early gastric cancer (in Japanese). Gastroenterol Endosc 4:4–14
10. Borrmann R (1926) Geschwulste des Magens und Duodenums. In: Handbuch der speziellen pathologischen Anatomie und Histologie, vol 4. Springer, Berlin, pp 812–1054
11. Murakami T, Nagayo T, Kanai S, et al (1963) Macroscopic classification of early gastric cancer and histopathological examination (in Japanese). Shoukakibyou no Rinshou 5:703–711
12. Inoue Y (1936) Lymphatic system of gastroduodenum, pancreas and diaphragma (in Japanese). Kaibougakuzasshi 9:35–123
13. Ayabe M (1949) So-called early gastric cancer (in Japanese). Rinshou to Kenkyu 26:514–525
14. Schlemper R, Itabashi M, Kato Y, et al (1997) Differences in diagnostic criteria for gastric carcinoma between Japanese and western pathologists. Lancet 349:1725–1729
15. Kato Y (1999) International concern to early gastric cancer—attempt to standardization of histological diagnosis (in Japanese). Dig Endosc 11:295–299
16. Sugano H, Kato Y (1996) Historical aspect of pathology. In: Gastric cancer in Japan (in Japanese). Kanehara Shuppan, Tokyo, pp 625–641
17. Kuipers E (1999) Review article: exploring the link between *Helicobacter pylori* and gastric cancer. Aliment Pharmacol Ther 13:3–11
18. Kawamata K (1871) History of gastric cancer (in Japanese). Igakutosho Shuppan, Tokyo
19. Takahama T, Wada T (1996) Surgical treatment. In: Gastric cancer in Japan (in Japanese). Kanehara Shuppan, Tokyo, pp 371–395
20. Kondo T (1899) An experiment in gastric cancer surgery (in Japanese). Nihon Gekagakkai Zasshi 1:234–252
21. Miyake H (1914) Treatment result of gastric cancer with surgery (in Japanese). Chugai Igakushinpo 823:901–902
22. Mutou M (1965) Surgical aspect of gastric cancer (in Japanese). Kanehara Shuppan, Tokyo
23. Tomoda M (1953) Surgery of gastric cancer (in Japanese). Rinshou to Kenkyu 30:300–308
24. Pichlmayr R, van Alste E (1976) Die totale Gastrektomie als Regeloperation beim operablen Magencarcinom. Langenbecks Arch Klin Chir 342:227–231
25. Kuru M (1935) Statistical consideration of radical surgery for gastric cancer (in Japanese). Rinshou IIgaku 23:390–390
26. Kajitani T (1944) Lymph node metastasis of gastric cancer (in Japanese). Nihon Gekagakkai Zassi 45:15–16
27. Jinnai D (1961) Extended radical operation of gastric cancer, with special emphasis on the lymph node dissection (in Japanese). Gekashinryou 3:556–556

28. Nakayama K (1949) Gastrectomy with fixation of posterior gastric wall to the pancreas (in Japanese). Shujutu 3:51–56
29. Miyagi J (1928) A variation of gastrectomy. Nihon Gekagakkai Zasshi 29:786–786
30. Gouzi J, Huguier M, Fagniez P, et al (1989) Total versus subtotal gastrectomy for adenocarcinoma of the gastric antrum. A French prospective controlled study. Ann Surg 209:162–166
31. Bozzetti F, Marubini E, Bonfanti G, et al (1999) Subtotal versus total gastrectomy for gastric cancer: five-year survival rates in a multicenter randomized Italian trial. Ann Surg 230:170–178
32. Miwa K (1996) Nationwide registry of gastric cancer and statistics. In: Gastric cancer in Japan (in Japanese). Kanehara Shuppan, Tokyo, pp 465–506
33. Weinberg J, Greaney E (1950) Identification of regional lymph nodes by means of a vital dye during surgery of gastric cancer. Surg Gynecol Obstet 90:561–567
34. Kajitani T, Yamada S (1955) Clinical application of vital lymph node staining with sky blue to radical surgery for gastric cancer (in Japanese). Gan no Rinsho 1:513–516
35. Uchida H (1971) A study on lymphography regional to the stomach and adjacent organs (in Japanese). Nihon Igakuhoushasen Gakkaishi 31:259–277
36. Hauser W, Atkins H, Richards P (1969) Lymph node scanning with ^{99m}Tc-sulfur colloid. Radiology 92:1369–1371
37. Aikou T, Saihara T, Nishi M (1983) Lymph flow at the cardia and lymphatic metastasis of cardiac cancer with special reference to the use of radio-isotope lymphography (in Japanese). Rinpagaku 6:248–252
38. Takahashi S, Takahashi T, Hagiwara A, et al (1987) Lymph node dissection according to the location of gastric cancer with staining of lymph nodes with micro-active carbon particles (in Japanese). Shoukakigeka Gakkai Zasshi 20:720–725
39. Siewert J, Bottcher K, Roder J, et al (1993) Prognostic relevance of systemic lymph node dissection in gastric carcinoma. German Gastric Carcinoma Study Group. Br J Surg 80:1015–1018
40. Pacelli F, Doglietto G, Bellantone R, Alfieri S, Sgadari A, Crucitti F (1993) Extensive versus limited lymph node dissection for gastric cancer: a comparative study of 320 patients. Br J Surg 80:1153–1156
41. Roukos D (1999) Current advances and changes in treatment strategy may improve survival and quality of life in patients with potentially curable gastric cancer. Ann Surg Oncol 6:46–56
42. Sierra A, Regueira F, Hernandez-Lizoain J, et al (2003) Role of the extended lymphadenectomy in gastric cancer surgery: experience in a single institution. Ann Surg Oncol 10:219–226
43. Bunt A, Hermans J, Boon M, et al (1994) Evaluation of the extent of lymphadenectomy in a randomized trial of Western- versus Japanese-type surgery in gastric cancer. J Clin Oncol 12:417–422
44. Cuschieri A, Weeden S, Fielding J, et al (1999) Patient survival after D1 and D2 resections for gastric cancer: long-term results of the MRC randomized surgical trial. Surgical Co-operative Group. Br J Cancer 79:1522–1530
45. Bonenkamp J, Hermans J, Sasako M, et al (1999) Extended lymph-node dissection for gastric cancer. Dutch Gastric Cancer Group. N Engl J Med 340:908–914
46. Pacelli F, Sgadari A, Doglietto G (1999) Surgery for gastric cancer. N Engl J Med 341:538–538
47. Brennan M (1999) Lymph-node dissection for gastric cancer. N Engl J Med 340:956–958
48. Marubini E, Bozzetti F, Bonfanti G, et al Gastrointestinal Tumor Study Group (2002) Lymphadenectomy in gastric cancer: prognostic role and therapeutic implications. Eur J Surg Oncol 28:406–412
49. Yoshioka H, Miyazaki S (1952) A case report of gastric cancer treated with pancreatoduodenectomy (in Japanese). Rinshou Geka 7:231–235

50. Kajitani T, Hoshino T, (1952) An experience of pancreatoduodenectomy (in Japanese). Rinshougeka 7:231–235
51. Appleby L (1953) The coeliac axis in the expansion of the operation for gastric carcinoma. Cancer (Phila) 6:704–707
52. Wada T, Katayama K, et al (1978) Extent of lymph node dissection in gastric cancer (in Japanese). Geka 40:154–159
53. Ohashi I, Takagi K, Konishi T, et al (1976) 5 year survivors of gastric cancer patients with para-aortic lymph node metastasis (in Japanese). Nihon Shoukakigeka Gakkaishi 9:507–512
54. Aikou T, Yoshinaka H, Shimazu H (1988) Significance and indication of para-aortic lymph node metastasis from esophago-gastric cancer (in Japanese). Gan no Rinshou 34:1677–1683
55. Yamada S, Okajima K, Isozaki H, et al (1989) Evaluation on the indication of para-aortic lymph node dissection in gastric cancer surgery (in Japanese). Nihon Gekagakkaishi 90:1314–1317
56. Takahashi S (1990) Study on the pattern of lymph node metastasis based on the analysis of gastric cancer patients treated with para-aortic dissection (in Japanese). Nihon Gekagakkaishi 91:29–35
57. Keighley M, Moore J, Roginski C, et al (1984) Incidence and prognosis of N4 node involvement in gastric cancer. Br J Surg 71:863–866
58. Ohashi I, Takagi K, Kajitani T (1984) Indication and method of left upper abdominal evisceration for advanced gastric cancer (in Japanese). Shoukakigeka 7:1535–1542
59. Ohyama S, Nakajima T, Ohta K, et al (1994) Left upper abdominal evisceration (in Japanese). Gan to Kagakuryouhou 21:1781–1786
60. Japanese Gastric Cancer Association (2001, 2004) Treatment guidelines of gastric cancer, 1st and 2nd edns (in Japanese). Kanehara Shuppan, Tokyo
61. Takekoshi T, Tajiri H, Ohashi K, et al (1981) Comparative study of biopsy specimen and histological examination: usefulness of endoscopic double snare polypectomy (in Japanese). Nihon Ganchiryougakkaishi 16:395
62. Hirao M, Takakuwa R, Kawashima H, et al (1988) Endoscopic mucosal resection with local injection of hyper saline solution for early gastric cancer (in Japanese). I to Chou 23:399–409
63. Tada M, Murata M, Murakami F, et al (1984) Developing strip-off biopsy (in Japanese). Shoukaki Naishikyou 26:833–836
64. Takeshita K, Inoue H, Honda T, et al (1993) Endoscopic mucosal resection of gastric cancer (in Japanese). Shujutu 47:1537–1546
65. Goh P, Tekant Y, Kum C, et al (1992) Totally intra-abdominal laparoscopic Billroth II gastrectomy. Surg Endosc 6:160
66. Kitano S, Iso Y, Moriyama M, et al (1994) Laparpscopy-assisted Billroth I gastrectomy. Surg Laparoscop Endoscop 4:146–148
67. Uyama I, Ogiwara H, Takahara T, et al (1994) Laparoscopic and minilaparotomy Billroth I gastrectomy for gastric ulcer using an abdominal wall-lifting method. J Laparoscop Surg 4:441–445
68. Japanese Gastric Cancer Association (2001) Commentary of gastric cancer treatment guidelines (in Japanese). JGCA, Tokyo
69. Japanese Gastric Cancer Association (1995) Japanese classification of gastric carcinoma. Kanehara, Tokyo
70. Kurihara M, Nakajima T (1981) Chemotherapy for gastric cancer (in Japanese). Shinkouigaku Shuppan, Tokyo
71. Furue H (1996) Chemotherapy. In: Gastric cancer in Japan (in Japanese). Kanehara Shuppan, Tokyo, pp 423–457
72. Ishidate M, Sakurai Y, Yoshida T, et al (1952) Experimental study of chemotherapy using Yoshida Sarcoma(III); suppression effect of nitrogen-mustard N-oxide (in Japanese). Gann 43:171–174

73. Macdonald JS, Woolley PV, Smythe T, et al (1979) 5-Fluorouracil, adriamycin, and mitomycin C (FAM) combination chemotherapy in the treatment of advanced gastric cancer. Cancer (Phila) 44:42–47
74. Sakata Y, Ohtsu A, Horikoshi N, et al (1998) Late phase II study of novel oral fluoropyrimidine anticancer drug S-1(1 M tegafur-0.4 M gimestat-1 M otastat potassium) in advanced gastric cancer patients. Eur J Cancer 34:1715–1720
75. Hyodo I, Nishina T, Moriwaki T, et al (2003) A phase I study of S-1 combined with weekly cisplatin for metastatic gastric cancer in an outpatient setting. Eur J Cancer 39:2328–2333
76. Yoshida K, Hirabayashi N, Takiyama W, et al (2004) Phase I study of combination therapy wtih S-1 and docetaxel(TXT) for advanced or recurrent gastric cancer. Anticancer Res 24:1843–1851
77. Mitachi Y, Sakata Y, Ohtsu A, et al (2002) Docetaxel and cisplatin in patients with advanced or recurrent gastric cancer: a multicenter phase I/II study. Gastric Cancer 5:160–167
78. Shirao K, Shimada Y, Kondo H, et al (1997) Phase I-II study of irinotecan hydrochloride combined with cisplatin in patients with advanced gastric cancer. J Clin Oncol 15:921–927
79. Yoshida M, Boku N, Ohtsu A, et al (2001) Combination chemotherapy of irinotecan plus cisplatin for advanced gastric cancer: efficacy and feasibility in clinical practice. Gastric Cancer 4:144–149
80. Skipper H, Schable FJ, Wilcox W (1964) Experimental evaluation of potential anticancer agent. XIII. On the criteria and kinetics associated with curability of experimental leukemia. Cancer Chemother Rep 35:1–111
81. Foley J, Kessinger M, Lemon H (1980) Treatment of breast cancer with oral four-drug chemotherapy. J Surg Oncol 14:67–72
82. Tucker R, Ferguson A, Van Wyk C, et al (1978) Chemotherapy of small cell carcinoma of the lung with V.P.16 213. Cancer (Phila) 41:1710–1714
83. Hahn R, Moertel C, Schutt A, et al (1975) A double-blind comparison of intensive course 5-fluorouracil by oral vs intravenous route in the treatment of colorectal carcinoma. Cancer (Phila) 35:1031–1035
84. Chlebowski R, Paroly W, Pugh R, et al (1979) Treatment of advanced gastric carcinoma with 5-fluorouracil: randomized comparison of two routes of delivery. Cancer Treat Rep 63:1979–1981
85. Bedikian A, Staab R, Livingston R, et al (1978) Chemotherapy for colorectal cancer with 5-fluorouracil, cyclophosphamide, and CCNU: comparison of oral and continuous iv administration of 5-fluorouracil. Cancer Treat Rep 62:1603–1605
86. Carmichael J, Popiela T, Radstone D, et al (2002) Randomized comparative study of Tegafur/Uracil and oral leucovorin versus parenteral fluorouracil and leucovorin in patients with previously untreated metastatic colorectal cancer. J Clin Oncol 20:3617–3627
87. Douillard J-Y, Hoff P, Skillings J, et al (2002) Multicenter phase III study of Uracil/Tegafur and oral leucovorin versus fluorouracil and leucovorin in patients with previously untreated metastatic colorectal cancer. J Clin Oncol 20:3605–3616
88. Shirao K, Hoff P, Ohtsu A, et al (2004) Comparison of the efficacy, toxicity and pharmacokinetics of a Uracil/Tegafur(UFT) plus oral leucovorin(LV) regimen between Japanese and American patients with advanced colorectal cancer: Joint United State and Japan Study of UFT/LV. J Clin Oncol 22:3466–3474
89. Feliu S, Gonzalez Baron M, Garcia-Giron C, et al (1996) Treatment of patients with advanced gastric carcinoma with the combination of etoposide plus oral tegafur modulated by uracil and leucovorin. Cancer (Phila) 78:211–216
90. Koizumi W, Kurihara M, Sasai T, et al (1993) A phase II study of combination therapy with 5′-deoxy-5-fluorouridine and cisplatin in the treatment of advanced gastric cancer with primary foci. Cancer (Phila) 72:658–662
91. Koizumi W, Kurihara M, Hasegawa K, et al (1996) Combination therapy with cisplatin,5′-deoxy-5-fluorouridine(5′-DFUR) and mitomycin (MMC) in patients with inoperable, advanced gastric cancer: a randomized trial comparing two dosage regimens. Oncol Rep 3:255–260

92. Koizumi W, Kurihara M, Nakano S, et al (2000) Phase II study of S-1, a novel oral derivative of 5-fluorouracil, in advanced gastric cancer. Oncology 58:191–197
93. Koizumi W, Tanabe S, Ohtsu A, et al (2003) Phase I/II study of S-1 combined with cisplatin in patients with advanced gastric cancer. Br J Cancer 89:2207–2212
94. Hoff P, Pazdur R, Benner S, et al (1998) UFT and leucovorin: a review of its clinical development and therapeutic potential in the oral treatment of cancer. Anti-cancer Drugs 9:479–490
95. Inokuchi K, Akiyoshi T (1962) Catheterization into the caeliac artery for local chemotherapy (in Japanese). Shujutu 16:601–604
96. Watkins E Jr, Sullivan R (1964) Cancer chemotherapy by prolonged arterial infusion. Surg Gynecol Obstet 118:3–19
97. Miura K, Sugiura M, Ishida S, et al (1966) Intra-arterial chemotherapy with Watkins' portable infusion pump (in Japanese). Ikakikaigaku Zasshi 36:504–508
98. Miura K, Wada T, Haida H, et al (1982) Subdermal implantable continuous infusion pump: Infusaid (in Japanese). Shujutu 36:1449–1458
99. Stephens FO, Adams BG, Crea P (1986) Intra-arterial chemotherapy given preoperatively in the management of carcinoma of the stomach. Surg Gynecol Obstet 162:370–374
100. Arai Y, Kido C, Endo T, et al (1989) Intra-arterial FAM chemotherapy for gastric cancer patients with liver metastasis (in Japanese). Gan to Kagakuryouhou 15:2433–2436
101. Aigner KR, Benthin F, Muler H (1991) Celiac axis infusion (CAI) chemotherapy for advanced gastric cancer. In: Sugarbaker PH (ed) Management of gastric cancer. Kluwer, Boston, pp 357–362
102. Nakajima T, Ota K, Ishihara S, et al (1997) Combined intensive chemotherapy and radical surgery for incurable gastric cancer. Ann Surg Oncol 4:203–208
103. Takahashi Y, Mai M, Taguchi T, et al (2000) Prolonged stable disease effects survival in patients with solid gastric tumor: analysis of phase II studies of doxifluridine. Int J Oncol 17:285–289
104. Takahashi Y, Nishioka K (1995) Survival without tumor shrinkage: re-evaluation of survival gain by cytostatic effect of chemotherapy. J Natl Cancer Inst 87:1262–1263
105. Japanese Society of Clinical Oncology (1986) Response evaluation criteria of chemotherapy for solid cancer (in Japanese). J Jpn Soc Clin Oncol 21:929–942
106. Therasse P, Arbuch S, Eisenhauer E, et al (2000) New guideline to evaluate the response to treatment in solid tumors. J Natl Cancer Inst 92:205–216
107. JCOG (1999) NCI-CTC (in Japanese). Gan to Kagakuryouhou 26:1084–1144
108. Nakajima T, Nishi M (1988) Adjuvant chemotherapy, immunochemotherapy, and neoadjuvant therapy for gastric cancer in Japan. In: Douglass HO Jr (ed) Gastric cancer, vol 8. Churchill Livingstone, New York, pp 125–143
109. Nakajima T (1990) Adjuvant chemotherapy for gastric cancer in Japan: present status and suggestions for rational clinical trials. Jpn J Clin Oncol 20:30–42
110. Sano T, Sasako M, Katai H, et al (1999) Randomized controlled trials on adjuvant therapy for gastric cancer: Japanese experience. In: Nakajima T, Yamaguchi T (eds) Multimodality therapy for gastric cancer. Springer-Verlag, Tokyo, pp 7–16
111. Imanaga H, Nakazato H (1977) Results of surgery for gastric cancer and effect of adjuvant mitomycin C on cancer recurrence. World J Surg 1:213–221
112. Nakajima T, Fukami A, Ohashi I, et al (1978) Long-term follow-up study of gastric cancer patients treated with surgery and adjuvant chemotherapy with mitomycin C. Int J Clin Pharmacol 16:209–216
113. Nakajima T, Fukami A, Takagi K, et al (1980) Adjuvant chemotherapy with mitomycin C, and with a multi-drug combination of mitomycin C, 5-fluorouracil and cytosine arabinoside after curative resection of gastric cancer. Jpn J Clin Oncol 10:187–194
114. Inokuchi K, Hattori T, Taguchi T, et al (1984) Postoperative adjuvant chemotherapy for gastric carcinoma. Analysis of data on 1805 patients followed for 5 years. Cancer (Phila) 53:2393–2397

115. Nakazato H, Koike A, Saji S, Ogawa N, Sakamoto J (1994) Efficacy of immunochemotherapy as adjuvant treatment after curative resection of gastric cancer. Lancet 343:1122–1126
116. Arima S, Ohsato K, Hisatsugu T, Shimura H (1994) Multicenter randomized study of adjuvant chemotherapy with mitomycin c and tegafur or tegafur-uracil in gastric cancer. Eur J Surg 160:227–232
117. Furukawa H, Iwanaga T, Nakajima T, et al (1995) Randomized study with mitomycin C + 5-fluorouracil, cytosine arabinoside (MFC) + 5-fluorouracil, MFC + Tegafur and Uracil (UFT), and MF + UFT in advanced gastric cancer: interinstitutional differences in a multicenter study in Japan. J Surg Oncol 60:59–64
118. Sugimachi K, Maehara Y, Ogawa M, et al (1997) Dose intensity of uracil and tegafur in postoperative chemotherapy for patients with poorly differentiated gastric cancer. Cancer Chemother Pharmacol 40:233–238
119. Nakajima T, Nashimoto A, Kitamura M, et al (1999) Adjuvant mitomycin and fluorouracil followed by oral uracil plus tegafur in serosa-negative gastric cancer: a randomized trial. Lancet 354:273–277
120. Nakajima T (2000) Evaluation of adjuvant UFT for gastric cancer. Oncology 14:82–86
121. Nashimoto A, Nakajima T, Furukawa H, et al (2003) Randomized trial of adjuvant chemotherapy with mitomycin, fluorouracil, and cytosine arabinoside followed by oral fluorouracil in serosa-negative gastric cancer: Japan Clinical Oncology Group 9206-1. J Clin Oncol 21:2282–2287
122. Hermans J, Bonenkamp H (1994) In reply to the editor. J Clin Oncol 12:879–880
123. Nakajima T, Ohta K, Ishihara S, et al (1994) Evaluation of adjuvant chemotherapy in gastric cancer with meta-analysis. Cancer Chemother 21:1800–1805
124. Nakajima T, Ohta K, Ohyama S, et al (1999) Meta-analysis of adjuvant chemotherapy trials for gastric cancer at the Cancer Institute Hospital, Tokyo. In: Nakajima T, Yamaguchi T (eds) Multimodality therapy for gastric cancer. Springer-Verlag, Tokyo, pp 27–31
125. Earle C, Maroun J (1999) Adjuvant chemotherapy after curative resection for gastric cancer in non-Asian patients: revisiting a meta-analysis of randomized trials. Eur J Cancer 35:1059–1064
126. Mari E, Floriani I, Tinassi A, et al (2000) Efficacy of adjuvant chemotherapy after curative resection for gastric cancer: a meta-analysis of published randomized trials. Ann Oncol 11:837–843
127. Panzini I, Gianni L, Fattori P, et al (2002) Adjuvant chemotherapy in gastric cancer: a meta-analysis of randomized trials and a comparison with previous meta-analyses. Tumori 88:21–27
128. Frei E, Miller ID, Clark JR, et al (1986) Clinical and scientific considerations in preoperative (neoadjuvant) chemotherapy. Recent Results Cancer Res 103:1–5
129. Yonemura Y, Sawa T, Kinoshita K, et al (1993) Neoadjuvant chemotherapy for high-grade advanced gastric cancer. World J Surg 17:256–261
130. Suga S, Iwase H, Shimada M, et al (1996) Neoadjuvant chemotherapy in scirrhous cancer of the stomach using uracil and tegafur and cisplatin. Intern Med 35:930–936
131. Tei Y, Yamashita Y, Nakada B, et al (1995) Clinical effect of continuous iv 5-FU and low-dose daily CDDP regimen for advanced and recurrent gastric cancer (in Japanese). Gan to Kagakuryouhou 22:149–151
132. Kondou T, Murase M, Yokoyama T, et al (1996) Preoperative chemotherapy with continuous 5-FU and low-dose daily CDDP regimen for advanced and recurrent gastric cancer (in Japanese). Gan to Kagakuryouhou 23:1299–1303
133. Chung Y, Yamashita Y, Inoue T (1997) Continuous infusion of 5-fluorouracil and low dose cisplatin infusion for the treatment of advanced and recurrent gastric adenocarcinoma. Cancer 80:1–7
134. Saikawa Y, Kanai T, Kawano Y, et al (2002) An experience of TS-1, low-dose CDDP regimen for gastric cancer patients with liver metastasis (in Japanese). Gan to Kagakuryouhou 29:1241–1245

135. Kelsen D, Ginsberg R, Pajak T, et al (1998) Chemotherapy followed by surgery compared with surgery alone for localized esophageal cancer. N Engl J Med 339:1979–1984
136. Songun I, Keizer H, Hermans J, et al (1999) Chemotherapy for operable gastric cancer: results of the Dutch randomized FAMTX trial. Eur J Cancer 35:558–562
137. Yamamoto T, Komechi T, Nishioka K, et al (1956) Cell agar plate (CAP) method as a chemosensitivity test (in Japanese). Gann 47:424–426
138. Nishioka K, Takehiko T, Yamamoto T, et al (1959) Chemo-sensitivity test for human anticancer virus and drugs (in Japanese). Nihon Rinshou 15:23–34
139. Ishibashi Y, Fujii G, Okada S (1957) Screening test for anti-cancer drugs with human cancer tissues (in Japanese). Rinshou no Nihon 3:141–149
140. Kondou T, Ichihashi H, Imamura T, et al (1964) Screening test of anti-cancer drugs (in Japanese). Gan no Rinshou 10:17–21
141. Ohsawa N (1975) Chemotherapy to the xenograft of human cancer tissue in nude mouse (in Japanese). Rinshou Seijinbyou 5:1039–1045
142. Tanigawa N (2004) Chemotherapy for gastrointestinal cancer (in Japanese). Nihon Medical Center, Tokyo, pp 7–57
143. Kubota T, Sasano N, Abe O (1995) Potential of the histoculture drug-responce assay to contribute to cancer patients survival. Clin Cancer Res 1:1537–1543

Part 2

Recent Advances in Molecular Carcinogenesis in Gastric Carcinoma

Recent Advances in Molecular Pathobiology of Gastric Carcinoma

Wataru Yasui[1], Naohide Oue[1], Yasuhiko Kitadai[2], and Hirofumi Nakayama[1]

Introduction

Cancer is a chronic proliferative disease with multiple genetic and epigenetic alterations, namely, disease with altered gene expression. Integrated research in molecular pathology over the past 15 years has uncovered the molecular mechanism of the development and progression of gastric cancer [1–5]. Multiple genetic and epigenetic alterations involve inactivation of tumor suppressor genes, activation of oncogenes, abnormalities of DNA repair genes, cell-cycle regulators, cell adhesion molecules, growth factors/receptors, matrix metalloproteinases, and so on. Gastric carcinoma is histologically classified into two types, well-differentiated and poorly differentiated types, and the former can be further classified into those with gastric and intestinal phenotypes. Some of these alterations occur commonly in both well-differentiated and poorly differentiated types whereas some differ depending on the histological types or mucin phenotypes. Recent advances in genomic science have enabled revealing the molecular mechanism of stomach carcinogenesis more in detail; these include global analysis of gene expression by microarray or other techniques and study of the association of genetic polymorphism with cancer risk. A better knowledge of the molecular bases of gastric cancer may lead to new approaches to diagnosis, treatment, and prevention.

This chapter presents an overview of the classical pathway of molecular stomach carcinogenesis, mechanism of epigenetic alterations, importance of genetic polymorphism, search for novel genes specific in gastric carcinoma through global analysis of gene expression, and the clinical implications.

[1]Department of Molecular Pathology, [2]Department of Medicine and Molecular Science, Hiroshima University Graduate School of Biomedical Sciences, 1-2-3 Kasumi, Minami-ku, Hiroshima 734-8551, Japan
e-mail: wyasui@hiroshima-u.ac.jp

TABLE 1. Footprint of molecular research on gastric cancer

Cancer in general		Gastric carcinoma	
1911	Rous sarcoma virus	1983	*Helicobacter pylori*
1914	Fijinami sarcoma virus		
1953	DNA double helix structure		
1956	Viral transformation	1984	c-*myc* amplification
1969	Oncogene theory	1985	Establishment of TMK-1
	Normal phenotype by cell fusion	1986	EGF overexpression
1970	Reverse transcriptase		H-*ras* altered expression
1971	Knudson's two-hit theory	1986	Identification of *HST-1*
1972	Epidermal growth factor (EGF)	1988	EGFR overexpression
	Apoptosis		*HER-2*/c-*erb*B2 amplification
1973	DNA transfection	1990	K-*sam* amplification
1975	Southern blot analysis	1991	Loss of E-cadherin
1976	Proto-oncogene c-*src*		Multiple loss of heterozygosity (LOH)
1979	Transformation by cellular DNA	1992	*p53*/*APC* mutations
	c-*src* encodes tyrosine kinase		c-*met* amplification
1982	Human H-*ras* oncogene		Cancer–stromal interaction
1983	Polymerase chain reaction (PCR) method	1993	Genetic changes in intestinal metaplasia
	Platelet-derived growth factor (PDGF) as c-*sis*, EGFR as v-*erb*B		Interleukin 1 (IL-1) as an autocrine growth factor
1986	*Rb* as a tumor suppressor gene		Molecular diagnosis
	Transcription factor Sp1	1994	Microsatellite instability in multiple cancer
1987	Cell adhesion molecule E-cadherin	1995	Increased telomerase activity

1988	Vogelstein's model for colon cancer
1989	*p53* as a tumor suppressor
1990	Cell-cycle regulator $p34^{CDC2}$
	Microsatellite assay
	Gene therapy for melanoma
1991	*APC* as a causative gene for famalial adenomatous polyposis (FAP)
	Angiogenesis: VEGF
1993	*hMSH2* as a causative gene for hereditary nonpolyposis colorectal carcinoma (HNPCC)
	p53 as transcription factor for p21
1994	TRAP assay for telomerase
1995	DNA microarrray technology
	Serial analysis of gene expression
	CpG island methylation of p16
1996	Laser capture microdissection
1997	Histone deacetylation
	Human telomerase reverse transcriptase (hTERT)
1999	DNA demethylase
	Chrosome 22 whole genome sequence
2001	Draft sequence of human genome
2003	Complete sequence of human genome
	Era of Post-Genome and Genomic Medicine
	Cyclin E gene amplification
1996	Reduced p21 expression
	Microsatellite instability in precancerous lesion
1997	Reduced p27 expression
1998	E-cadherin germline mutation
	hTERT expression
	IL-8 and VEGF expression
1999	*hMLH1* hypermethylation
	p73 genomic imbalance
2000	Hypoacetylation of histones
2002	23040 gene expression profile by microarray
2004	Serial analysis of gene expression (SAGE) libraries of gastric cancer

Overview of the Classical Pathway of Molecular Stomach Carcinogenesis

Footprint of Molecular Research on Gastric Carcinoma

We have learned from the footprint of cancer research that the history of cancer research is a repetition of establishment of hypothesis, development of new technologies, and discovery of novel findings (Table 1). For instance, Todaro and Huebner [6] hypothesized the oncogene theory in 1969 and Knudson [7] proposed the two-hit theory in 1971. After several years, methods of DNA transfection, Southern blotting, and polymerase chain reaction (PCR) amplification were developed and enabled them to verify and identify *c-src* as an oncogene and *Rb* as a tumor suppressor gene. Microarray is a powerful technique to reveal gene expression profiles of individual cancers. As of April 2003, the human genome sequence has been completed, and this is now the era of postgenome sequence and genomic medicine.

The history of molecular research on gastric carcinoma began only 20 years ago when c-*myc* amplification was found in primary gastric carcinoma in 1984 [8]. The first oncogene of gastric carcinoma, *HST-1*, was isolated from a primary gastric cancer in 1986 in the National Cancer Center in Tokyo [9]. In the late 1980s and 1990s, extensive analyses of molecular pathogenesis had been performed and the role and significance of novel genes and molecules, identified in other tumors or systems, had been clarified in gastric carcinoma with minimal time lag [4]. Examples include epidermal growth factor (EGF), EGF receptor (EGFR), E-cadherin, *p53*, cyclin E, $p27^{Kip1}$, human telomerase reverse transcriptase (*hTERT*), and *hMLH*1. The importance of DNA methylation and genetic instability during stomach carcinogenesis was also proved. In 1993, a routine system of molecular diagnosis on pathology specimens was established and this useful information was given to clinics [2,10]. Furthermore, the molecular mechanism of cancer–stromal interaction and genetic changes in intestinal metaplasia was explored, and the HGF/c-*met* system and mutations of *p53* and *APC*, respectively, were found to be involved [4]. Recently, dissection of gene expression profiles has been carried out using miroarray or other technology, and vast amounts of information regarding carcinogenesis, biological behavior, and chemosensitivity have been obtained, information that is directly connected with diagnosis and treatment.

Outline of Molecular Stomach Carcinogenesis

A variety of genetic and epigenetic alterations occur during multistep stomach carcinogenesis (Fig. 1) [1–5]; these include activation of oncogenes and growth factors/receptors, inactivation of tumor suppressor genes, DNA repair genes, and cell adhesion molecules, and abnormalities of cell-cycle regulators. Genetic alterations found in gastric carcinoma are gene amplification, point mutation, and loss of heterozygosity, whereas representative epigenetic changes are gene silencing by DNA methylation and overexpression at the transcriptional level [5]. Some alterations are found in both well- and poorly differentiated types, and others are unique depending on the histological type. The former may confer development of cancer whereas the latter may participate in tumor morphogenesis and biological behavior. Genetic polymorphism predisposes to an endogenous cause and alters cancer susceptibility. Genetic instability, cytosine p guanine (CpG) island methylation, telomerase activation, and *p53* mutation commonly participate in the early steps of stomach carcinogenesis. Amplification and overexpression of the c-*met* and cyclin E genes are frequently associated with the advanced stage. Reduced expression of $p27^{Kip1}$ participates in both development and progression of gastric carcinoma. Overexpression of growth factors/cytokines confers progression through multiple autocrine loops. On the other hand, K-*ras* mutations, *HER-2*/c-*erb*B2 amplification, and *APC* mutation preferentially occur in the well-differentiated type. Precancerous lesions such as intestinal metaplasia and adenoma share alterations similar to those of the well-differentiated carcinomas. Loss of heterozygosity (LOH) of the *p73* gene occurs specifically in well-differentiated gastric carcinomas with foveolar epithelial phenotype. Inactivation of cadherins and catenins and amplification of the K-*sam* and c-*met* are frequently associated with poorly differentiated or scirrhous-type carcinomas.

Telomeric Repeats and Telomerase

The DNA sequence at telomeres consists of tandem repeats of TTAGGG, which protects chromosome ends from recombination and fusion and stabilizes the chromosome structure. Maintenance of the telomere by telomerase activation induces cellular immortalization [11]. Strong telomerase activity associated with hTERT expression is present in a majority of gastric carcinomas regardless of histological type and tumor staging [4]. Some intestinal metaplasia and adenomas express telomerase acvitity at certain levels. Telomerase activity is found in half of gastric adenomas at a level of activity about 10% of that in gastric carcinomas [12]. Hyperplasia of epithelial "stem cells" expressing hTERT and telomerase activity in precancerous lesion may be triggered by *Helicobacter pylori* (*H. pylori*) infection.

PINX1, a telomeric-repeat binding factor (TRF)1-binding protein, binds hTERT and inhibits its activity directly [13]. Reduced expression of PINX1 is detected in 70% of gastric carcinomas that show higher telomerase activity [13]. LOH of *PINX1* locus (8p23) is found in 33% of gastric carcinoma and is correlated significantly with reduced PINX1 expression. There are cases with reduced PINX1 expression but without LOH. Treatment with histone deacetylase inhibitor (HDAC) induces PINX1 expression, enhances histone H4 acetylation, and inhibits telomerase activity in gastric carcinoma cell lines. Therefore, reduced expression of PINX1 by LOH of PINX locus and hypoacetylation of histone H4 cause telomerase activation, resulting in cancer development.

POT1, a telomere end-binding protein, is proposed not only to cap telomeres but also to recruit telomerase to the ends of chromosomes [14]. POT1 expression levels are significantly higher in gastric carcinomas of advanced stage, and downregulation is frequently observed in those of early stage [14]. Reduced expression of POT1 is associated with telomere shortening and decreased telomerase activity. Inhibition of *POIT1* by antisense oligonucleotides increases telomere shortening, inhibits telomerase activity, and increases anaphase bridging, a sign of telomere dysfunction. Therefore, POT1 may play an important role in regulation of telomere length and that inhibition of POT1 may induce telomere dysfunction. Changes in POT1 expression levels may be associated with development and progression of gastric carcinoma.

Microsatellite Instability

Genomic instability is broadly classified into microsatellite instability associated with mutator phenotype and chromosome instability recognized by gross chromosomal abnormalities. A defect in DNA mismatch repair (MMR) is responsible for hereditary nonpolyposis colorectal carcinoma (HNPCC). Target genes for microsatellite instability (MSI) include *TGFBRII*, *IGFIIR*, *BAX*, *hMSH3*, *hMSH6*, and *MBD4* [4]. MSI or genetic instability causes accumulation of genetic alterations and participates in pathogenesis of sporadic gastric carcinomas as well [4]. The frequency of MSI is estimated to be about 30% of gastric carcinoma; the frequency is especially high in well-differentiated gastric carcinoma of foveolar phenotype with papillary morphology. Some intestinal metaplasias and adenomas also show MSI, and these should be considered "true precancerous lesions." Another important aspect of genetic instability is that multiple primary cancers frequently display MSI. Representative reports demonstrating the relation between MSI and tumor multiplicity are shown in Table 2. Although the frequency of MSI differs depending on the number and site of microsatellites, all show that the frequency of MSI is significantly higher in cases with multiple primary cancers. This finding indicates that the detection of MSI in a cancer may serve as a good molecular marker for the assessment of the risk of a second cancer in the same patient. CpG island hypermethylation of *hMLH1* and loss of expression is the main mechanism of MSI in sporadic gastric carcinoma [15].

Cell-Cycle Regulators

Cell-cycle checkpoints are regulatory pathway that control cell-cycle transitions and ensure that DNA replication and chromosome segregation are completed with high fidelity. The checkpoints also respond to damage by arresting the cell cycle to provide time for repair. Imbalance in cell-cycle regulators results in genomic instability and unbridled cell proliferation and is implicated in stomach carcinogenesis [2,4]. Table 3 shows representative abnormalities of cell-cycle regulators found in gastric carcinoma. The cyclin E gene is amplified in 15%–20% of gastric carcinoma, and the over-

Table 2. Representative reports of Microsatellite instability (MSI) and multiple primary gastric carcinomas

Multiple vs. solitary		MSI cases	Reference
Early gastric cancer	Multiple cancer	21/63 (33%)	Takahashi H, Endo T, Yamashita K, et al. (2002) Int J Cancer 100:419–424
	Solitary cancer	3/39 (8%)	
Synchronous gastric cancer + adenoma	Multiple cancer	9/18 (50%)	Lee HS, Lee BL, Woo DK, et al. (2001) Int J Cancer 91:619–624
	Solitary cancer	14/149 (9%)	
Gastric cancer	Multiple cancer	11/14 (79%)	Nakashima H, Honda M, Inoue H, et al. (1995) Int J Cancer 64:239–242
	Solitary cancer	5/24 (21%)	
Gastrointestinal and biliary cancer	Multiple cancer	34/38 (89%)	Horii A, Han JHJ, Shimada M, et al. (1994) Cancer Res 54:3373–3375
	Solitary cancer	19/174 (11%)	

TABLE 3. Abnormalities in cell-cycle regulators found in gastric carcinoma

Cell-cycle regulators	Method[a]	Incidence	Role[b]	References
CDC2 high kinase activity	Kinase	92%	D	Yasui W, Ayhan A, Kitadai Y et al. (1993) Int J Cancer 53:36–41
Cyclin E gene amplification	Southern	16%	P	Akama Y, Yasui W, Yokozaki H, et al. (1995) Jpn J Cancer Res 86:617–621
Cyclin E overexpression	IHC	27%	D/P	Yasui W, Yokozaki H, Shimamoto F, et al. (1999) Pathol Int 49:763–774
CDC25A overexpression	Northern	38%	D	Kudo Y, Yasui W, Ue T, et al. (1997) Jpn J Cancer Res 88:947–952
CDC25B overexpression	Northern	70%	D/P	Kudo Y, Yasui W, Ue T, et al. (1997) Jpn J Cancer Res 88:947–952
p21 reduced expression	Northern	53%	D	Akama Y, Yasui W, Kuniyasu H, et al. (1996) Mol Cell Differ 4:187–198
p21 reduced expression	IHC	46%	D	Yasui W, Akama Y, Kuniyasu H, et al. (1996) J Pathol 180:122–128
p27 reduced expression	IHC	56%	D/P	Yasui W, Kudo Y, Semba S, et al. (1997) Jpn J Cancer Res 88:625–629
E2F-1 overexpression	Northern	40%	D	Suzuki T, Yasui W, Yokozaki H, et al. (1999) Int J Cancer 81:535–538
E2F-3 reduced expression	Northern	70%	D	Suzuki T, Yasui W, Yokozaki H, et al. (1999) Int J Cancer 81:535–538
Chk1 overexpression	Western	71%	D	Shigeishi H, Yokozaki H, Oue N, et al. (2002) Int J Cancer 99:58–62
Chk2 overexpression	Western	78%	D	Shigeishi H, Yokozaki H, Oue N, et al. (2002) Int J Cancer 99:58–62

[a] Kinase, kinase assay; Southern, Southern blotting; Northern, Northern blotting; IHC, immunohistochemistry; Western, Western blotting
[b] Participation in tumor development (D) or progression (P)

expression of cyclin E tends to correlate with tumor invasion and advanced stage. The overexpression of CDC25B is found in 70% of gastric carcinoma that is associated with invasion and metastasis. On the other hand, reduction in the expression of $p27^{Kip1}$ is associated with both development and progression of gastric carcinoma. An important downsteam target of cyclins/CDKs at G_1/S transition is a family of transcription factor E2F. E2F-1 is overexpressed in 40% of gastric carcinoma and 70% of gastric carcinomas show reduced expression of E2F-3, suggesting that E2F family members may have a distinct role in stomach carcinogenesis. Chk1 and Chk2 are DNA damage-activated kinases involved in the G_2/M checkpoint. Both Chk1 and Chk2 are overexpressed in more than 70% of gastric carcinoma. The overexpression is associated with *p53* mutations. Therefore, Chk1 and Chk2 may play a role in checkpoint function in gastric carcinoma harboring *p53* mutation when their functions are preserved to prevent cell-cycle progression.

Angiogenic Factors

Angiogenesis, which is a prerequisite for tumor growth and metastasis, depends on the production of angiogenic factors by host and tumor cells (Fig. 2). Increased vascularity enhances the growth of primary neoplasms and provides an avenue for hematogenous metastasis. In gastric carcinoma, increasing microvessel counts correlate with lymph node metastasis, hepatic metastasis, and poor prognosis. Several growth factors have been identified that regulate angiogenesis in gastric carcinoma [4]. Gastric carcinoma cells produce various angiogenic factors, including vascular endothelial growth factor (VEGF), interleukin (IL)-8, basic fibroblast growth factor (bFGF), and platelet-derived endothelial cell growth factor (PD-ECGF) [4,16–18]. Takahashi et al. [16] have found that the angiogenic phenotype differs between the well-differentiated type and poorly differentiated type of gastric carcinoma. Well-differentiated-type tumors, but not the poorly differentiated type, highly express VEGF, whose levels significantly correlate with vessel counts. bFGF expression was higher in the poorly differentiated type, especially scirrhous-type carcinoma. A majority of gastric carcinomas express IL-8/receptor systems, and the expression levels of IL-8 directly correlate with tumor vascularity [17]. Gastric carcinoma cells transfected with the IL-8 gene produce rapidly growing and highly vascular neoplasms at the orthotopic site (gastric wall) in nude mice [19]. Furthermore, IL-8 increases the expression of EGFR, VEGF, and IL-8 itself by the tumor cells themselves [20].

The microenvironment may influence the angiogenic phenotype of gastric carcinoma. In our in vitro study, *H. pylori* infection, a candidate promoter for gastric carcinoma, increased expression of mRNA encoding IL-8, VEGF, and angiogenin by tumor cells [21]. In addition to the neoplastic cells, various interstitial cells in the tumor microenvironment may be involved in angiogenesis. Macrophage infiltration into gastric carcinoma correlates significantly with tumor vascularity and monocyte chemoattractant protein (MCP)-1 expression by tumor cells. Because the activated macrophage is a producer for VEGF, IL-8, and PD-ECGF, MCP-1 expressed by gastric carcinoma cells plays a role in angiogenesis via macrophage recruitment and activation.

Molecular Bases of Gastric and Intestinal Phenotype Gastric Carcinoma

Well-differentiated gastric carcinoma is classified into those with gastric and intestinal phenotypes by mucin histochemistry and immunohistochemistry [22]. Gastric carcinoma cells can be differentiated into a gastric epithelial cell (G) type, resembling pyloric glands and foveolar epithelia, and an intestinal epithelial cell (I) type, such as goblet and intestinal absorpitive cells, by analyzing phenotypic expression. The *p53* gene abnormalities are frequently associated with I-type carcinoma, whereas LOH of the *p73* gene, a homologue of *p53*, occurs specifically in G type with foveolar epithelial phenotype [23,24]. Caudal-type homeobox (*CDX*) 1 and *CDX2* are members of the caudal-related homeobox gene family, and CDX proteins act as intestine-specific transcription factors [25]. CDX2 upregulates goblet-specific *MUC2* gene expression [26]. I-type carcinomas express CDX1 and CDX2 at high levels [25]. Liver-intestine (LI) cadherin, also known as cadherin 17 (CDH17), is overexpressed in I-type carcinoma that is correlated with tumor invasion and metastasis [27–29]. It has been shown that CDX2 binds to the promoter of *CDH17* and upregulates gene expression [30]. On the other hand, the expression of SOX2, a member of transcription factor family containing an *Sry*-like high-mobility group box, is well preserved in G-type carcinoma and down-regulated in I-type carcinoma [22]. MSI associated with *hMLH1* hypermethylation is frequent in G-type carcinoma [23]. Details of the molecular bases of gastric carcinoma with foveolar epithelial phenotype are described in chapter by Yokozaki et al. (this volume).

Epigenetic Alterations of Tumor-Related Genes

DNA Methylation

Many lines of evidence indicate that DNA methylation is important in differential control of gene expression. The abnormal methylation of CpG islands associated with tumor suppressor genes can lead to transcriptional silencing, inactivating the gene and participating in tumorigenesis. In gastric carcinoma, aberrant methylation is involved in the inactivation of various important genes such as $p16^{MTS1/INK4A}$, *CDH1* (E-cadherin), *hMLH1*, *RAR-beta*, *RUNX3*, *MGMT* (O^6-methylguanine methyltransferase), *TSP1* (thrombospondin-1), *HLTF* (helicase-like transcription factor), *RIZ1* (retinoblastoma protein-interacting zinc finger gene-1), and *CHFR* [4,31–36]. The incidence of DNA hypermethylation and inactivation of these genes in gastric carcinoma ranges from 10% to 70%. The expression is restored by treatment of 5-aza-2′-deoxyxytidine (5-aza-dC), a DNA methyltransferase inhibitor. Because these genes have respective functions, the inactivation participates in stomach carcinogenesis through abnormalities in cell-cycle regulation, cell adhesion property, signal transduction, gene regulation, DNA repair, and so on. Carcinomas frequently have the CpG island methylator phenotype (CIMP) [37]. Gastric carcinomas showing methylation at more than three of the five loci of *methylated in tumors* (MINT) were designated as CIMP positive. Significant association is found between the CIMP-positive and promoter hypermethylation of *hMLH1*, *p16*, *CDH1*, and *RAR-beta*. By a genome scanning technique, methylation-sensitive representational difference analysis, Kaneda et al. [38] found that nine CpG islands (CGIs) in the 5′-regions of nine genes, *LOX*, *HRASLS*, *bA305P22.2.3*, *FLNc* (gamma-filamin/ABPL), *HAND1*, a homologue of *RIKEN 2210016F16*, *FLJ32130*, *PGAR* (*HFARP/ANGPTL4/ARP4*), and thrombomodulin, were methylated in gastric carcinoma cell lines but unmethylated in the normal samples. These genes may include important genes in gastric carcinoma development and would be useful to identify a distinct subset of gastric carcinomas.

Alterations in DNA methylation patterns sometimes differ depending on histological type of gastric carcinoma [39,40]. Hypermethylation of *hMLH1* is frequent in papillary subtype (foveolar phenotype) of well-differentiated adenocarcinomas [23]. On the other hand, CpG island methylation of *CDH-1* and reduced E-cadherin expression is commonly observed in poorly differentiated adenocarcinoma of nonsolid (scirrhous) type [39]. Methylation of *CDH1* promoter is known as the second genetic hit in hereditary scirrhous gastric carcinoma. Furthermore, CIMP and *p16* methylation are frequent in well-differentiated type or poorly differentiated solid type, whereas *RAR-beta* methylation is common in the poorly differentiated nonsolid type [40].

In addition to tumor-specific DNA methylation, some gene promoters become hypermethylated in nonneoplastic condition during aging. Alternatively, the incidence of promoter hypermethylation of *hMLH1* and *p16* is more frequent in nonneoplastic gastric mucosa of gastric carcinoma patients than in those of noncancer individuals. Although hypermethylation of *hMLH1*, *p16*, *TSP1*, and *TIMP-3* sometimes occurs in intestinal metaplasia and adenomas, the number of methylated genes increases from normal mucosa to intestinal metaplasia to adenoma to carcinoma [41]. These observations indicate that DNA methylation occurs early and accumulates along the multistep stomach carcinogenesis.

Although DNA methyltransferase and demethylase are enzymes potentially affecting promoter methylation status, tumor-specific hypermethylation is not fully understood and does not simply depend on the expression levels of promethylating (DNMT1, DNMT3A, DNMT3B) and antimethylating (MBD2) enzymes. It has been shown that DNMT1 and DNMT3B cooperate to silence genes and that DNMT1 is required to maintain CpG methylation and aberrant gene silencing in human cancers [42,43].

Histone Modification and Chromatin Remodeling

Histone acetylation and chromatin remodeling linked with CpG island methylation play a major role in the epigenetic regulation of gene expression [44]. Acetylation of histones through an imbalance of histone acetyltransferases and deacetylases disrupts nucleosome structure, which leads to DNA relaxation and a subsequent increase in accessibility for transcription factors. There is a tight association between histone acetylation and DNA methylation. Histone deacetylase-1 (HDAC1) can form a complex with both methyl-CpG-binding proteins (MeCP) and DNMT1 to silence the gene expression. In contrast, methylation of histone tails is alternately linked to activation and repression, depending on the residue methylated [45]. The expression of acetylated histone H4 is reduced in 70% of gastric carcinomas, 40% of gastric adenomas, and some of the intestinal metaplasia adjacent to carcinoma, suggesting that a low level of global histone acetylation may occur even in precancerous cells [5]. Furthermore, reduced histone acetylation is significantly associated with depth of tumor invasion and nodal metastasis of gastric carcinoma. Hypoacetylation of histones H3 and H4 in the $p21^{WAF1/Cip1}$ promoter region is observed in more than 50% of gastric cancer tissues by chromatin immunoprecipitation (ChIP). Hypoacetylation of histone H3 in the promoter is associated with reduced expression of p21 regardless of *p53* gene status. A HDAC inhibitor, trichostatin A (TSA), induces growth arrest and apoptosis and suppresses invasion of gastric carcinoma cells [5]. TSA increases the expression of p21, CBP, Bak, and cyclin E, while it reduces the expression of E2F-1, E2F-4, HDAC-1, and the phosphorylated form of Rb protein [5]. TSA also induces the expression of many suppressor genes of invasion and metastasis including TIMPs and nm23H1/H2. These findings suggest that histone deacethylation may participate not only in tumorigenesis but also in invasion and metastasis through modifying a variety of gene expression. Therefore, histone acetylation should be a promising target for cancer therapy, especially against invasive and metastatic disease.

Histone hypoacetylation and DNA hypermethylation occur concordantly in transcriptional regulation of several genes. For instance, HLTF is a homologue to SWI/SNFs, which are ATP-dependent chromatin remodeling enzymes [34]. Half of gastric cancers show DNA methylation of *HLTF* gene, whereas no gastric mucosa from healthy subjects show the methylation. Loss of HLTF expression in gastric carcinoma cells is rectified by 5-aza-dC and TSA. The acetylation levels of histones H3 and H4 in the CpG island of the HLTF are inversely associated with DNA methylation status.

Genetic Polymorphism and Gastric Carcinoma Risk

Genetic polymorphism is an important determinant for the endogenous cause of cancer. Individual variations in cancer risk are associated with genetic polymorphisms (specific variant alleles of different genes) that are present in a significant proportion of the normal population. Gonzalez et al. [46] has described an overview of genetic susceptibility and gastric carcinoma risk. Genetic susceptibility must be crucial in various processes relevant to stomach carcinogenesis, including (1) mucosal protection against *H. pylori* infection or other carcinogens; (2) the inflammatory response that conditions the maintenance, severity, and outcome of the *H. pylori* infection; (3) the functioninig of carcinogen detoxification and antioxidant protection; (4) the intrinsic variability of DNA repair processes; and (5) cell proliferation activity. Representative reports of the association between genetic polymorphism and gastric carcinoma risk are shown in Table 4. IL-1beta gene (*IL1B*) and the IL-1 receptor angagonist gene (*IL1RN*) variants *IL1B* (-31 T genotype) and *IL1RN* IVS 86 bp VNTR (2/2 genotype), thought to increase IL-1beta production and to inhibit gastric acid secretion, are associated with an increased risk of chronic hypochlorhydric response to *H. pylori* infection and an increased gastric carcinoma risk. *NAT1* is responsible for *N*-acetyltransferase activity, which catalyzes acetylation and modification of aromatic and heterocyclic amine carcinogens. A significant increase of gastric carcinoma risk is associated with genotypes of NAT1 (1088 T > A, 1095 C > A). In the Japanese population, gastric cancer risk is particularly high in well-differentiated carcinoma and in heavy smokers, suggesting the involvement of NAT1 in smoking-induced stomach carcinogenesis.

As to the relation between polymorphism of tumor-related genes and cancer risk, several studies have been performed. Single nucleotide polymorphism (SNP) (A > G, *Ile* > *Val*) is present in the transmembrane domain of the *HER-2*/c-*erb*B2. Our case-control study has demonstrated that the *Val* genotype is significantly more frequent in gastric carcinoma patients than in controls. In patients, gastric carcinomas of advanced stage are more frequent in patients with *Val* genotype than those with *Ile*

Table 4. Association of genetic polymorphism with gastric carcinoma risk and progression

Gene and molecule	Site of single nucleotide polymorphism (SNP)	Role	Reference
MUC1	Coding VNTR	Risk Portuguese	Carvalho F, Seruca R, David L, et al. (1997) Glycoconj J 14:107–111
Interleukin 1 beta (*IL1B*)	Promoter −31 C/T	Risk	El-Omar EM, Carrington M, Chow WH, et al. (2000) Nature (Lond) 404:398–402
Interleukin 1 receptor antagonist (*IL1RN*)	IVS2 86-bp VNTR	Risk	El-Omar EM, Carrington M, Chow WH, et al. (2000) Nature (Lond) 404:398–402
N-Acetyltransferase 1 [*NAT1*]	1088 T/A, 1095 C/A	Risk	Katoh T, Boissy RJ, Nagata N, et al. (2000) Int J Cancer 85:46–49
Cytochrome P450 2E1 (*CYP2E1*)	−1053 C/T	Risk Brazilians	Nishimoto IN, Hanaoka T, Sugimura H, et al. (2000) Cancer Epidemiol Biomark Prev 9:675–680
Glutathione *S*-transferase P1 (*GSTP1*)	Coding Ile105Val	Risk?	Katoh T, Kaneko S, Takasawa S, et al. (1999) Pharmacogenetics 9:165–169
Methylenetetrahydrofolate reductase (*MTHFR*)	Coding Ala677Val	Risk Chinese	Shen H, Xu Y, Zheng Y, et al. (2001) Int J Cancer 95:332–336
HER-2/c-*erb*B2	Coding Ile 665 Val	Risk	Kuraoka K, Oue M, Matsumura S, et al. (2003) Int J Cancer 107:593–596
MMP-1	Promoter −1607 G/GG	Histology	Matsumura S, Oue N, Kitadai Y, et al. (2004) J Cancer Res lin Oncol 130:259–265

genotype, suggesting that this SNP could modulate gastric cancer risk and serve as a predictor of risk for a malignant phenotype. Matrix metalloproteinase-1 (MMP-1) plays a key role in cancer invasion and metastasis. There is 1G/2G SNP in the promoter region of the *MMP-1* affecting the transcriptional activity. Although no difference has been found in the frequency of 1G/2G genotype between gastric carcinoma patients and controls, a significant association is detected with histological differentiation. The 2G genotype is more frequent in poorly differentiated gastric carcinoma than in well-differentiated tumors. Controversial observations have been reported in the association between *CDH1* (E-cadherin) promoter (−160 C > A) polymorphism and the risk of gastric carcinoma. One report indicates that individuals with A/A genotype have a decreased risk of gastric carcinoma [47], whereas another shows no difference in genotype frequencies between gastric carcinoma cases and controls [48]. The important limitations in case-control studies that preclude definitive conclusions are lack of appropriate control, low number of cases analyzed, and lack of concomitant analysis with exposure to relevant cofactors such as *H. pylori* infection and smoking. Proper association studies between genetic polymorphism and cancer risk and genotype information in individuals must be important because those factors directly connect with personalized cancer prevention. Furthermore, genetic polymorphisms have been associated with therapeutic efficacy and toxicity of anticancer drugs [49]. For instance, polymorphism of VNTR in the promoter region of thymidylate synthase influences response to 5-fluorouracil. Polymorphism (difference in number of TA repeats) in the promoter region of the UDP-glucuronosyltransferase 1A1 gene affects severity of toxicity during irinotecan (CPT-11) therapy.

Novel Genetic Markers Identified by Gene Expression Profile

Microarray Study

Cancer is accompanied by multiple genetic and epigenetic alterations, including mutation, gene amplification, LOH, gene silencing by DNA methylation, and loss of imprinting, all of which modify gene expression profiles. Therefore, genome-wide study of gene expression is greatly important to uncover the precise mechanism of development and progression of cancer. Microarray technology provides high-throughput analysis of gene expression profiles by means of small-array slides. cDNA microarray, array slides spotted with cDNAs, is commonly used to detect differences between tumor and normal cells among various histologies and clinical outcomes, for example. The use of laser capture microdissection and T7-based RNA amplification helps to study gene expression profile in a small amount of sample with minimal contamination of other components than those of interest.

Several microarray studies have been performed on gastric carcinoma. El-Rifai et al. [50] examined the gene expression profile of gastric carcinoma using cDNA microarray with 1200 genes and found that S100A4, CDK4, MMP14, and beta catenin are the most upregulated in gastric carcinoma. Hippo et al. [28] studied the expression profile of 6800 genes and identified 162 that were highly expressed in gastric carcinoma tissues; these included genes related to cell cycle, growth factor, cell motility, cell adhesion, and matrix remodeling. They also found several genes associated with metastasis, including Oct-2, a POU domain transcription factor, or intestinal histology, including CDH17 and LI-cadherin. Hasegawa et al. [51] performed genome-wide analysis of gene expression in well-differentiated gastric cancer using a cDNA microarray representing 23 040 genes and reported that 61 genes and 63 genes were commonly up-regulated and downregulated, respectively, in gastric carcinoma. Altered expression of 12 genes including *DDOST*, *GNS*, *NEDD8*, *LOC51096*, and *AIM2* was found to be associated with lymph node metastasis. Hasegawa et al. developed a "predictive score" based on the expression profiles of these five genes that could distinguish cancers with metastasis from those without metastasis. A similar approach has been carried out by Inoue et al. [52] to develop a prognostic scoring system using cDNA microarray. They selected 78 genes that were differentially expressed between aggressive and nonaggressive groups with respect to conventional pathological parameters and determined a coefficient for each gene. The prognostic score, calculated by summing up the value for each gene, could predict stage of disease and the patient's prognosis. Those strategies can be applicable to identify genes associated with sensitivity of cancer to anticancer drugs [53]. These observations indicate that the gene expression profile and a scoring system based on microarray analysis have great potential for dissecting the character of gene expression in individual cancers and predicting biological behavior and chemosensitivity.

Serial Analysis of Gene Expression (SAGE)

Besides microarray technique, serial analysis of gene expression (SAGE) is a powerful technique to allow global analysis of gene expression in a quantitative manner without prior knowledge of the sequence of the genes [54]. SAGE is based on the following principles. A short nucleotide sequence tag (about 10 base pairs) is sufficient to uniquely identify a transcript, provided it is isolated from a defined position within the transcript. Concentration of short sequence tags allows the efficient analysis of transcripts in a serial manner by the sequencing of multiple tags within a single clone. Because the SAGE tag numbers directly reflect the abundance of the mRNA, SAGE data are highly accurate and quantitative, and completion of the human genome sequence has facilitated the mapping of specific genes to individual tags. Up to now, four SAGE studies of gastric carcinoma, including ours, have been reported that identified several upregulated and downregulated genes [55–58]. Our SAGE study on five samples of gastric carcinoma of different stages and histology from four patients generated a total of 137 706 tags including 38 903 unique tags [58]. Our SAGE libraries are the largest gastric carcinoma libraries in the world, and sequence data from our SAGE libraries are publicly available at SAGEmap (GEO accession number GSE 545, SAGE Hiroshima gastric cancer tissue) (*http://www.ncbi.nlm.nih.gov/SAGE/*).

Comparison between SAGE tags from gastric carcinoma and those from normal gastric epithelia identifies upregulated and downregulated genes that may participate in stomach carcinogenesis (Table 5) [29,58]. If SAGE libraries are compared between early cancer and advanced cancer or between primary tumor and metastatic tumor, candidate genes involved in invasion and metastasis can be identified. The upregulated genes in gastric carcinoma include *APOC1*, *NDUF2*, *TEBP*, *COL1A1*, and so on, in addition to *TFF3* and *S100A4*, which are known to be upregulated in gastric carcinoma [58]. Quantitative real-time reverse transcription-PCR (RT-PCR) confirmed that *APOC1*, *CEACAM6*, and *YF13H12* are frequently overexpressed. The downregulated gene cluster includes *LIPF* (gastric lipase), *CHIA*, *ATP4B*, *MBD3*, and many unknown genes. By comparing gene expression profiles between gastric carcinomas at early and advanced stages, several differentially expressed genes by tumor stage were also identified, including *FUS*, *CDH17*, *COL1A1*, and *COL1A2*, that should be novel genetic markers for high-grade malignancy. *FUS* is a tumor-associated fusion gene, especially in myxoid liposarcoma, and its possible role is supposed to be to regulate transcription and maintain chromosomal stability [59]. Regarding genes involved in metastasis, the 20 most upregulated tags and corresponding genes in the

TABLE 5. Upregulated and downregulated tags and genes in gastric carcinoma obtained by serial analysis of gene expression (SAGE)

Commonly upregulated and downregulated tags and genes in gastric carcinoma in comparison with normal gastric epithelia	
Upregulated	APOC1, S100A4, NDUF2, TEBP, COL1A2, SUFU, SYAP1, KIAA0930, KIAA1694, TFF3, CEACAM6, FLJ20249, FLJ2167, EIF4A1, COLPH2, G3BP, YF13H12, KRT7, SH3BP2, COL1A1, LOC284371
Downregulated	CAGCGCTTCT (no match), CACCTCCCCA (no match), AGCCTCCCCA (no match), ACCCTCCCCA (no match), LIPF, AACCTCCCCC (no match), CHIA, TAGTGCTTCT (no match), TACAAGGTCC (no match), GTGGTCAGCT (no match), ATP4B, FLJ20410, MBD3, CAGTGCTTTT (no match), Hs.199360, Hs.353061
The 20 most upregulated and downregulated tags and genes in advanced carcinoma in comparison with early carcinoma[a]	
Upregulated	TCCCCGTAAA (no match), TCCCGTACAT (no match), CDH17, FUS, PRO1073, FLJ36926, FLJ30146, PAI-RBP1, COL1A2, TCCTATTAAG (no match), COL1A1, GRAP2, HNRPL, NUTF2, ERP70, PES1, CYP2J2, DAG1, IQGAP1, IL16, FXYD3, COQ4, LOC91966, CTBP1, TTCGGTTGGT (no match), alpha4GnT, Hs.290723, AKT3, CCT3, HMG20A
Downregulated	Hs.216636, LOC116228, SH3MD2, NAB1, TTCCCCCAAA (no match), DDX5, VMP1, LOC51123, LZK1, CGCAGATCAG (no match), IFRD2, Hs.284464, RPS4Y, RPS4Y2, UAP1, Hs.180804, CATTAAATTA (no match), IKBKAP, ARPC3, NAGA, UBE3A, TRAG3, PNN, CTAATTCTTT (no match), TCCATCGTCC (no match)
The 20 most upregulated and downregulated tags and genes in metastatic tumor in comparison with primary tumor of gastric carcinoma[a]	
Upregulated	SCAND1, RGS5, S100A11, RNPC2, APOE, FLJ10815, RNASE1, H3F3B, P24B, LOC151103, CLDN3, MRPL14, PRexl, TCCCCTATTA (no match), Hs.105379, ATP5G1, NPD007, MGC3180, WDR11, ARPC1B, ABTB2, DNAJB1, HMGN2, KIAA1393, RAP1B, FLJ12150, STUB1
Downregulated	ERdj5, RPL27A, DHRS3, E2IG5, USP7, CTSL, KRTHB1, KRTHB3, TGCACTACCC (no match), ALG12, S100A9, CTAGCTTTTA (no match), ELOVL5, LOC375463, GGGGGAGTTT (no match), ACTGCCCTCA (no match), SPC18, CTNND1, CYP20A1, FLJ11151, RPS17, ZYX, RPS16, GCTTTCTCAC (no match), BCL2L2

Symbol of gene is described; UniGene ID is described if symbol is not present
No match, tag sequence is not matched to known gene
[a] Because some genes share the same SAGE tag, gene numbers are more than 20

metastatic tumor of gastric carcinoma included *SCAN D1*, *RGS5*, *S100A11*, *RNPC2*, and *APOE* [58]. *APOE* (apolipoprotein E) expression is associated with T grade, N grade, and advanced stage.

SAGE is also useful to isolate novel biomarkers of gastric carcinoma. The ideal biomarker should be overexpressed in a majority of gastric carcinoma and expressed on the cell surface or secreted to facilitate its detection. Moreover, if the function of the gene product is involved in the neoplastic process, the gene is not just a biomarker but can be a therapeutic target. One example is *REGIV* (regenerating gene type IV), which is identified by comparing the expressed tags of poorly differentiated nonsolid type (scirrhous-type) gastric carcinoma with those of normal gastric epithelia [58,60]. About half of gastric carcinomas overexpress *REGIV* mRNA regardless of tumor stage and histological differentiation. In vitro studies using *RegIV*-transfected cells revealed that RegIV is secreted by carcinoma cells and that RegIV inhibits apoptosis, suggesting that RegIV may serve as a novel biomarker and therapeutic target for gastric carcinoma. Other examples include *GW112* and *MIA*, both of which encode secreting proteins [61,62]. GW112 demonstrates strong antiapoptotic effects in cancer cells treated with stress exposures and forced expression of GW112 leads to more rapid tumor formation, indicating that GW112 plays an important role in tumor cell survival and growth and should be a good therapeutic target [61].

Clinical Implication of Global Gene Expression Analysis

A strategy to clinical applications of global analysis of gene expression such as diagnostics, treatment, and prevention is shown in Fig. 3. According to gene expression profiles among gastric carcinomas or with those in normal gastric tissue obtained by microarray study or SAGE, specifically upregulated or downregulated genes are identified. The expression of these genes is confirmed in a large number of cases by real-time RT-PCR and immunohistochemistry if antibodies are available. With the specific genes identified by SAGE, known genes participating in the development and progression of gastric carcinoma and known genetic markers for chemosensitivity, a custom-made cDNA microarray is prepared. If the specific gene encodes secretory protein, this may be detected in the blood and should be a novel biomarker of gastric carcinoma. For such molecules, DNA/RNA aptamer or antibody is produced to establish a measuring system such as enzyme-limited immunosorbent assay (ELISA) in blood sample. These methods can be applied for clinical diagnosis and cancer detection. Polymorphism of genes, highly altered in their expression in gastric carcinoma, may be candidates of novel risk factors, and this information will be used for cancer prevention. By functional analysis, the molecular mechanism of stomach carcinogenesis can be understood in more detail and the possibility whether the genes are novel therapeutic targets can be revealed. Combination of these testings not only can attain cancer detection but also can clarify the character of an individual tumor and person, which is directly connected with personalized medicine and cancer prevention.

Conclusion

In the course of multistep carcinogenesis of the stomach, various alterations of oncogenes, tumor suppressor genes, DNA repair genes, growth factors/receptors, cell-cycle regulators, and cell adhesion molecules are accumulated. Some of these changes occur commonly in both well-differentiated and poorly differentiated types and some differ depending on the histological types. Among various epigenetic alterations, modified gene expression through DNA methylation and chromatin remodeling by histone modification are the most important events. Genetic polymorphism is a crucial endogenous cause and fundamental factor of cancer risk. Using genomic science including novel techniques for global analysis of gene expression and bioinformatics, the individual character of each person and cancer can be dissected precisely, which is directly connected to personalized medicine and cancer prevention. Understanding of the diversity of gastric cancer must be critical in the era of genomic medicine at the clinical setting.

References

1. Tahara E (1993) Molecular mechanism of stomach carcinogenesis. J Cancer Res Clin Oncol 119:265–272
2. Yasui W, Oue N, Kuniyasu H, et al (2001) Molecular diagnosis of gastric cancer: present and future. Gastric Cancer 4:113–121
3. Ohgaki H, Yasui W, Yokota J (2003) Genetic pathway to human cancer. In: Vainio H, Hietanen E (eds) Handbook of experimental pharmacology. Mechanisms in carcinogenesis and cancer research. Springer, Heidelberg, pp 25–39
4. Yokozaki H, Yasui W, Tahara E (2001) Genetic and epigenetic changes in stomach cancer. Int Rev Cytol 204:49–95
5. Yasui W, Oue N, Ono S, et al (2003) Histone acetylation and gastrointestinal carcinogenesis. Ann NY Acad Sci 983:220–231
6. Todaro GJ, Huebner RJ (1972) N.A.S. symposium: new evidence as the basis for increased efforts in cancer research. Proc Natl Acad Sci U S A 69:1009–1015
7. Knudson AG Jr (1971) Mutation and cancer: statistical study of retinoblastoma. Proc Natl Acad Sci U S A 68:820–823
8. Nakasato F, Sakamoto H, Mori M, et al (1984) Amplification of the c-myc oncogene in human stomach cancers. Gann (Jpn J Cancer Res) 75:737–742
9. Sakamoto H, Mori M, Taira M, et al (1986) Transforming gene from human stomach cancers and a noncancerous portion of stomach mucosa. Proc Natl Acad Sci U S A 83:3997–4001
10. Yasui W, Yokozaki H, Shimamoto F, et al (1999) Molecular-pathological diagnosis of gastrointestinal tissues and its contribution to cancer histopathology. Pathol Int 49:763–774
11. Kim NW, Piatyszek MA, Prowse KR, et al (1994) Specific association of human telomerase activity with immortal cells and cancer. Science 266:2011–2015
12. Yasui W, Tahara E, Tahara E, et al (1999) Immunohistochemical detection of human telomeraase reverse transcriptase in normal and precancerous lesions of the stomach. Jpn J Cancer Res 90:589–595
13. Kondo T, Oue N, Mitani Y, et al (2005) Loss of heterozygosity and histone hypoacetylation of the PINX1 gene are associated with reduced expression in gastric carcinoma. Oncogene 24:157–164
14. Kondo T, Oue N, Yoshida K, et al (2004) Expression of POT1 is associated with tumor stage and telomere length in gastric carcinoma. Cancer Res 64:523–529
15. Fleisher AS, Esteller M, Wang S, et al (1999) Hypermethylation of the *hMLH1* promoter in human gastric cancers with microsatellite instability. Cancer Res 59:1090–1095
16. Takahashi Y, Cleary KR, Mai M, et al (1996) Significance of vessel count and vascular endothelial growth factor and its receptor (KDR) in intestinal-type gastric cancer. Clin Cancer Res 2:1679–1684

17. Kitadai Y, Haruma K, Sumii K, et al (1998) Expression of IL-8 correlates with vascularity in human gastric carcinomas. Am J Pathol 152:93–100
18. Takahashi Y, Bucana CD, Akagi Y, et al (1998) Significance of platelet-derived endothelial cell growth factor in the angiogenesis of human gastric cancer. Clin Cancer Res 4:429–434
19. Kitadai Y, Takahashi Y, Haruma K, et al (1999) Transfection of interleukin-8 increases angiogenesis and tumorigenesis of human gastric carcinoma cells in nude mice. Br J Cancer 81: 647–653
20. Kitadai Y, Haruma K, Mukaida N, et al (2000) Regulation of disease-progression genes in human gastric carcinoma cells by interleukin-8. Clin. Cancer Res 6:2735–2740
21. Kitadai Y, Sasaki A, Ito M, et al (2003) *Helicobacter pylori* infection influences expression of genes related to angiogenesis and invasion in human gastric carcinoma cells. Biochem Biophys Res Commun 311:809–814
22. Tatematsu M, Tsukamoto T, Inada K (2003) Stem cells and gastric cancer: role of gastric and intestinal mixed intestinal metaplasia. Cancer Sci 94:135–141
23. Ohmura K, Tamura G, Endoh Y, et al (2000) Microsatellite alterations in differentiated-type adenocarcinomas and precancerous lesions of the stomach with special reference to cellular phenotype. Hum Pathol 31:1031–1035
24. Yokozaki H, Shitara Y, Fujimoto J, et al (1999) Alterations of p73 preferentially occur in gastric adenocarcinomas with foveolar epithelial phenotype. Int J Cancer 83:192–196
25. Almeida R, Silva E, Santos-Silva F, et al (2003) Expression of intestine-specific transcription factors, CDX1 and CDX2, in intestinal metaplasia and gastric carcinomas. J Pathol 199:36–40
26. Yamamoto H, Bai YQ, Yuasa Y (2003) Homeodomain protein CDX2 regulates goblet-specific MUC2 gene expression. Biochem Biophys Res Commun 300:813–818
27. Grotzinger C, Kneifel J, Patschan D, et al (2001) LI-cadherin: a marker of gastric metaplasia and neoplasia. Gut 49:73–81
28. Hippo Y, Taniguchi H, Tsutsumi S, et al (2002) Global gene expression analysis of gastric cancer by oligonucleotide microarrays. Cancer Res 62:233–240
29. Yasui W, Oue N, Ito R, et al (2004) Search for new biomarkers of gastric cancer through serial analysis of gene expression and its clinical implications. Cancer Sci 95:385–392
30. Hinoi T, Lucas PC, Kuick R, et al (2002) CDX2 regulates liver intestine-cadherin expression in normal and malignant colon epithelium and intestinal metaplasia. Gastroenterology 123: 1565–1577
31. Oshimo Y, Oue N, Mitani Y, et al (2004) Frequent loss of RUNX3 expression by promoter hypermethylation in gastric carcinoma. Pathobiology 71:137–143
32. Oue N, Shigeishi H, Kuniyasu H, et al (2001) Promoter methylation of MGMT is associated with protein loss in gastric carcinomas. Int J Cancer 93:805–809
33. Oue N, Matsumura S, Nakayama H, et al (2003) Expression of theTSP-1 gene and its association with promoter hypermethylation in gastric carcinomas. Oncology 64:423–429
34. Hamai Y, Oue N, Mitani Y, et al (2003) DNA methylation and histone acetylation status of HLTF gene are associated with reduced expression in gastric carcinoma. Cancer Sci 94:692–698
35. Oshimo Y, Oue N, Mitani Y, et al (2004) Frequent epigenetic inactivation of RIZ1 by promoter hypermethylation in human gastric carcinoma. Int J Cancer 110:212–218
36. Satoh A, Toyota M, Itoh F, et al (2003) Epigenetic inactivation of CHFR and sensitivity to microtubule inhibitors in gastric cancer. Cancer Res 63:8606–8613
37. Toyota M, Ahuja N, Suzuki H, et al (1999) Aberrant methylation in gastric cancer associated with the CpG island methylator phenotype. Cancer Res 59:5438–5442
38. Kaneda A, Kaminishi M, Yanagihara K, et al (2002) Identification of silencing of nine genes in human gastric cancers. Cancer Res 62:6645–6650
39. Oue N, Motoshita J, Yokozaki H, et al (2002) Distinct promoter hypermethylation of p16ink4a, CDH1, and RAR-beta in intestinal, diffuse-adherent, and diffuse-scattered type gastric carcinoma. J Pathol 198:55–59
40. Oue N, Oshimo Y, Mitani Y, et al (2003) DNA methylation of multiple genes in gastric carcinoma: association with histological type and CpG island methylator phenotype. Cancer Sci 94:901–905

41. Kang GH, Shim Y-H, Jung H-Y, et al (2001) CpG island methylation in premalignant stages of gastric carcinoma. Cancer Res 61:2847–2851
42. Rhee I, Bachman KE, Park BH, et al (2002) DNMT1 and DNMT3b cooperate to silence genes in human cancer cells. Nature (Lond) 416:552–556
43. Robert M-F, Morin S, Beaulieu N, et al (2003) DNMT1 is required to maintain CpG methylation and aberrant gene silencing in human cancer cells. Nat Genet 33:61–65
44. Kouzarides T (1999) Histone acetylases and deacetylases in cell proliferation. Curr Opin Genet Dev 9:40–48
45. Kouzarides T (2002) Histone methylation in transcriptional control. Curr Opin Genet Dev 12:198–209
46. Gonzalez CA, Sala N, Capella G (2002) Genetic susceptibility and gastric cancer risk. Int J Cancer 100:249–260
47. Wu M-S, Huang S-P, Chang Y-T, et al (2002) Association of the −160 C → A promoter polymorphism of the *E-cadherin* gene with gastric carcinoma risk. Cancer (Phila) 94:1443–1448
48. Pharoah PDP, Oliveira C, Machado JC, et al (2002) *CDH1* c-160a promoter polymorphism is not associated with risk of stomach cancer. Int J Cancer 101:196–197
49. Watters JW, McLeod HL (2003) Cancer pharmacogenomics: current and future applications. Biochim Biophys Acta 1603:99–111
50. El-Rifai W, Frierson HF Jr, Harper JC, et al (2001) Expression profiling of gastric adenocarcinoma using cDNA array. Int J Cancer 92:832–838
51. Hasegawa S, Furukawa Y, Li M, et al (2002) Genome-wide analysis of gene expression in intestinal-type gastric cancers using a complementary DNA microarray representing 23 040 genes. Cancer Res 62:7012–7017
52. Inoue H, Matsuyama A, Mimori K, et al (2002) Prognostic score of gastric cancer determined by cDNA microarray. Clin Cancer Res 8:3475–3479
53. Zembutsu H, Ohnishi Y, Tsunoda T, et al (2002) Genome-wide cDNA microarray screening to correlate gene expression profiles with sensitivity of 85 human cancer xenografts to anticancer drugs. Cancer Res 62:518–527
54. Velculescu VE, Zhang L, Vogelstein B, et al (1995) Serial analysis of gene expression. Science 270:484–487
55. El-Rafai W, Moskaluk CA, Abdrabbo MK, et al (2002) Gastric cancers overexpress S100A calcium-binding proteins. Cancer Res 62:6823–6826
56. Oien KA, Vass JK, Downie I, et al (2003) Profiling, comparison and validation of gene expression in gastric carcinoma and normal stomach. Oncogene 22:4287–4300
57. Lee J-Y, Eom E-M, Kim D-S, et al (2003) Analysis of gene expression profiles of gastric normal and cancer tissues by SAGE. Genomics 82:78–85
58. Oue N, Hamai Y, Mitani Y, et al (2004) Gene expression profile of gastric carcinoma; identification of genes and tags potentially involved in invasion, metastasis, and carcinogenesis by serial analysis of gene expression. Cancer Res 64:2397–2405
59. Hicks GG, Singh N, Nashabi A, et al (2000) Fus deficiency in mice results in defective B-lymphocyte development and activation, high levels of chromosomal instability and perinatal death. Nat Genet 24:175–179
60. Hartupee JC, Zhang H, Bonaldo MF, et al (2001) Isolation and characterization of a cDNA encoding a novel member of the human generating protein family. Biochim Biophys Acta 1518:287–293
61. Zhang X, Huang Q, Yang Z, et al (2004) GW112, a novel antiapoptotic protein that promotes tumor growth. Cancer Res 64:2474–2481
62. Krupnik VE, Sharp JD, Jiang C, et al (1999) Functional and structural diversity of the human Dickkopf gene family. Gene (Amst) 238:301–313

Color Plates to appear on the following pages.

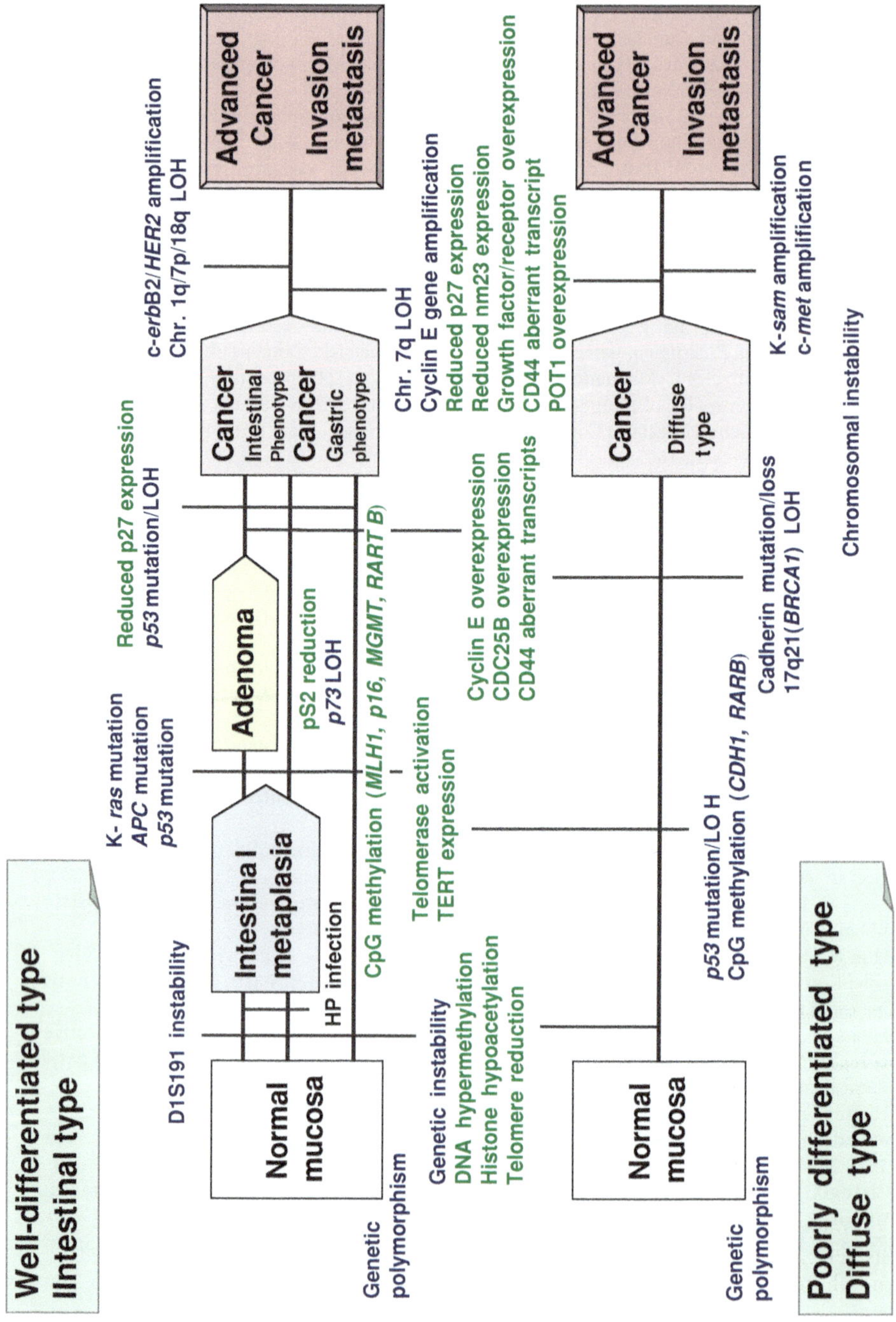

Fig. 1. Multiple genetic and epigenetic alterations during stomach carcinogenesis. Words printed in *dark blue* represent genetic alterations and those in *green* represent epigenetic alterations

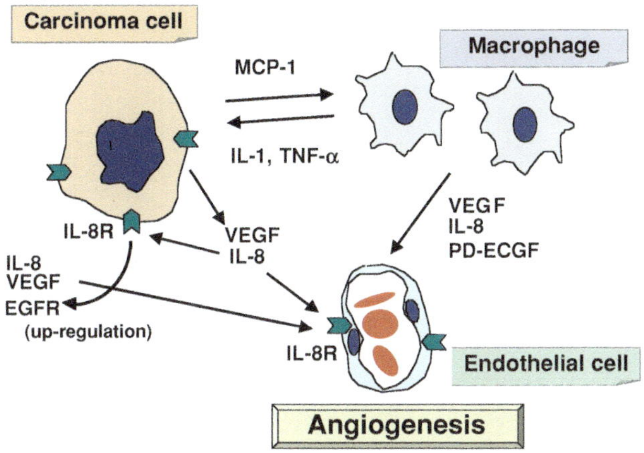

FIG. 2. Schematic illustration of cancer cells and macrophages in angiogenesis. *MCP-1*, monocyte chemoattractant protein-1; *IL*, interleukin; *TNF-α*, tumor necrosis factor-alpha; *VEGF*, vascular endothelial growth factor; *EGFR*, epidermal growth factor receptor; *PD-ECGF*, platelet-derived endothelial cell growth factor; *IL-8R*, IL-8 receptor

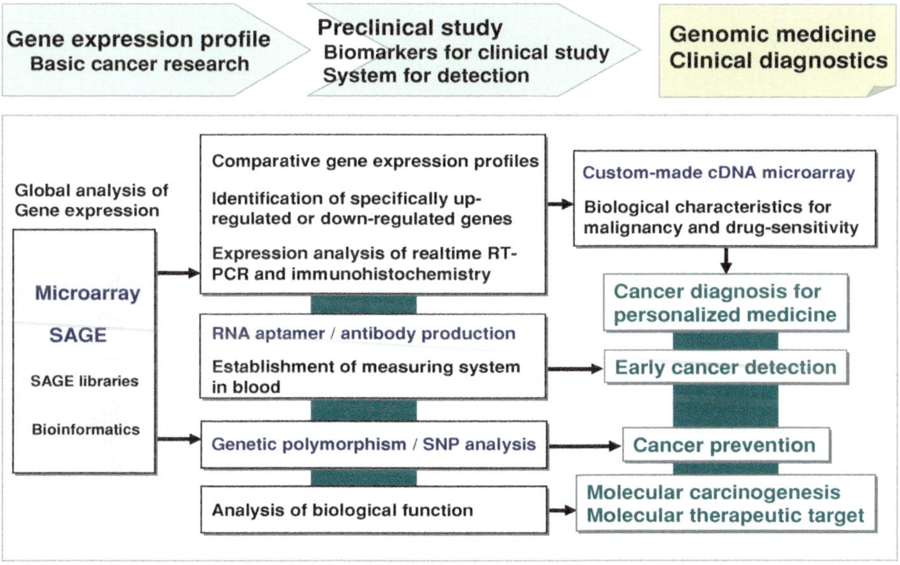

FIG. 3. Strategy to search for novel genes of gastric cancer through gene expression profiles and its clinical implication. *SAGE*, serial analysis of gene expression; *SNP*, single nucleotide polymorphism

Part 3
Pathogenesis and Pathology

Helicobacter pylori and Gastric Carcinoma

Nobuyuki Shimizu[1,2], Masae Tatematsu[2], Michio Kaminishi[1]

Introduction

A large amount of epidemiological evidence has accumulated indicating a significant relationship between *Helicobacter pylori* (Hp) infection and chronic gastritis [1,2], peptic ulcers [3], intestinal metaplasia [4,5], and adenocarcinoma [6–8] or lymphoma [9] development. In 1994, the World Health Organization/International Agency for Research on Cancer concluded that "Hp is a definite carcinogen" based on the epidemiological findings [10]. Hp infection almost always results in chronic antral gastritis, but only a proportion of patients develop stomach cancer, so it is clear that the bacterium cannot be the only causative factor. To demonstrate a "causal link" between Hp infection and stomach carcinogenesis, as well as intervention studies, it is essential to establish an experimental animal model. In Mongolian gerbils (MGs), Hp infection, chronic active gastritis, peptic ulcers, and intestinal metaplasia closely mimic those in man [11]. In this chapter, epidemiological and experimental evidence associated with Hp infection and gastric carcinogenesis is reviewed.

Before the Discovery of Hp

Many kinds of stomach diseases and conditions were considered as "precancerous lesion" before the relationship between Hp infection and gastric cancer development was investigated (Table 1) [12]. According to development of endoscopy in the 1970s, many reports described the findings of gastric mucosa and discussed the precancerous condition.

Peptic Ulcers

From the early 20th century, chronic peptic ulcer has been thought to be one of the most possible candidates for precancerous lesions of gastric cancer. The fact that sur-

[1]Department of Gastrointestinal Surgery, The University of Tokyo Graduate School of Medicine, 7-3-1 Hongo, Bunkyo-ku, Tokyo 113-8655, Japan
[2]Division of Oncological Pathology, Aichi Cancer Center Research Institute, 1-1 Kanokoden, Chikusa-ku, Nagoya 464-8681, Japan
e-mail: e05009-tky@umin.ac.jp

Table 1. "Precancerous lesion" of the stomach

Candidate	Reference number
Chronic peptic ulcer	13, 14
Gastric adenoma	15, 16, 17
Intestinal metaplasia	18, 19, 20
Remnant stomach	21, 22
Chronic gastritis	23, 24

gical specimens resected from patients suffering from gastric ulcer often contained gastric cancer supported this hypothesis [13]. It was reported that recurring ulceration in the rat stomach enhanced gastric carcinogenesis induced by a chemical carcinogen [14]. This report also implied that the regeneration of gastric mucosa might play a role in gastric carcinogenesis.

Gastric Adenoma

Gastric "adenoma" has been used for a lesion that is classified in pathological "dysplasia" and is difficult to judge by morphology whether it is a benign or malignant lesion. Some investigators reported that about a tenth of adenomas developed into adenocarcinomas and a quarter of adenomas with colonic phenotype would grow adenocarcinomas [15,16]. Flat-type adenomas were reported to turn into gastric cancers twice as frequently as elevated-type adenomas [17]. It was also reported that stomachs possessing adenomas tended to possess a differentiated adenocarcinoma. Therefore, stomachs with adenomas are at least high-risk mucosa, if not precancerous lesions.

Intestinal Metaplasia

The hypothesis that most gastric cancer, especially differentiated-type adenocarcinoma, grows from intestinal metaplasia is commonly accepted [18], although no experimental data have demonstrated this hypothesis. The hypothesis has been supported by the pathological findings that many differentiated gastric cancers were surrounded by or next to intestinal metaplasias. Tatematsu et al. reported that almost all gastric cancers had a gastric phenotype and acquired an intestinal phenotype according to their development, and that gastric cancers mainly developed in the gastric mucosa [19]. An experimental gastric carcinogenesis model employing rats induced by chemical carcinogens also showed that early-stage cancers had a gastric phenotype and that there was no intestinal metaplasia in the mucosa surrounding the cancers [20]. Intestinal metaplasia should not be thought of as a "precancerous lesion."

Remnant Stomach

Remnant stomachs develop gastric cancers more frequently than ordinary stomachs. Surgical procedures may make many changes in the stomach mucosal condition, such as decrease of blood flow, denervation, and reflux of duodenal juice [21]. Kaminishi et al. demonstrated that rats subjected to Billroth II operation developed adenocarcinoma more frequently than rats subjected to Billroth I operation, and adding vagotomy increased the incidence of gastric cancer [22].

Chronic Gastritis

Atrophic gastritis is also thought to be one candidate of precancerous lesions of gastric cancer [23,24]. This hypothesis was supported by pathological findings that were observed in surgical specimens from patients suffering from gastric cancer. Up to the present, there have been no experimental data sufficiently supporting this hypothesis.

Helicobacter pylori Infection and Gastric Diseases in Humans

In 1953, it was reported that there was no bacterium in the human stomach from observation of more than 1000 clinical materials [25]. This report was widely accepted, and few reports concerning stomach bacterial flora was discussed. Since 1983, when infection with Hp was first described by Warren and Marshall [1], there have been a very large number of reports on the relevance of this bacterium to disease in humans. Thus, associations between *H. pylori* infection and chronic gastritis [1,2], peptic ulcers [3], intestinal metaplasia [4,5], adenocarcinomas [6–8], and lymphoma [9] development have been noted.

In addition to these epidemiological studies, Uemura et al. reported that gastric cancer developed in Hp-positive patients whose early gastric cancers were treated with endoscopical mucosal resection more frequently than in Hp-negative patients [26]. Gastric mucosa in which adenocarcinoma had developed might be initiated, so this report strongly suggested that infection with Hp had enhancing effects for gastric canrcinogenesis.

Helicobacter pylori and Gastric Carcinogenesis Employing an Animal Model

Colonization of the stomach mucosa by Hp has been reported in dogs [27], ferrets [28], monkeys [29], and mice [30]. However, few studies on stomach carcinogenesis in animal models have been documented so far. Hirayama et al. first established the Hp infection model in MGs and described the development of chronic active gastritis, peptic ulcers, and intestinal metaplasia (Figs. 1, 2) [11]. MGs resemble humans in their susceptibility and response to Hp infection. Therefore, the MG model appears admirably suited for investigating the role of Hp in human stomach disorders. It is clear, however, that most persons infected with Hp will never develop stomach cancer, and the bacterium cannot be the only causative factor.

We subsequently established glandular stomach carcinogenesis models using *N*-methyl-*N'*-nitro-*N*-nitorosoguanigine (MNNG) and *N*-metyl-*N*-nitorosourea (MNU) in MGs [31].

Carcinogenesis Model Employing MGs

In a multistep carcinogenesis protocol, we demonstrated that Hp infection enhanced glandular stomach carcinogenesis in MGs treated with MNU [32] and MNNG [33].

TABLE 2. Summary of stomach carcinogenesis model employing Mongolian gerbils

Chemical carcinogen	Conc (ppm)	Duration (week)	Hp infection	Incidence of gastric cancer (%)
MNU	10	20	pre	36.8
	10	20	(–)	0.0
	30	10	post	33.3
	30	10	(–)	0.0
MNNG	60	10	post	24.0
	60	10	(–)	0.0
	300	10	post	44.4
	300	10	(–)	5.3
	20	30	post	60.0
	20	30	(–)	5.0

MNU, *N*-methyl-*N*-nitrosourea; MNNG, *N*-methyl-*N′*-nitro-*N*-nitrosoguanidine; conc, concentration of chemical carcinogens; duration, duration of chemical carcinogen administration; pre, *Helicobacter pylori* (Hp) infection followed by chemical carcinogen administration; post, Hp infection following chemical carcinogen administration

Briefly, Hp infection followed by chemical carcinogen (MNU or MNNG) administration or following chemical carcinogen administration could increase the incidence of induced gastric cancer (Table 2). We previously demonstrated that the proportion of undifferentiated-type lesions depends on the concentration of carcinogen given in mice [34]. In the MG Hp infection model, animals treated with a high concentration of MNNG tended to develop poorly differentiated adenocarcinomas [33]. This result suggests that the histological type of cancer depends on the genotoxic acting chemical carcinogen rather than the Hp infection. It has been proposed that chronic inflammation enhances cell proliferation [35], which may enhance carcinogenesis by increasing the turnover of initiated cells.

In these studies, we observed signet-ring cell carcinomas as well as poorly differentiated and well-differentiated adenocarcinomas (Fig. 3). This variety of induced stomach cancers as well as response to Hp infection similar to that in humans suggests advantages of this model for research on stomach carcinogenesis in humans [36]. It has been considered that Hp infection causes atrophic gastritis followed by development of intestinal metaplasia and well-differentiated adenocarcinomas [37]. However, a meta-analysis indicated that Hp infection is equally associated with differentiated and poorly differentiated types of gastric cancer [38], in agreement with our findings. Intestinal metaplasia in humans has been considered a preneoplastic change for well-differentiated adenocarcinomas [18], but in the present experiment, no relationship between intestinal metaplasia and glandular stomach cancers induced by Hp infection and chemical carcinogen administration in MGs was found.

To explore the influence of Hp infection according to time at which Hp infection is established, we modified our protocol [39]. MGs were infected with Hp at 4, 18, and 32 weeks of age, and thereafter they were administrated low doses of chemical carcinogen (MNU). In this protocol, animals infected with Hp at a younger age showed higher incidence of induced gastric cancers and higher titers of serum anti-Hp anti-

TABLE 3. Age of acquisition of Hp infection and cancer risk

MNU administration	Age (weeks) at Hp infection	Incidence of induced cancer (%)
+	4	60.0
+	18	18.2
+	32	10.0
−	4	0.0
−	18	0.0
−	32	0.0
+	−	14.8
−	−	0.0

MNU was administrated 2 weeks after Hp infection with a dose of 10 ppm for 20 weeks

TABLE 4. Eradication of Hp and gastric cancer incidence

MNU treatment	Hp infection (week)	Eradication (week)	Incidence of induced cancer (%)	
30 ppm × 10 weeks	11	—	65.2	at week 50
30 ppm × 10 weeks	11	21	20.8	
30 ppm × 10 weeks	—	—	6.7	
10 ppm × 20 weeks	0	—	34.6	
10 ppm × 20 weeks	0	21	9.1	
10 ppm × 20 weeks	—	—	5.6	
30 ppm × 10 weeks	10	15	6.7	at week 75
30 ppm × 10 weeks	10	35	27.3	
30 ppm × 10 weeks	10	55	38.2	
30 ppm × 10 weeks	10	—	56.3	
30 ppm × 10 weeks	—	—	6.3	
—	10	—	0.0	
—	—	—	0.0	

body (Table 3). The results implied that Hp infection in childhood might have stronger enhancing effect on stomach cancer development than that in adulthood and that host response to Hp might be also important for pathogenicity.

Eradication of Hp

With regard to cancer prevention, we reported that Hp eradication could diminish the enhancing effect of Hp infection on stomach carcinogenesis [40]. MGs infected with Hp followed by or following MNU administration showed enhancing effect on gastric carcinogenesis, but adding eradication diminished this enhancing effect (Table 4). This study provides direct evidence that Hp eradication may be useful as a prevention approach. Recently, many clinicians have been prescribing Hp eradication for medical care of patients suffering not only from peptic ulcers [41] and MALT lymphomas [42, 43] but also from dyspepsia [44]. However, after complete clearance of the bacteria, reflux esophagitis may occur [45], and this side effect is thought to be an important risk factor for esophageal adenocarcinoma development [46]. Therefore, establishment of criteria for Hp eradication is now a top priority.

For application of Hp eradication to humans, time will presumably be of essential significance. In the study, we eradicated Hp in the period of active chronic gastritis but before intestinal metaplasia or atrophic gastritis had appeared. The early phase might be expected to be most amenable to intervention. To explore the effectiveness of Hp eradication in later phases, we modified our protocol [47]. MGs were given chemical carcinogen (MNU) followed by Hp infection. In this study, earlier eradication of Hp diminished the enhancing effect of Hp on gastric cancer development more effectively. This result may imply that clinically Hp eradication at an earlier time is more effective than at a later time and that eradication at the later time also diminishes the incidence of stomach cancer development to some degree. Concerning the effect of Hp infection on gastric carcinogenesis, it is natural to understand that Hp infection has a promoting effect on carcinogenesis but does not itself possess carcinogenicity.

High-Salt Diet

A high-salt diet has been also considered as a risk factor of gastric cancer [48], and we could obtain a solution of the pathogenicity of a high-salt diet using the MG model. We carried out experiments on MGs using a high-salt diet, chemical carcinogen, and Hp infection [49]. In this study, a high-salt diet, which had not showed an enhancing effect on stomach cancer development induced by chemical carcinogen alone could enhance carcinogenesis induced by chemical carcinogen and Hp infection (Table 5). It was also observed that the titer of serum anti-Hp antibody and the level of serum gastrin concentration increased, so it might imply that a high-salt diet enhanced host response to Hp and consequently the development of stomach cancer.

TABLE 5. High salt diet and Hp infection

MNU treatment[a]	Hp infection[b]	High salt diet[c]	Incidence of cancer (%)	Anti-Hp titer (A.I.)
+	+	+	32.1	337.5
+	+	−	11.8	254.7
+	−	+	0.0	1.7
+	−	−	0.0	2.1
−	+	+	0.0	283.9
−	+	−	0.0	121.0
−	−	+	0.0	1.5
−	−	−	0.0	2.1

A.I., arbitrary index
[a] MNU treatment: 20 ppm × 10 weeks
[b] Hp infection at experimental week 10
[c] High salt diet contained 10% (w/w) sodium chloride

Mechanism of Gastric Carcinogenesis Related to Hp

To determine the pathogenic role of Hp, it is necessary to investigate the interaction between parasite and host. Important roles have been demonstrated for cagA and vacA genes in the pathogenicity of Hp [50]. As Tomb et al. elucidated the complete genome sequence of Hp in 1997 [51], it is likely that a fuller understanding will be generated in the near future.

One interesting point in the MG model is the reason for persistent Hp infection in the stomachs of MG, which is not found in mice and rats. The organism obviously prefers to colonize the layer of surface mucous cell type mucins in the human stomach [52]. The decreased rate of Hp infection with aging and with stomach mucosal damage by MNNG in MGs as noted in the above study and increase in Hp infection related to stomach mucosal damage by MNU or a salty diet in mice [53] imply important roles for mucous conditions of the stomach mucosa for Hp infection. It is essential to clarify this point to develop effective prevention strategies.

Concerning host interaction, it was demonstrated that T-helper 1 cellular immune responses contribute to *Helicobacter*-associated gastritis in mice [54] and humans [55], and D'Elios et al. showed that Hp-specific T-helper 1 effectors might play a role in peptic ulcers in humans [56]. In our study, although overlap of titer levels between groups was observed, the titers of anti-Hp antibodies of the tumor-bearing animals were higher than in tumor-free animals treated in the same manner [33]. The data imply that humoral immunity, which may mean T-helper 2 response, is dominant with regard to neoplasia, in contrast to the T-helper 1 dominance in sufferers from peptic ulcers. The Hp infection model employing MGs, without doubt, may give us information concerning treatment of Hp infection in human and suggestions for experiments in vitro, so it was reported that this model would become a main animal model to investigate the pathogenicity of Hp infection [36].

Concerning Hp itself, the cagA gene is thought to be one of the most virulent factors to gastric mucosa. The function of CagA protein has been investigated for a long time, and it became clear that cagA gene is an indirect marker for cag pathogenicity island (cagPAI). This lesion codes for the genes concerning type IV secretion [57]. Through the type IV secretion system, Hp transfers many virulent proteins, including CagA, into the host cells. In host cells, CagA protein is phosphorylated and activated, binds to the SHP-2 and consequently the complex induces hummingbird morphology [58,59]. It may imply that CagA protein can function as a growth factor. Another mechanism was also reported, that CagA binds to growth factor receptor bound 2 (Grb2), one of the intrasignaling molecules, and the CagA-Grb2 complex activates Ras/MEK/ERK cascade [60]. Therefore, CagA might be a key molecule of pathogenicity of Hp, if not having direct carcinogenicity [61].

Conclusion

Clinical diversity of Hp infection may be caused by variation of Hp itself and host reaction, other factors such as food intake, and interaction of these factors. The present carcinogenesis model employing MGs and epidemiological study have demonstrated a causal link of Hp infection and gastric cancer development. In vitro experiments have showed the mechanisms by which Hp infection inflict injury on gastric mucosal cells. From the point of view of "tailor-made medicine," these in vivo and in vitro experiments may contribute to the development of more effective treatment for Hp infection.

References

1. Warren JR, Marshall B (1983) Unidentified curved bacilli on gastric epithelium in active chronic gastritis. Lancet 1:1273–1275
2. Marshall B, Warren JR (1984) Unidentified curved bacilli in the stomach of patients with gastritis and peptic ulceration. Lancet 1:1311–1315
3. Hu PJ, Li YY, Zhou MH, et al. (1995) *Helicobacter pylori* associated with a high prevalence of duodenal ulcer disease and a low prevalence of gastric cancer in a developing nation. Gut 36:198–202
4. Craanen ME, Dekker W, Blok P, et al. (1992) Intestinal metaplasia and *Helicobacter pylori*: an endoscopic bioptic study of the gastric antrum. Gut 33:16–20
5. Rugge M, Cassaro M, Leandro G, et al. (1996) *Helicobacter pylori* in promotion of gastric carcinogenesis. Dig Dis Sci 41:950–955
6. Nomura A, Stemmermann GN, Chyou PH, et al. (1991) *Helicobacter pylori* infection and gastric carcinoma among Japanese Americans in Hawaii. N Engl J Med 325:1132–1136
7. Parsonnet J, Friedman GD, Vandersteen DP, et al. (1991) *Helicobacter pylori* infection and the risk of gastric carcinoma. N Engl J Med 325:1127–1131
8. Forman D, Newell DG, Fullerton F, et al. (1991) Association between infection with *Helicobacter pylori* and risk of gastric cancer: evidence from a prospective investigation. BMJ 302:1302–1305
9. Parsonnet J, Hansen S, Rodriguez L, et al. (1994) *Helicobacter pylori* infection and gastric lymphoma. N Engl J Med 330:1267–1271
10. IARC Working Group on the Evaluation of Carcinogenic Risks to Humans (1994) *Helicobacter pylori*. In: Schistosomes, liver flukes, and *Helicobacter pylori*. Views and expert opinions of an IARC working group on the evaluation of carcinogenic risks to human. IARC, Lyon, pp 177–241
11. Hirayama F, Takagi S, Yokoyama Y, et al. (1996) Establishment of gastric *Helicobacter pylori* infection in Mongolian gerbils. J Gastroenterol 31:24–28
12. Kawaguchi T, Kurisu M, Numanyu N, et al. (1976) Precancerous changes in the stomach. Cancer Res 36:2673–2677
13. Wada T, Fukuda M, Ibayashi J, et al. (1964) Clinical consideration of chronic ulcer of the stomach; on its significance in the precancerous pathogenesis of stomach cancer. Gan No Rinsho 10:600–606
14. Takahashi M, Shirai T, Fukushima S, et al. (1976) Effect of fundic ulcers induced by iodoacetamide on development of gastric tumors in rats treated with *N*-methyl-*N*′-nitro-*N*-nitrosoguanidine. Gann 67:47–54
15. Kamiya T, Morishita T, Asakura H, et al. (1982) Long-term follow-up study on gastric adenoma and its relation to gastric protruded carcinoma. Cancer (Phila) 50:2496–2503
16. Nakamura T, Nakano G. (1985) Histopathological classification and malignant change in gastric polyps. J Clin Pathol 38:754–764
17. Nakamura K, Sakaguchi H, Enjoji N (1988) Depressed adenoma of the stomach. Cancer (Phila) 62:2197–2202
18. Morson BC (1955) Carcinoma arising from area of intestinal metaplasia of the gastric mucosa. Br J Cancer 9:377–385

19. Tatematsu M, Ichinose M, Miki K, et al. (1990) Gastric and intestinal phenotypic expression of human stomach cancers as revealed by pepsinogen immunohistochemistry and mucin histochemistry. Acta Pathol Jpn 40:494–504
20. Tatematsu M, Furihata C, Katsuyama T, et al. (1983) Independent induction of intestinal metaplasia and gastric cancer in rats treated with *N*-methyl-*N'*-nitro-*N*-nitrosoguanidin. Cancer Res 43:1335–1341
21. Kaminishi M, Shimizu N, Yamaguchi H, et al. (1996) Different carcinogenesis in the gastric remnant after gastrectomy for gastric cancer. Cancer (Phila) 77:S1646–S1653
22. Kaminishi M, Shimizu N, Shimoyama S, et al. (1995) Etiology of gastric remnant cancer with special reference to the effects of denervation of the gastric mucosa. Cancer (Phila) 75:S1490–S1496
23. Walker IR, Stickland RG, Ungar B, et al. (1971) Simple atrophic gastritis and gastric carcinoma. Gut 12:906–911
24. Maaroos HI, Salupere V, Uibo R (1981) Gastric ulcer, gastritis and gastric carcinoma. Ann Clin Res 13:151–153
25. Palmer ED (1954) Investigation of the gastric mucosa spirochetes of the human. Gastroenterology 27:218–220
26. Uemura N, Mukai T, Okamoto S, et al. (1997) Effect of *Helicobacter pylori* eradication on subsequent development of cancer after endoscopic resection of early gastric cancer. Cancer Epidemiol Biomarkers Prev 6:639–642
27. Radin MJ, Eaton KA, Krakowka S, et al. (1990) *Helicobacter pylori* gastric infection in gnotobiotic beagle dogs. Infect Immun 58:2606–2612
28. Fox JG (1994) Gastric disease in ferrets: effects of *Helicobacter mustelae*, nitrosamines and reconstructive gastric surgery. Eur J Gastroenterol Hepatol 6:S57–S65
29. Shuto R, Fujioka T, Kubota T, et al. (1993) Experimental gastritis induced by *Helicobacter pylori* in Japanese monkeys. Infect Immun 61:933–939
30. Karita M, Kouchiyama T, Okita K, et al. (1991) New small animal model for human gastric *Helicobacter pylori* infection: success in both nude and euthymic mice. Am J Gastroenterol 86:1596–1603
31. Tatematsu M, Yamamoto M, Shimizu N, et al. (1998) Induction of glandular stomach cancers in *Helicobacter pylori*-sensitive Mongolian gerbils treated with *N*-methyl-*N*-nitrosourea and *N*-methyl-*N'*-nitro-*N*-nitrosoguanidine in drinking water. Jpn J Cancer Res 89:97–104
32. Sugiyama A, Maruta F, Ikeno T, et al. (1998) *Helicobacter pylori* infection enhances *N*-methyl-*N*-nitrosourea-induced stomach carcinogenesis in the Mongolian gerbil. Cancer Res 58:2067–2069
33. Shimizu N, Inada K, Nakanishi H, et al. (1999) *Helicobacter pylori* infection enhances glandular stomach carcinogenesis in Mongolian gerbils treated with chemical carcinogens. Carcinogenesis (Oxf) 20:669–676
34. Yamachika T, Nakanishi H, Inada K, et al. (1998) *N*-methyl-*N*-nitrosourea concentration-dependent, rather than total intake-dependent, induction of adenocarcinomas in the glandular stomach of BALB/c mice. Jpn J Cancer Res 89:385–391
35. Biozzi G, Ribeiro OG, Saran A, et al. (1998) Effect of genetic modification of acute inflammatory responsiveness on tumorigenesis in the mouse. Carcinogenesis (Oxf) 19:337–346
36. Lee A (2000) Animal models of gastroduodenal ulcer disease. Best Pract Res Clin Gastroenterol Baillieres 14:75–96
37. Correa P (1996) *Helicobacter pylori* and gastric cancer: state of the art. Cancer Epidemiol Biomarkers Prev 5:477–481
38. Huang JQ, Sridhar S, Chen Y, et al. (1998) Meta-analysis of the relationship between *Helicobacter pylori* seropositivity and gastric cancer. Gastroenterology 114:1169–1179
39. Cao X, Tsukamoto T, Nozaki K, et al. (2002) Earlier *Helicobacter pylori* infection increases the risk for the *N*-methyl-*N*-nitrosourea-induced stomach carcinogenesis in Mongolian gerbils. Jpn J Cancer Res 93:1293–1298

40. Shimizu N, Ikehara Y, Inada K, et al. (2000) Eradication diminishes enhancing effects of *Helicobacter pylori* infection on glandular stomach carcinogenesis in Mongolian gerbils. Cancer Res 60:1512–1514
41. Peek RM Jr, Blaser MJ (1997) Pathophysiology of *Helicobacter pylori*-induced gastritis and peptic ulcer disease. Am J Med 102:200–207
42. Neubauer A, Thiede C, Morgner A, et al. (1997) Cure of *Helicobacter pylori* infection and duration of remission of low-grade gastric mucosa-associated lymphoid tissue lymphoma. J Natl Cancer Inst 89:1350–1355
43. Sackmann M, Morgner A, Rudolph B, et al. (1997) Regression of gastric MALT lymphoma after eradication of *Helicobacter pylori* is predicted by endosonographic staging. MALT Lymphoma Study Group. Gastroenterology 113:1087–1090
44. Agreus L, Talley NJ (1998) Dyspepsia: current understanding and management. Annu Rev Med 49:475–493
45. Labenz J, Blum AL, Bayerdorffer E, et al. (1997) Curing *Helicobacter pylori* infection in patients with duodenal ulcer may provoke reflux esophagitis. Gastroenterology 112:1442–1447
46. Naef AP, Savary M, Ozzello L (1975) Columnar-lined lower esophagus: an acquired lesion with malignant predisposition. Report on 140 cases of Barrett's esophagus with 12 adenocarcinomas. J Thorac Cardiovasc Surg 70:826–835
47. Nozaki K, Shimizu N, Ikehara Y, et al. (2003) Effect of early eradication on *Helicobacter pylori*-related gastric carcinogenesis in Mongolian gerbils. Cancer Sci 94:235–239
48. Tajima K, Tominaga S (1985) Dietary habits and gastrointestinal cancers: a comparative case-control study of stomach and large intestinal cancers in Nagoya, Japan. Jpn J Cancer Res 76:705–716
49. Nozaki K, Shimizu N, Inada K, et al. (2002) Synergistic promoting effects of *Helicobacter pylori* infection and high-salt diet on gastric carcinogenesis in Mongolian gerbils. Jpn J Cancer Res 93:1083–1089
50. Parsonnet J, Friedman GD, Orentreich N, et al. (1997) Risk for gastric cancer in people with CagA positive or CagA negative *Helicobacter pylori* infection. Gut 40:297–301
51. Tomb JF, White O, Kerlavage AR, et al. (1997) The complete genome sequence of the gastric pathogen *Helicobacter pylori*. Nature (Lond) 388:539–547
52. Shimizu T, Akamatsu T, Sugiyama A, et al. (1996) *Helicobacter pylori* and the surface mucous gel layer of the human stomach. Helicobacter 1:207–218
53. Shimizu N, Kaminishi M, Tatematsu M, et al. (1998) *Helicobacter pylori* promotes development of pepsinogen-altered pyloric glands, a preneoplastic lesion of glandular stomach of BALB/c mice pretreated with *N*-methyl-*N*-nitrosourea. Cancer Lett 123:63–69
54. Mohammadi M, Nedrud J, Redline R, et al. (1997) Murine CD4 T-cell response to *Helicobacter* infection: TH1 cells enhance gastritis and TH2 cells reduce bacterial load. Gastroenterology 113:1848–1857
55. Bamford KB, Fan X, Crowe SE, et al. (1998) Lymphocytes in the human gastric mucosa during *Helicobacter pylori* have a T helper cell 1 phenotype. Gastroenterology 114:482–492
56. D'Elios MM, Manghetti M, De Carli M, et al. (1997) T helper 1 effector cells specific for *Helicobacter pylori* in the gastric antrum of patients with peptic ulcer disease. J Immunol 158:962–967
57. Odenbreit S, Puls J, Sedlmaier B, et al. (2000) Translocation of *Helicobacter pylori* CagA into gastric epithelial cells by type IV secretion. Science 287:1497–1500
58. Asahi M, Azuma T, Ito Y, et al. (2000) *Helicobacter pylori* CagA protein can be tyrosine phosphorylated in gastric epithelial cells. J Exp Med 191:593–602
59. Higashi H, Tsumi R, Muto S, et al. (2002) SHP-2 tyrosine phosphatase as an intracellular target of *Helicobacter pylori* CagA protein. Science 295:683–686
60. Mimuro H, Suzuki T, Tanaka J, et al. (2002) Grb2 is a key mediator of *H. pylori* CagA protein activities. Mol Cell 10:745–755
61. Sugiyama T, Asaka M (2004) *Helicobacter pylori* infection and gastric cancer. Med Electron Microsc 37:149–157

Color Plates

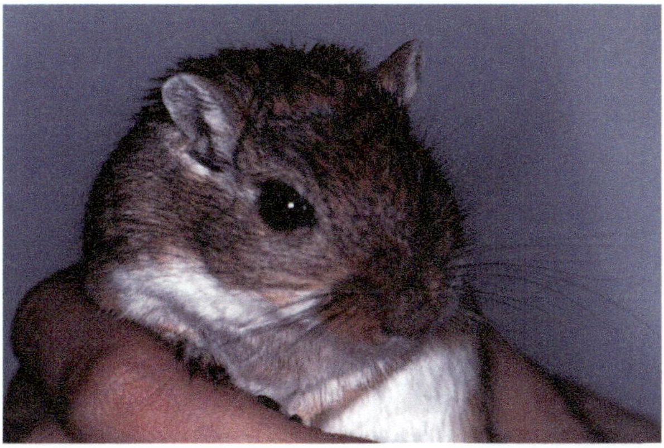

FIG. 1. Mongolian gerbil (*Meriones Unguiculatu*)

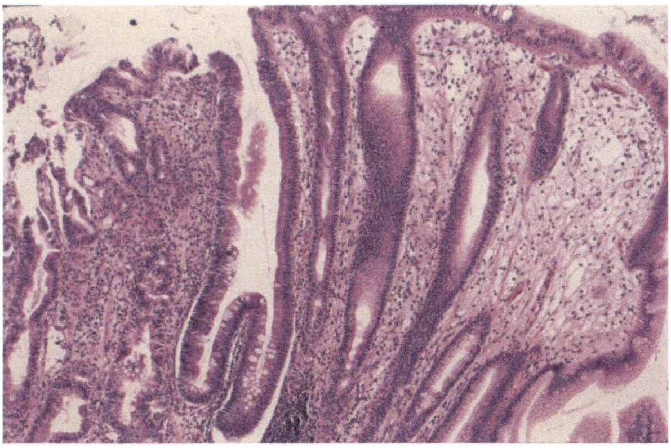

FIG. 2. Intestinal metaplasia observed in gerbil infected with *Helicobacter pylori* at week 50. H&E, ×100

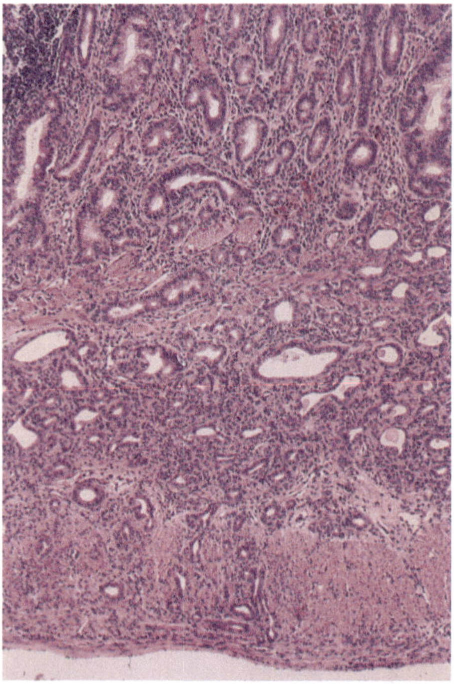

a

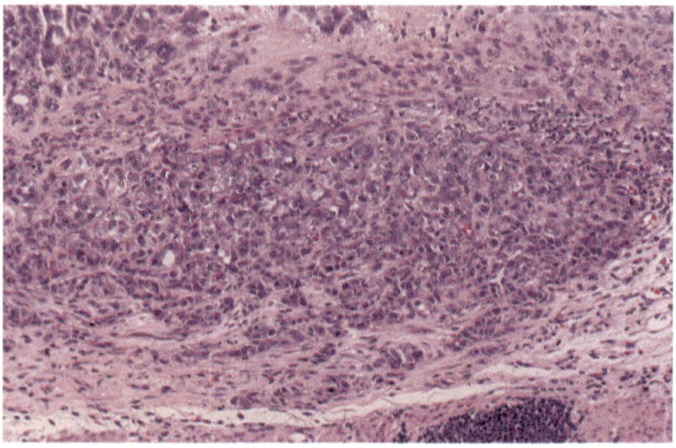

b

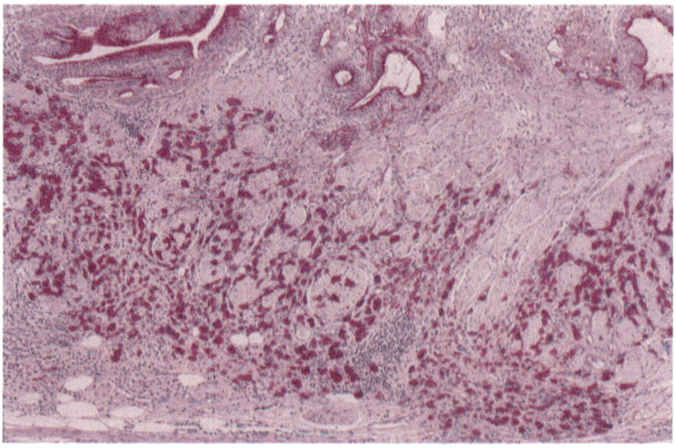

c

Fig. 3. Histological sections of gastric mucosa induced by *Helicobacter pylori* infection and *N*-Methyl-*N*′-nitro-*N*-nitrosoguanidine administration in Mongolian gerbils. **a** A well differentiated glandular stomach adenocarcinoma characterized by tubular structures with cellular atypia. H&E, ×400. **b** A poorly differentiated glandular stomach adenocarcinoma characterized by little tendency to form glandular structures with severe cellular atypia. H&E, ×500. **c** A signet ring cell carcinoma characterized by isolated tumor cells containing abundant amounts of mucin. AB-PAS, ×150

Fundic Mucosal Change Associated with Oxyntic Atrophy

Hirokazu Yamaguchi[1,2], Jeffrey R. Lee[2], James R. Goldenring[3], and Michio Kaminishi[1]

Introduction

The normal gastric fundic mucosa is assembled from a diverse group of cell lineages responsible for lumenal secretion of mucins, pepsinogen, intrinsic factor, and HCl. A number of investigations over the past decade have demonstrated that lineages in the normal fundic mucosa arise from a progenitor zone located in the glands [1]. In the gastric mucosa, the progenitor zone is located at two-thirds of the mucosa from the base, and this location is maintained by the differentiation of cell lineages with differing longevity. Short-lived surface mucous cells having a 4- to 6-day lifetime arise from the progenitor zone and migrate toward the lumen [2]. Although a minority of parietal cells migrate toward the luminal surface, the majority of parietal cells migrate toward the basal lamina [3]. Mucous neck cells arise from preneck cells, and it is thought that they redifferentiate into chief cells during migration toward the base [4]. Those cells have a long lifetime, such as 80 days in parietal cells and 200 days in chief cells. This process of differentiation of specific cell lineages from the progenitor zone is regulated by hormonal and paracrine regulators.

To maintain mucosal integrity, the gastric mucosa responds to both mechanical and caustic injuries. Chronic injury by *Helicobacter pylori* infection leads to oxyntic atrophy, foveolar hyperplasia, and mucous cell metaplasia [5,6]. Recent investigations have described TFF2/spasmolytic polypeptide expressing metaplasia (SPEM) in mice infected with *Helicobacter felis* [7], in humans with fundal predominant *H. pylori* gastritis [8], and in the mucosa adjacent to gastric adenocarcinoma [8–10]. The cells of this lineage recapitulate the morphology of duodenal Brunner's glands or the cells of the deep antral glands and immunostain for the trefoil polypeptide spasmolytic polypeptide (SP), also known as TFF2. SPEM was identified in a high percentage of gastric fundic biopsies with *H. pylori* gastritis, and within the adjacent mucosa in 91%

[1] Department of Gastrointestinal Surgery, The University of Tokyo Graduate School of Medicine, 7-3-1 Hongo, Bunkyo-ku, Tokyo 113-8655, Japan
[2] Institute of Molecular Medicine and Genetics, Medical College of Georgia, Augusta, GA, USA
[3] Nashville VA Medical Center and the Department of Surgery, Epithelial Biology Program, Vanderbilt-Ingram Cancer Center, Vanderbilt University School of Medicine, Nashville, TN, USA
e-mail: hiro-tky@umin.ac.jp

of gastric cancer resections. In addition, most of these sections demonstrated SP staining cells within dysplastic cells [8]. The association of SPEM with gastric adenocarcinoma and oxyntic atrophy suggested that SPEM may represent a candidate precursor to gastric adenocarcinoma.

In addition to its association with *Helicobacter* gastritis, SPEM is also observed in other animal models with oxyntic atrophy. Metallothionein-tumor necrosis factor (TGF)-α transgenic mice demonstrate not only expansion of the surface cell compartment of fundic glands but also marked decrease of parietal cells and emergence of SPEM at the base of fundic glands [11,12]. Another model is rats administrated with DMP-777 that leads to a reversible pharmacological ablation of parietal cells [13]. This drug is a cell permeant neutrophil elastase inhibitor that also acts as a parietal cell-specific protonophore. Treatment of rats with DMP-777 for 3 months induced oxyntic atrophy and expansion of the surface compartment as well as the emergence of SPEM from the base of fundic glands [13]. These results support the hypothesis that loss of parietal cells may be a primary event in evolution of the spectrum of lineage changes. Furthermore, the production of SPEM the base of fundic mucosa suggested the presence of a second cryptic progenitor zone at the base of the glands.

Previous gastric resection is a risk factor for the development of gastric remnant cancer [14]. Causative factors have been investigated, including duodenogastric bile reflux, intragastric bacterial flora overgrowth with an increase in carcinogenic *N*-nitroso compounds, denervation, and decreased vascularity [15]. Remnant stomachs show oxyntic atrophy, and remnant gastric cancer develops in the fundic glands; therefore, remnant gastric cancer is another good model for investigating the association between SPEM, oxyntic atrophy, and gastric cancer development.

Human Remnant Gastric Cancer

In a previous study, we reported SPEM in the remnant stomach with cancer [10]. We obtained archival tissue on 19 patients who underwent gastric resection or endoscopic mucosal resection of a remnant gastric adenocarcinoma at the Branch Hospital of the University of Tokyo and investigated SPEM expression through immunohistochemistry using a murine monoclonal IgM anti-TFF2 antibody.

The indications for primary gastric resection in this group were complications of peptic ulcer disease [9] or gastric cancer [10]. The mean age at the time of presentation of remnant gastric cancer was 65 years, and the time interval from primary resections to development of the remnant gastric cancer was 16 years on average. The time interval was longer in the ulcer group than in the cancer group. Eight malignancies were intestinal histologic type and 11 were diffuse. According to TMN classification, 8 cases were classified as pT1, 2 were pT2, and 9 were pT3 or pT4. The mucosa of the remnant stomachs demonstrated atrophic gastritis. Intestinal mataplasia was observed in 10 cases (52%). Gastritis cystica profunda (GCP) was seen in 5 cases (26%). All of the GCP demonstrated immunostaining for TFF2. SPEM was identified in the adjacent fundic mucosa to the cancer. SPEM expression did not appear to correlate with previous disease, time interval, or malignant histological type. In 4 of 16 cases (25%), TFF2 staining within the cells of malignancy was observed (Fig. 1).

Remnant Gastric Cancer Models in Rats

We have also reported SPEM in a postgastrectomy rat model. Using a well-established postgastrectomy rat model [16], we examined six groups of rats. Groups I and II received truncal vagotomy without or with duodenogastric reflux, groups III and IV received antrectomy and Billroth I anastomosis without or with truncal vagotomy, groups V and VI received nitrite carcinogen *N*-methyl-*N*′-nitro-*N*-nitrosoguanigine (MNNG) treatment before antrectomy and Billroth I anastomosis without or with truncal vagotomy. Untreated rats were also examined as a control group. Oxyntic atrophy was quantified in each group as loss of parietal cell mass. Progressive oxyntic atrophy correlated with the severity of operative procedure and carcinogen administration. There was an approximate 22% decrease in parietal cells from the control group to groups I and II, a 23% decrease from groups I and II to groups III and IV, and a 40% decrease from groups III and IV to groups V and VI (Fig. 2). GCP was not seen in groups I and II; however, it was seen in the more severe surgical group. Intestinal metaplasia was seen in groups V and VI (group V, 17%; group VI, 25%). Adenocarcinoma was identified in the carcinogen treatment groups (group V, 17%; group VI, 50%).

Immunohistochemistry using the anti-TFF2 antibody was performed. Truncal vagotomy with duodenogastric reflux induced scattered TFF2 immunoreactive glands at the base of the mucosa. Antrectomy with vagotomy caused a marked expansion of basally located TFF2 immunoreactive cells with early phenotypic changes toward SPEM. Animals receiving the carcinogen in groups V and VI demonstrated SPEM at the base of the atrophic fundic mucosa. group V demonstrated SPEM in 50% of cases, whereas group VI had SPEM in 100% (Fig. 3).

To investigate proliferating cells, immunostaining with antibodies against proliferating cell nuclear antigen (PCNA) was performed. In groups I, II, and III, PCNA-

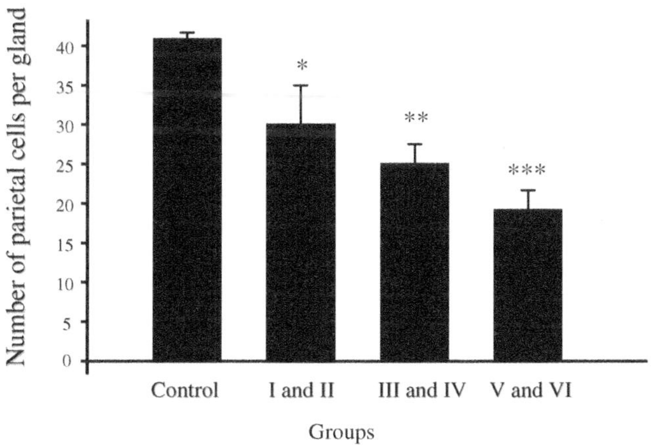

Fig. 2. Number of parietal cells per gland for each group. Control versus *, $P < 0.01$; * versus **, $P < 0.05$; ** versus ***, $P < 0.01$

labeled nuclei were observed in the normal progenitor zone; however, in group IV there was widening of the progenitor zone with increase of PCNA-labeled cells. With the addition of carcinogen, two distinct zones of PCNA immunostaining were observed. In addition to proliferative activity in cells at the physiological midgland zone, PCNA staining cells was observed in the base of the fundic mucosa. The distribution of deep gland PCNA-staining cells in the atrophic mucosa correlated with the appearance of SPEM at the base of the base of glands (Fig. 4).

Intrinsic factor is a marker for chief cells in rats. In rats without carcinogen (groups I to IV), intrinsic factor immunoreactivity was seen only in normal-appearing chief cells; however, in the carcinogen groups (Groups V and VI), intrinsic factor immunoreactivity was observed in metaplastic cells at the base of atrophic fundic glands that were also stained by anti-TFF2 antibodies. Double immunofluorescence for TFF2 and intrinsic factor revealed that SPEM cells were immunoreactive for both TFF2 and intrinsic factor at the base of the glands. The intracellular distribution of TFF2 and intrinsic factor in SPEM cells was distinct (Fig. 5).

Discussion

The normal gastric mucosa is assembled from a repertoire of short- and long-lived differentiated cell lineages [1–4]. All these lineages derive from the same primary progenitor population located in the two-thirds of the gland from the base. The short-lived surface cells differentiate from presurface cells and migrate toward the lumen [2]. Long-lived lineages populate the portions of the gland deep to the proliferative zone. The majority of parietal cells differentiate from preparietal cells and migrate toward the gland base [3]. It is thought that mucous neck cells differentiate from preneck cells and migrate toward the base, differentiating into chief cells [4]. Previous investigations have demonstrated that parietal cells are responsible for the secretion of a number of critical growth factors including TGF-α, amphiregullin, and heparin binding-epidermal growth factor (HB-EGF) [17,18]. Thus, loss of parietal cells may eliminate important agents required for appropriate differentiation of deeper gland lineages such as mucous neck and chief cells. *H. felis*-infected mice, MT-TGF-α transgenic mice, and DMP-777-treated rats that demonstrated SPEM also showed oxyntic atrophy at the background of the mucosa. SPEM was also identified in a high percentage of gastric fundic biopsies with *H. pylori* gastritis and within the adjacent mucosa of gastric cancer resection that demonstrated oxyntic atrophy. In the study of the remnant gastric cancer model with rats, oxyntic atrophy was quantified as loss of parietal cell mass and progressive oxyntic atrophy correlated with expansion of TFF2 staining and emergence of SPEM. The association between severity of oxyntic atrophy and SPEM emergence suggested that parietal cells may provide important agents required for appropriate differentiation of deeper gland lineages.

Immunohistochemistry with anti-PCNA antibodies revealed that loss of parietal cells was accompanied by the emergence of a second proliferative population located at the gland base that gave rise to SPEM. The findings indicate that the fundic mucosa responds to an injury resulting in parietal cell loss with induction of a novel mucous cell metaplasia with an antral/Brunner's gland phenotype.

Because parietal cell loss is associated with gastric cancer, an understanding of the changes in the gastric mucosa attendant with oxyntic atrophy is critical. In humans, a number of mucosal pathologies are associated with oxyntic atrophy. Foveolar hyperplasia, the expansion of normal-appearing surface cells, is often associated with oxyntic atrophy following either chronic *H. pylori* infection or following antrectomy [19].

A number of investigations have noted an association of goblet cell intestinal metaplasia with oxyntic atrophy [6]. We observed intestinal metaplasia in the rats receiving carcinogen and antrectomy; however, the incidence of SPEM in the rats with carcinogen and antrectomy was higher that that of intestinal metaplasia.

SPEM developed from the base of fundic glands coincident with the emergence of a proliferative cell population that appeared separate from the normal proliferative zone. Importantly, we also observed that a subpopulation of SPEM cells expressed intrinsic factor, normally a marker of the chief cell lineage in mice. Previous investigations have suggested that chief cells have a long lifetime [4]. Thus, dual intrinsic factor/TFF2 staining cells suggests the possibility that SPEM originates from transdifferentiation of chief cells. Given the role for parietal cells in growth factor secretion, it is possible that factors released from parietal cells are required for maintenance of chief cell differentiation. Alternatively, we have previously proposed that SPEM may arise from a cryptic progenitor cell population located at the base of the glands. Given the similarity of the SPEM lineage to deep antral cells, the SPEM phenotype is consistent with "antralization." Such a cryptic progenitor cell could be a remnant of mucosal cells from development before the emergence of parietal cells. Under this model, factors secreted from parietal cells would normally suppress the proliferation of the cryptic progenitor cells.

In summary, oxyntic atrophy in gastric mucosa has strong association with a TFF2/SP-expressing metaplasia (SPEM) from a basally located progenitor cell population. The dual labeling of a portion of the SPEM cells suggests that SPEM may derive from transdifferentiation of chief cells.

References

1. Karam SM, Leblond CP (1993) Dynamics of epithelial cells in the corpus of the mouse stomach. I. Identification of proliferative cell types and pinpointing of the stem cells. Anat Rec 236:259–279
2. Karam SM, Leblond CP (1993) Dynamics of epithelial cells in the corpus of the mouse stomach. II. Outward migration of pit cells. Anat Rec 236:280–296
3. Karam SM, Leblond CP (1993) Dynamics of epithelial cells in the corpus of the mouse stomach. IV. Bidirectional migration of parietal cells ending in their gradual degeneration and loss. Anat Rec 236:314–332
4. Karam SM, Leblond CP (1993) Dynamics of epithelial cells in the corpus of the mouse stomach. III. Inward migration of neck cells followed by progressive transformation into zymogenic cells. Anat Rec 236:297–313
5. Appelman H (1994) Gastritis: terminology, etiology, and clinicopathological correlations: another biased view. Hum Pathol 25:1006–1019
6. El-Zimaity HMT, Ramchatesingh J, Saeed MA, Graham DY (2001) Gastric intestinal metaplasia: subtypes and natural history. J Clin Pathol 54:679–683

7. Wang TC, Goldenring JR, Dangler C, et al. (1998) Mice lacking secretory phospholipase A2 show altered apoptosis and differentiation with *Helicobacter felis* infection. Gastroenterology 114:675–689
8. Schmidt PH, Lee JR, Joshi V, et al. (1999) Identification of a metaplastic cell lineage associated with human gastric adenocarcinoma. Lab Invest 79:639–646
9. Halldorsdottir AM, Sigurdardottir M, Jonasson JG, et al. (2003) Spasmolytic polypeptide expressing metaplasia (SPEM) associated with gastric cancer in Iceland. Dig Dis Sci 48:431–441
10. Yamaguchi H, Goldenring JR, Kaminishi M, et al. (2001) Identification of spasmolytic polypeptide expressing metaplasia (SPEM) in remnant gastric cancer and surveillance postgastrectomy biopsies. Dig Dis Sci 47:573–578
11. Goldenring JR, Poulsom R, Ray GS, et al. (1996) Expression of trefoil peptides in the gastric mucosa of transgenic mice overexpressing transforming growth factor-α. Growth Factors 13:111–119
12. Goldenring JR, Ray GS, Soroka CJ, et al. (1996) Overexpression of transforming growth factor-alpha alters differentiation of gastric cell lineages. Dig Dis Sci 41:773–784
13. Goldenring JR, Ray GS, Coffey RJ, et al. (2000) Reversible drug-induced oxyntic atrophy in rats. Gastroenterology 118:1080–1093
14. Kaminishi M, Simizu N, Shimoyama S, et al. (1995) Etiology of gastric remnant cancer with special reference to the effects of denervation of the gastric mucosa. Cancer (Phila) 75: 1490–1496
15. Kaminishi M, Shimizu N, Shimoyama S, et al. (1997) Denervation promotes the development of cancer-related lesion in the gastric remnant. J Clin Gastroenterol 25(suppl):129–134
16. Yamaguchi H, Goldenring JR, Kaminishi M, et al. (2002) Association of spasmolytic polypeptide expressing metaplasia (SPEM) with carcinogen administration and oxyntic atrophy in rats. Lab Invest 82:1045–1052
17. Karam SM, Leblond CP (1993) Dynamisc of epithelial cells in the corpus of the mouse stomach. V. Behavior of entero-endocrine and caveolated cells: general conclusions of cell kinetics in the oxyntic epithelium. Anat Rec 236:333–340
18. El-Zimaity HMT, Ota H, Graham DY, et al. (2002) Patterns of gastric atrophy in intestinal type gastric carcinoma. Cancer (Phila) 94:1428–1436
19. Ray GS, Jackson MW, Goldenring JR (1996) Foveolar hyperplasia following partial gastrectomy results from expansion of the surface mucous cell compartment. Dig Dis Sci 41: 2016–2024

Color Plates

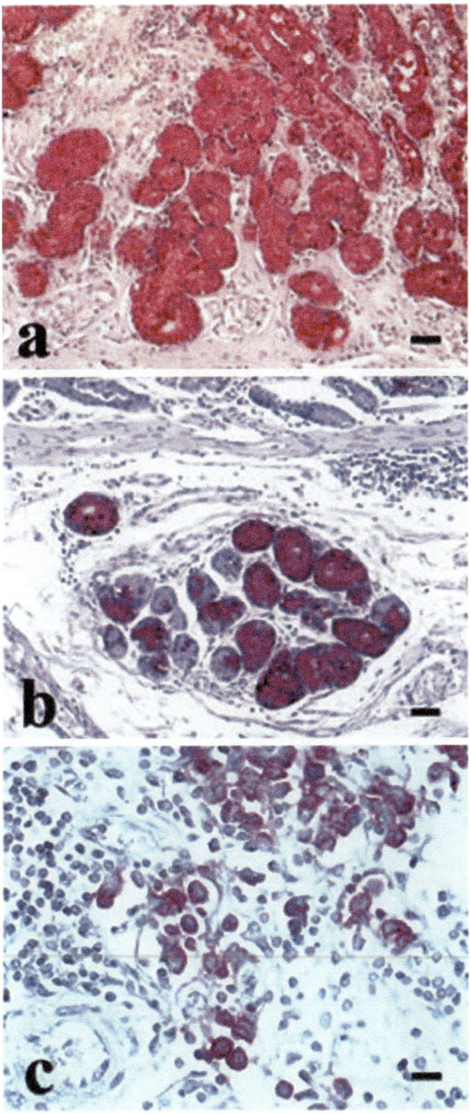

Fig. 1. **a** Spasmolytic polypeptide expressing metaplasia (SPEM) is observed above the muscularis mucosa at the base of atrophic fundic mucosa. **b** Glands of gastritis cystica profunda deep to the muscularis mucosa. TFF2 immunostaining is identical to SPEM. **c** TFF2 staining within malignant cells. *Bars* **a,b** 26 μm; **c** 12 μm

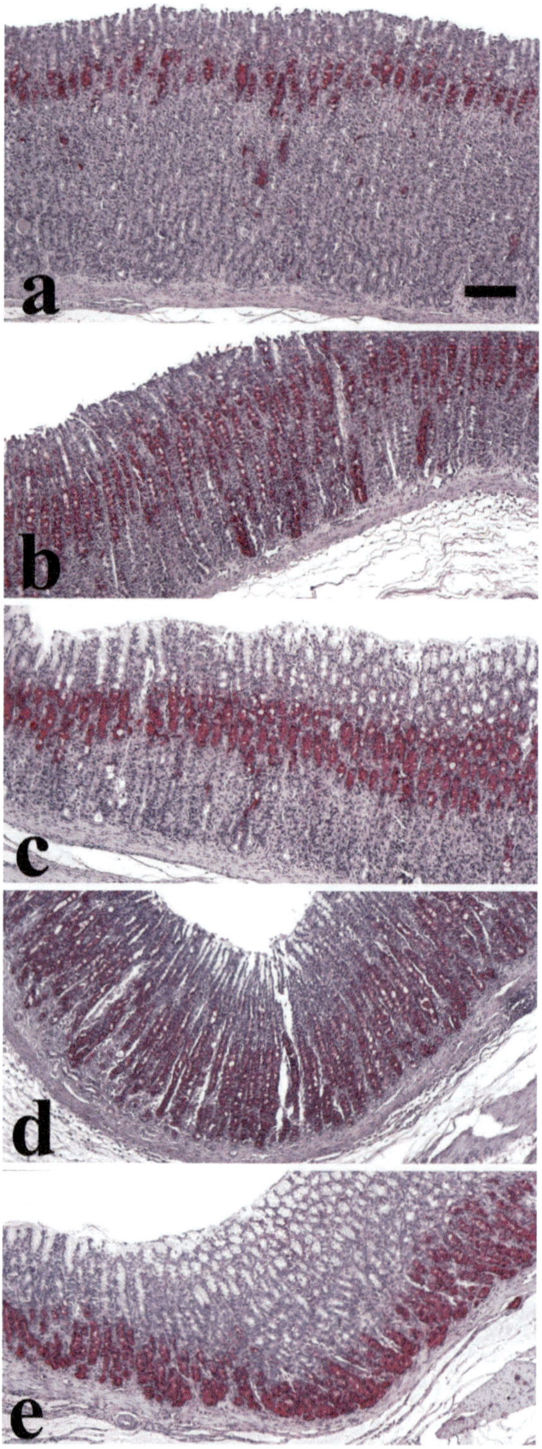

FIG. 3. SPEM in rat model. **a** Group I, physiological staining in mucous neck cells in midgland zone; **b** group II, scattered TFF2-positive staining at base of glands; **c** group III, expansion of midgland zone; **d** group IV, expansion of TFF2 staining to base of glands; **e** group VI, development of SPEM at the base of atrophic mucosa. *Bar* 100 μm

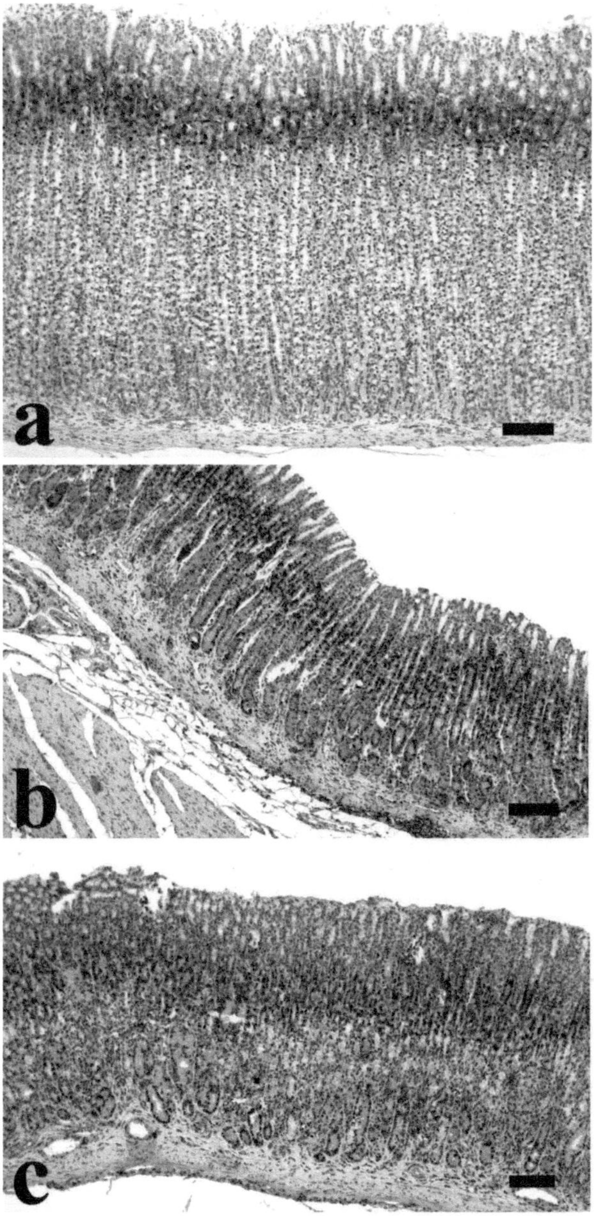

Fig. 4. Proliferating cell nuclear antigen (PCNA) immunostaining in rat model. **a** Group I, scattered proliferating cells at the base of glands; **b** group IV, scattered proliferative cells at base of glands; **c** group VI, distinct dual zones of proliferation at midgland and base of glands. *Bars* 100 µm

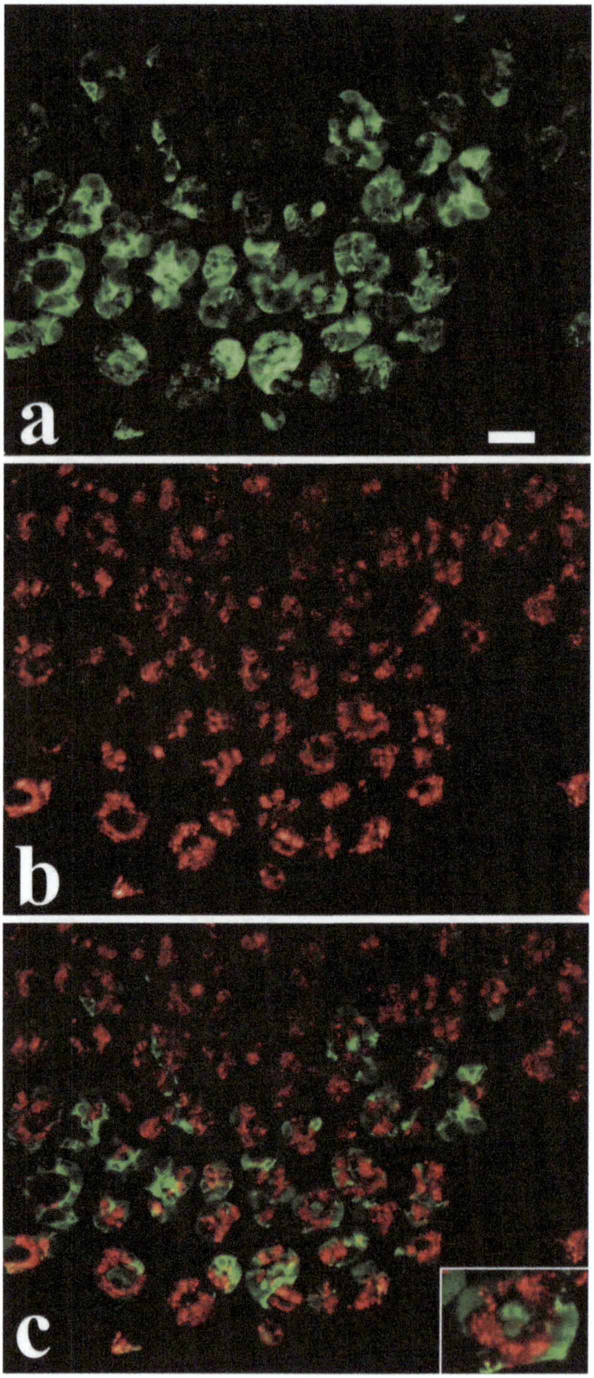

Fig. 5. Expression of intrinsic factor and TFF2/SP in SPEM cells (**a**, *green* = intrinsic factor; **b**, *red* = TFF2/SP). An overlay of dual staining (**c**) demonstrates the majority of the SPEM cells were dual labeled. Intracellular patterns of intrinsic factor and SP were different

DNA Methylation and Gastric Carcinoma

ATSUSHI KANEDA

Introduction

Gastric cancer is the second most common cancer in the world [1,2]. Epigenetic alteration, especially aberrant DNA methylation, is highly involved in gastric carcinogenesis [3–7]. Promoter methylation is the major inactivation mechanism of most cancer-related genes except *p53* in gastric cancers. Association of promoter methylation of some specific genes with histology of gastric cancers was reported. There is a subset of gastric cancers displaying frequent promoter methylations, and association of the frequent methylation with histology was also reported. There is another subset of gastric cancers displaying frequent promoter hypomethylation. Here, DNA methylation as involved in gastric carcinoma is reviewed.

Epigenetics and DNA Methylation

Epigenetics is defined as modifications of the genome, heritable during cell division, that do not involve a change in the DNA sequence [3,4,8]. There are several features distinguishing epigenetics from genetics such as reversibility, and the most common epigenetic modification is DNA methylation, a covalent modification by a methyl group at the C5 position of cytosine at CpG dinucleotides [8,9] (Fig. 1). The methylation status is stably maintained in DNA replication by DNA methyltransferases [10–14], and the fidelity of the methylation pattern in normal cells was reported to be as high as 99.85%–99.92%/site/generation [15].

Epigenetics play important roles in normal development and tissue differentiation [16,17]. Dynamic changes of DNA methylation are observed during embryonic development, and tissue-specific patterns of DNA methylation are observed in somatic tissues [18,19]. Aberrant epigenetic alteration may lead to diseases, including cancers [3,4,20].

Carcinogenesis Division, National Cancer Center Research Institute, 5-1-1 Tsukiji, Chuo-ku, Tokyo 104-0045, Japan
Present address: Johns Hopkins University School of Medicine, Ross 1018, 720 Rutland Avenue, Baltimore, MD 21205, USA
e-mail: akaneda@jhu.edu

Aberrant DNA Methylation in Cancer

Aberrant DNA methylation is present in various genomic regions in cancers. First, global hypomethylation, the decrease of 5-methylcytosine content in the whole genome, was reported in 1983 [21]. Hypomethylation was shown to involve coding regions of genes [22] and then repetitive sequences as well [23]. From the fact that 80% of CpG dinucleotides are present in repetitive sequences and they are mostly methylated [24,25], global hypomethylation is considered to be mainly the result of hypomethylation of the repetitive sequences. Second, hypomethylation is also observed in normally methylated CpG islands in promoter regions, and it induces aberrant expression of their downstream genes if transcription factors are available in cancer cells [26,27]. Known normally methylated promoter CpG islands are very limited and include some cancer-testis antigen genes, such as the *MAGE* genes [28–30]. Third, hypermethylation of normally unmethylated, that is, ordinary, CpG islands in promoter regions [31–33] is well known. Promoter CpG island methylation affects the basal transcriptional machinery by altering the DNA secondary structure and inducing chromosome remodeling through the methyl group-binding proteins and histone deacetylase, which leads to transcriptional silencing of the downstream gene [3,4,20] (Fig. 2). Gene silencing by aberrant promoter methylation in cancers was first pointed out in the *RB* gene in 1993 [34]. Since then, many tumor suppressor genes have been reported to be silenced, for example, *VHL* in renal carcinoma in 1994 [35], *E-cadherin* (*CDH1*) in hepatocellular carcinoma in 1995 [36], and *p16* in various cancers in 1995 [37]. Gene silencing is now regarded as one of the major mechanisms to inactivate tumor suppressor genes, along with gene mutations and deletions, and is causally involved in development and progression of cancers [3,4,20].

Silenced Genes in Gastric Cancers

One of the most well known tumor suppressor genes silenced by promoter methylation is *p16*, which is methylated in 25%–42% of gastric cancers [5,6,38,39]. It is known that mutations and deletions of *p16* are rare, and it is inactivated mainly by promoter methylation in primary human gastric cancers [38]. Microsatellite instability (MSI) is observed at incidences ranging between 31% and 67% [40,41]. Although mutations of DNA mismatch-repair genes such as *hMLH1* and *hMSH2* were rarely observed in gastric cancers [41,42], promoter methylation of *hMLH1* is known to be a major cause of MSI in gastric cancers [43,44]. *CDH1* is a gene responsible for familial diffuse-type gastric cancers in New Zealand by germline mutations [45], and its somatic mutations were also observed in 17%–56% of sporadic diffuse gastric cancers [46,47]. The second hit in *CDH1* mutations is generally caused by promoter methylation [48]. *RUNX3* was shown to be causally involved in human gastric cancers, and the major mechanism for its inactivation is also promoter methylation [49]. *TGF-β type I receptor* [50], *p57* [51], *MGMT* [52,53], *RASSF1A* [54], *TIMP3* [55], *14-3-3 sigma* [56], *HLTF* [57,58], *CHFR* [59], etc. were also reported to be methylated in gastric cancers.

Genome-Wide Search for Aberrant Promoter Methylation

Many known tumor suppressor genes have been reported to be inactivated also by promoter methylation. Based on the idea that novel genes involved in tumor suppression could be isolated by using aberrant promoter methylation as their marker, several genomic scanning methods have been developed, mainly since 1997 [60–66]. Those methods included restriction landmark genomic scanning (RLGS) in 1993 [60], methylation-sensitive-representational difference analysis (MS-RDA) in 1997 [61], methylation-sensitive arbitrarily primed polymerase chain reaction (MS-AP-PCR) in 1997 [62], methylation-sensitive restriction fingerprinting (MSRF) in 1997 [63], methylated CpG island amplification-representational difference analysis (MCA-RDA) in 1999 [64], differential methylation hybridization (DMH) in 1999 [65], and segregation of partly melted molecule-methylated CpG-binding domain column (MBD-SPM) in 1999 [66]. MS-RDA was applied to genome-wide analysis of aberrant methylation in human gastric cancers with some modifications, and silenced genes in cancers were newly identified as strong candidate cancer-related genes [6,67,68] (Fig. 3). Among those genes, *Lysyl Oxidase* and *HRAS-like suppressor* were reported to show growth suppressive activity in ras-transformed fibroblasts [69–71], and *Lysil Oxidase* was shown to be a tumor suppressor gene in gastric cancers [72]. *Thrombomodulin* showed growth suppressive activity in melanoma cells [73], and *PGAR/ARP4/ANGPTL4* showed antiangiogenetic activity [74]. Methylation-based genome scanning can be a useful strategy to identify novel cancer-related genes in gastric cancers.

Methylator Phenotype in Gastric Cancer

It is known that subsets of cancers display significantly higher frequencies of aberrant methylation (Fig. 4). A subset of cancers with frequent aberrant methylations of CpG islands was first described in colon cancers as the CpG island methylator phenotype (CIMP) [75]. CIMP was detected using CpG islands so-called type-C MINT (methylated in tumors) clones and was reported in gastric cancers as well [5]. Epstein–Barr virus (EBV) was reported to be positive in 7% (70/1000) of gastric cancers [76], and EBV-positive gastric cancers were reported to constitute CIMP-positive cancers [77]. The host cells are known to methylate foreign viral DNA inserted into the host genome and the adjacent host DNA as well [78,79]. Viral infection may be one of the triggers for frequent aberrant methylations of CpG islands. Using CpG islands in promoter regions, clustering of aberrant promoter methylations were also shown in EBV-positive gastric cancers [77,80]. These cancers were suggested to be involved in accumulation of gene silencing by promoter methylation, whereas others may be rather involved in genetic and chromosomal instabilities.

Aberrant Methylation and Histology of Gastric Cancer

Gastric cancers are classified histologically into two major types: intestinal (well differentiated) and diffuse (poorly differentiated) [81]. Diffuse-type gastric cancers can be classified into two subtypes: diffuse-adherent and diffuse-scattered [82].

Some genetic alterations are found type specifically, such as *CDH1* mutations in diffuse gastric cancers [46,47]. The major second hit of *CDH1* mutations is promoter methylation [48], and significant correlation between promoter methylation of *CDH1* and diffuse-scattered gastric cancers was also reported ($P = 0.0175$ and 0.008) [83,84]. Significant correlation between promoter methylation and diffuse-type histology was also pointed out in the *14-3-3 sigma* gene ($P = 0.006$) [56]. By analysis of nine silenced genes identified by MS-RDA, most of them were associated with diffuse gastric cancers, and the subset of gastric cancers with frequent promoter methylations was strongly correlated with diffuse-type histology ($P < 0.001$) [6]. Accumulation of aberrant promoter methylations was suggested to lead to diffuse-type histology of gastric cancers, at least in part. Or, some of these methylations that had been considered as "aberrant" may reflect the methylations that were present in the precursor cells of diffuse-type gastric cancers [6].

In contrast, aberrant methylation of the exon 1 region of *p16* was reported to correlate with intestinal gastric cancers ($P = 0.002$) [83]. CIMP analyzed using MINT CpG islands was reported to be more common in intestinal and diffuse-adherent gastric cancers than in diffuse-scattered gastric cancers ($P = 0.013$) [83]. Methylation at the promoter region of *p16*, not the exon 1 region, is known to play a causal role in its silencing [85], although methylation status of the exon 1 region may link to its promoter methylation. MINT CpG islands are not necessarily derived from promoter regions, although CIMP is reported to correlate with promoter methylation of genes such as *p16* and *hMLH1* [5,75]. Two possibilities can be argued about these discrepancies in correlations between methylation and gastric cancer histologies. One possibility is that correlation between promoter methylation and histology of gastric cancers is gene dependent and some promoter methylations may correlate with intestinal-type histology. Another possibility is that accumulation of promoter methylations correlates with diffuse-type histology but methylation of other regions, which does not affect gene transcription, may show different association with histology occasionally. Recently increased DNA methyltransferase 1 protein expression was shown to correlate with poorer differentiation and frequent methylation of CpG islands in gastric cancers, but it was also associated with EBV infection [86]. DNA methyltransferase 1 is an enzyme to target replication foci by binding to proliferating cell nuclear antigen and maintain methylated status of CpG sites by methylating hemimethylated CpG sites into fully methylated CpG sites in DNA replication [10,11]. DNA methyltransferase 1 was also reported to possess de novo methylation activity as well as maintenance activity [87]. Accumulation of methylation by increased DNA methyltransferase activity seems to cause diffuse-type histology, or etiological factors such as EBV infection may cause the histology and aberrant methylation in parallel. Further research should be directed to clarify the causal association between methylation and histology.

DNA Methylation as Clinical Markers of Gastric Cancer

Aberrant methylation of some genes, including *APC*, *RASSF1A*, and *CDH1*, was reported to correlate with poor prognosis of certain cancers and could be a prognostic marker for cancers with unfavorable outcome [88–91]. In gastric cancers, it was reported that *MGMT* was silenced by aberrant methylation and loss of *MGMT* correlated with poor prognosis [92]. On the other hand, methylation of *hMLH1* is known to cause MSI in gastric cancers [43,44], and MSI-positive gastric cancers were found to show relatively good prognosis [93,94]. Such results may suggest that aberrant promoter methylation of some genes possibly correlates with good prognosis of cancers, at least gastric cancers, and that epigenetic markers for both good and poor prognosis of gastric cancers could perhaps be developed.

Cancer-related aberrant DNA is known to circulate in the serum/plasma of cancer patients, and the circulating DNA can be detected as tumor markers in the serum/plasma [95,96]. Detection of aberrantly methylated DNA circulating in the serum/plasma not only leads to diagnosis of presence of cancers, but promoter methylation of some genes such as *APC* and *RASSF1A* was reported to possibly predict the prognosis of cancers [88,90]. Promoter methylation of *APC* was observed in 92% of tissue samples and 25% of plasma samples of 52 esophageal cancer patients, and high levels of methylated *APC* in the plasma were associated with reduced patient survival [88]. Analysis of promoter methylation of 39 genes in the serum DNA of breast cancer patients revealed that methylated *RASSF1A* and/or *APC* in the serum were associated with poor outcome [90]. In gastric cancers, it was reported that *p16* methylation was detected in 23 of 60 gastric cancer tissues and 6 serum samples of the 23 methylation-positive gastric cancer patients [97]. No association was detected between the aberrant *p16* methylation and clinicopathological features of gastric cancers [97]. Although the clinical relevance is still unclear, aberrantly methylated DNA circulating in the serum/plasma was shown to be detected in gastric cancer patients as well.

Hypomethylation in Gastric Cancer

Aberrant hypomethylation is also detected in gastric cancers. The first reported alteration of DNA methylation in cancers was global hypomethylation, detected by the high pressure liquid chromatography (HPLC) method [21]. Total genomic DNA methylation refers to the overall content of 5-methyl cytosine in the whole genome [98]. In human DNA of normal somatic cells, 70%–90% of CpGs are methylated depending on the tissues [99,100]. This amount translates into 3%–4% of all cytosine residues, because the CpG dinucleotide is represented much less than the other dinucleotides, and 0.76%–1.00% of all bases in the genome [25,98]. In gastric epithelial tissues, the 5-methyl cytosine content was 0.82% $\pm$ 0.07% (mean $\pm$ SD) [101] (Fig. 5). In gastric cancers, some showed slightly lower levels of 5-methyl cytosine, 0.74% $\pm$ 0.03%, and some showed much lower levels, 0.55% $\pm$ 0.10% (overall, 0.65% $\pm$ 0.12%) [101].

Hypomethylation potentially promotes cancer via a number of mechanisms: activation of protooncogenes [102,103], chromosomal instability [104–106], reactivation of transposable elements [107,108], and loss of imprinting [20,109,110]. Although hypomethylation in gastric cancers has not been well analyzed, global hypomethylation in gastric cancers was shown to correlates with hypomethylation of repetitive sequences and hypomethylation of normally methylated promoter CpG islands, which induced aberrant gene expressions [101]. These hypomethylations in gastric cancers were shown to occur independently from promoter methylation, designated as CpG island hypomethylator phenotype (CHOP) [6]. CHOP-positive gastric cancers showed frequent promoter hypomethylations and constituted a different subset from those with frequent promoter methylations, but did not correlate with histology, tumor depth, or status of lymph node metastasis [101]. Further research is necessary to clarify the roles of hypomethylation in development and progression of these cancers.

References

1. Fuchs CS, Mayer RJ (1995) Gastric carcinoma. N Engl J Med 333:32–41
2. Parkin DM, Pisani P, Ferlay J (1999) Estimates of the worldwide incidence of 25 major cancers in 1990. Int J Cancer 80:827–841
3. Jones PA, Baylin SB (2002) The fundamental role of epigenetic events in cancer. Nat Rev Genet 3:415–428
4. Baylin SB, Herman JG (2000) DNA hypermethylation in tumorigenesis: epigenetics joins genetics. Trends Genet 16:168–174
5. Toyota M, Ahuja N, Suzuki H, et al (1999) Aberrant methylation in gastric cancer associated with the CpG island methylator phenotype. Cancer Res 59:5438–5442
6. Kaneda A, Kaminishi M, Yanagihara K, et al (2002) Identification of silencing of nine genes in human gastric cancers. Cancer Res 62:6645–6650
7. Ushijima T, Sasako M (2004) Focus on gastric cancer. Cancer Cell 5:121–125
8. Feinberg AP (2001) Cancer epigenetics takes center stage. Proc Natl Acad Sci USA 98: 392–394
9. Laird PW, Jaenisch R (1996) The role of DNA methylation in cancer genetic and epigenetics. Annu Rev Genet 30:441–464
10. Bestor T, Laudano A, Mattaliano R, et al (1988) Cloning and sequencing of a cDNA encoding DNA methyltransferase of mouse cells. The carboxyl-terminal domain of the mammalian enzymes is related to bacterial restriction methyltransferases. J Mol Biol 203:971–983
11. Chuang LS, Ian HI, Koh TW, et al (1997) Human DNA-(cytosine-5) methyltransferase-PCNA complex as a target for p21WAF1. Science 277:1996–2000
12. Okano M, Bell DW, Haber DA, et al (1999) DNA methyltransferases Dnmt3a and Dnmt3b are essential for de novo methylation and mammalian development. Cell 99:247–257
13. Rhee I, Jair KW, Yen RW, et al (2000) CpG methylation is maintained in human cancer cells lacking DNMT1. Nature (Lond) 404:1003–1007
14. Robert MF, Morin S, Beaulieu N, et al (2003) DNMT1 is required to maintain CpG methylation and aberrant gene silencing in human cancer cells. Nat Genet 33:61–65
15. Ushijima T, Watanabe N, Okochi E, et al (2003) Fidelity of the methylation pattern and its variation in the genome. Genome Res 13:868–874
16. Jaenisch R, Bird A (2003) Epigenetic regulation of gene expression: how the genome integrates intrinsic and environmental signals. Nat Genet 33(suppl):245–254
17. Li E (2002) Chromatin modification and epigenetic reprogramming in mammalian development. Nat Rev Genet 3:662–673
18. Reik W, Dean W, Walter J (2001) Epigenetic reprogramming in mammalian development. Science 293:1089–1093
19. Futscher BW, Oshiro MM, Wozniak RJ, et al (2002) Role for DNA methylation in the control of cell type-specific maspin expression. Nat Genet 31:175–179
20. Feinberg AP, Tycko B (2004) The history of cancer epigenetics. Nat Rev Cancer 4:143–153
21. Gama-Sosa MA, Slagel VA, Trewyn RW, et al (1983) The 5-methylcytosine content of DNA from human tumors. Nucleic Acids Res 11:6883–6894
22. Feinberg AP, Vogelstein B (1983) Hypomethylation distinguishes genes of some human cancers from their normal counterparts. Nature (Lond) 301:89–92

23. Jurgens B, Schmitz-Drager BJ, Schulz WA (1996) Hypomethylation of L1 LINE sequences prevailing in human urothelial carcinoma. Cancer Res 56:5698–5703
24. Dunn BK (2003) Hypomethylation: one side of a larger picture. Ann N Y Acad Sci 983:28–42
25. Esteller M, Herman JG (2002) Cancer as an epigenetic disease: DNA methylation and chromatin alterations in human tumours. J Pathol 196:1–7
26. Weber J, Salgaller M, Samid D, et al (1994) Expression of the MAGE-1 tumor antigen is up-regulated by the demethylating agent 5-aza-2′-deoxycytidine. Cancer Res 54:1766–1771
27. De Smet C, Lurquin C, Lethe B, et al (1999) DNA methylation is the primary silencing mechanism for a set of germ line- and tumor-specific genes with a CpG-rich promoter. Mol Cell Biol 19:7327–7335
28. van der Bruggen P, Traversari C, Chomez P, et al (1991) A gene encoding an antigen recognized by cytolytic T lymphocytes on a human melanoma. Science 254:1643–1647
29. Traversari C, van der Bruggen P, Luescher IF, et al (1992) A nonapeptide encoded by human gene MAGE-1 is recognized on HLA-A1 by cytolytic T lymphocytes directed against tumor antigen MZ2-E. J Exp Med 176:1453–1457
30. Takahashi K, Shichijo S, Noguchi M, et al (1995) Identification of MAGE-1 and MAGE-4 proteins in spermatogonia and primary spermatocytes of testis. Cancer Res 55:3478–3482
31. Bird AP (1986) CpG-rich islands and the function of DNA methylation. Nature (Lond) 321:209–213
32. Gardiner-Garden M, Frommer M (1987) CpG islands in vertebrate genomes. J Mol Biol 196:261–282
33. Takai D, Jones PA (2002) Comprehensive analysis of CpG islands in human chromosomes 21 and 22. Proc Natl Acad Sci USA 99:3740–3745
34. Ohtani-Fujita N, Fujita T, Aoike A, et al (1993) CpG methylation inactivates the promoter activity of the human retinoblastoma tumor-suppressor gene. Oncogene 8:1063–1067
35. Herman JG, Latif F, Weng Y, et al (1994) Silencing of the VHL tumor-suppressor gene by DNA methylation in renal carcinoma. Proc Natl Acad Sci U S A 91:9700–9704
36. Yoshiura K, Kanai Y, Ochiai A, et al (1995) Silencing of the E-cadherin invasion-suppressor gene by CpG methylation in human carcinomas. Proc Natl Acad Sci U S A 92:7416–7419
37. Merlo A, Herman JG, Mao L, et al (1995) 5′ CpG island methylation is associated with transcriptional silencing of the tumour suppressor p16/CDKN2/MTS1 in human cancers. Nat Med 1:686–692
38. Lee YY, Kang SH, Seo JY, et al (1997) Alterations of $p16^{INK4A}$ and $p15^{INK4B}$ genes in gastric carcinomas. Cancer (Phila) 80:1889–1896
39. Shim YH, Kang GH, Ro JY (2000) Correlation of p16 hypermethylation with p16 protein loss in sporadic gastric carcinomas. Lab Invest 80:689–695
40. Rhyu MG, Park WS, Meltzer SJ (1994) Microsatellite instability occurs frequently in human gastric carcinoma. Oncogene 9:29–32
41. Akiyama Y, Nakasaki H, Nihei Z, et al (1996) Frequent microsatellite instabilities and analyses of the related genes in familial gastric cancers. Jpn J Cancer Res 87:595–601
42. Keller G, Grimm V, Vogelsang H, et al (1996) Analysis for microsatellite instability and mutations of the DNA mismatch repair gene hMLH1 in familial gastric cancer. Int J Cancer 68:571–576
43. Leung SY, Yuen ST, Chung LP, et al (1999) *hMLH1* promoter methylation and lack of *hMLH1* expression in sporadic gastric carcinomas with high-frequency microsatellite instability. Cancer Res 59:159–164
44. Fleisher AS, Esteller M, Wang S, et al (1999) Hypermethylation of the *hMLH1* gene promoter in human gastric cancers with microsatellite instability. Cancer Res 59:1090–1095
45. Guilford P, Hopkins J, Harraway J, et al (1998) E-cadherin germline mutations in familial gastric cancer. Nature (Lond) 392:402–405

46. Becker KF, Atkinson MJ, Reich U, et al (1994) E-cadherin gene mutations provide clues to diffuse type gastric carcinomas. Cancer Res 54:3845–3852
47. Muta H, Noguchi M, Kanai Y, et al (1996) E-cadherin gene mutations in signet ring cell carcinoma of the stomach. Jpn J Cancer Res 87:843–848
48. Machado JC, Oliveira C, Carvalho R, et al (2001) E-cadherin gene (*CDH1*) promoter methylation as the second hit in sporadic diffuse gastric carcinoma. Oncogene 20:1525–1528
49. Li QL, Ito K, Sakakura C, et al (2002) Causal relationship between the loss of *RUNX3* expression and gastric cancer. Cell 109:113–124
50. Kang SH, Bang YJ, Im YH, et al (1999) Transcriptional repression of the transforming growth factor-beta type I receptor gene by DNA methylation results in the development of TGF-beta resistance in human gastric cancer. Oncogene 18:7280–7286
51. Shin JY, Kim HS, Park J, et al (2000) Mechanism for inactivation of the KIP family cyclin-dependent kinase inhibitor genes in gastric cancer cells. Cancer Res 60:262–265
52. Oue N, Shigeishi H, Kuniyasu H, et al (2001) Promoter hypermethylation of MGMT is associated with protein loss in gastric carcinoma. Int J Cancer 93:805–809
53. Park TJ, Han SU, Cho YK, et al (2001) Methylation of O(6)-methylguanine-DNA methyltransferase gene is associated significantly with K-*ras* mutation, lymph node invasion, tumor staging, and disease free survival in patients with gastric carcinoma. Cancer (Phila) 92:2760–2768
54. Byun DS, Lee MG, Chae KS, et al (2001) Frequent epigenetic inactivation of RASSF1A by aberrant promoter hypermethylation in human gastric adenocarcinoma. Cancer Res 61:7034–7038
55. Kang GH, Lee HJ, Hwang KS, et al (2003) Aberrant CpG island hypermethylation of chronic gastritis, in relation to aging, gender, intestinal metaplasia, and chronic inflammation. Am J Pathol 163:1551–1556
56. Suzuki H, Itoh F, Toyota M, et al (2000) Inactivation of the 14-3-3 sigma gene is associated with 5′ CpG island hypermethylation in human cancers. Cancer Res 60:4353–4357
57. Hibi K, Nakayama H, Kanyama Y, et al (2003) Methylation pattern of HLTF gene in digestive tract cancers. Int J Cancer 104:433–436
58. Hamai Y, Oue N, Mitani Y, et al (2003) DNA hypermethylation and histone hypoacetylation of the HLTF gene are associated with reduced expression in gastric carcinoma. Cancer Sci 94:692–698
59. Satoh A, Toyota M, Itoh F, et al (2003) Epigenetic inactivation of CHFR and sensitivity to microtubule inhibitors in gastric cancer. Cancer Res 63:8606–8613
60. Hayashizaki Y, Hirotsune S, Okazaki Y, et al (1993) Restriction landmark genomic scanning method and its various applications. Electrophoresis 14:251–258
61. Ushijima T, Morimura K, Hosoya Y, et al (1997) Establishment of methylation-sensitive-representational difference analysis and isolation of hypo- and hypermethylated genomic fragments in mouse liver tumors. Proc Natl Acad Sci USA 94:2284–2289
62. Gonzalgo ML, Liang G, Spruck CH III, et al (1997) Identification and characterization of differentially methylated regions of genomic DNA by methylation-sensitive arbitrarily primed PCR. Cancer Res 57:594–599
63. Huang TH, Laux DE, Hamlin BC, et al (1997) Identification of DNA methylation markers for human breast carcinomas using the methylation-sensitive restriction fingerprinting technique. Cancer Res 57:1030–1034
64. Toyota M, Ho C, Ahuja N, et al (1999) Identification of differentially methylated sequences in colorectal cancer by methylated CpG island amplification. Cancer Res 59:2307–2312
65. Huang TH, Perry MR, Laux DE (1999) Methylation profiling of CpG islands in human breast cancer cells. Hum Mol Genet 8:459–470
66. Shiraishi M, Chuu YH, Sekiya T (1999) Isolation of DNA fragments associated with methylated CpG islands in human adenocarcinomas of the lung using a methylated DNA binding column and denaturing gradient gel electrophoresis. Proc Natl Acad Sci USA 96:2913–2918

67. Kaneda A, Kaminishi M, Nakanishi Y, et al (2002) Reduced expression of the *insulin-induced protein 1* and *p41 Arp2/3 complex* genes in human gastric cancers. Int J Cancer 100:57–62
68. Kaneda A, Takai D, Kaminishi M, et al (2003) Methylation-sensitive representational difference analysis and its application to cancer research. Ann N Y Acad Sci 983:131–141
69. Contente S, Kenyon K, Rimoldi D, et al (1990) Expression of gene *rrg* is associated with reversion of NIH 3T3 transformed by LTR-c-H-*ras*. Science 249:796–798
70. Kenyon K, Contente S, Trackman PC, et al (1991) Lysyl oxidase and *rrg* messenger RNA. Science 253:802
71. Akiyama H, Hiraki Y, Noda M, et al (1999) Molecular cloning and biological activity of a novel Ha-Ras suppressor gene predominantly expressed in skeletal muscle, heart, brain, and bone marrow by differential display using clonal mouse EC cells, ATDC5. J Biol Chem 274:32192–32197
72. Kaneda A, Wakazono K, Tsukamoto T, et al (2004) *Lysyl Oxidase* is a tumor-suppressor gene inactivated by methylation and loss of heterozygosity in human gastric cancers. Cancer Res 64:6410–6415
73. Zhang Y, Weiler-Guettler H, Chen J, et al (1998) Thrombomodulin modulates growth of tumor cells independent of its anticoagulant activity. J Clin Invest 101:1301–1309
74. Ito Y, Oike Y, Yasunaga K, et al (2003) Inhibition of angiogenesis and vascular leakiness by angiopoietin-related protein 4. Cancer Res 63:6651–6657
75. Toyota M, Ahuja N, Ohe-Toyota M, et al (1999) CpG island methylator phenotype in colorectal cancer. Proc Natl Acad Sci U S A 96:8681–8686
76. Imai S, Koizumi S, Sugiura M, et al (1994) Gastric carcinoma: monoclonal epithelial malignant cells expressing Epstein-Barr virus latent infection protein. Proc Natl Acad Sci U S A 91:9131–9135
77. Kang GH, Lee S, Kim WH, et al (2002) Epstein-Barr virus-positive gastric carcinoma demonstrates frequent aberrant methylation of multiple genes and constitutes CpG island methylator phenotype-positive gastric carcinoma. Am J Pathol 160:787–794
78. Remus R, Kammer C, Heller H, et al (1999) Insertion of foreign DNA into an established mammalian genome can alter the methylation of cellular DNA sequences. J Virol 73: 1010–1022
79. Heller H, Kammer C, Wilgenbus P, et al (1995) Chromosomal insertion of foreign (adenovirus type 12, plasmid, or bacteriophage lambda) DNA is associated with enhanced methylation of cellular DNA segments. Proc Natl Acad Sci U S A 92:5515–5519
80. Chong JM, Sakuma K, Sudo M, et al (2003) Global and non-random CpG-island methylation in gastric carcinoma associated with Epstein-Barr virus. Cancer Sci 94:76–80
81. Lauren P (1965) The two histological main types of gastric carcinoma. Diffuse and so-called intestinal type carcinoma: an attempt at histological classification. Acta Pathol Microbiol Scand 64:31–49
82. Shimoyama Y, Hirohashi S (1991) Expression of E- and P-cadherin in gastric carcinomas. Cancer Res 51:2185–2192
83. Oue N, Motoshita J, Yokozaki H, et al (2002) Distinct promoter hypermethylation of p16INK4a, CDH1, and RAR-beta in intestinal, diffuse-adherent, and diffuse-scattered type gastric carcinomas. J Pathol 198:55–59
84. Oue N, Oshimo Y, Nakayama H, et al (2003) DNA methylation of multiple genes in gastric carcinoma: association with histological type and CpG island methylator phenotype. Cancer Sci 94:901–905
85. Gonzalgo ML, Hayashida T, Bender CM, et al (1998) The role of DNA methylation in expression of the p19/p16 locus in human bladder cancer cell lines. Cancer Res 58:1245–1252
86. Etoh T, Kanai Y, Ushijima S, et al (2004) Increased DNA methyltransferase 1 (DNMT1) protein expression correlates significantly with poorer tumor differentiation and frequent DNA hypermethylation of multiple CpG islands in gastric cancers. Am J Pathol 164:689–699

87. Rhee I, Bachman KE, Park BH, et al (2002) DNMT1 and DNMT3b cooperate to silence genes in human cancer cells. Nature (Lond) 416:552–556
88. Kawakami K, Brabender J, Lord RV, et al (2000) Hypermethylated APC DNA in plasma and prognosis of patients with esophageal adenocarcinoma. J Natl Cancer Inst 92:1805–1811
89. Kim DH, Kim JS, Ji YI, et al (2003) Hypermethylation of RASSF1A promoter is associated with the age at starting smoking and a poor prognosis in primary non-small cell lung cancer. Cancer Res 63:3743–3746
90. Muller HM, Widschwendter A, Fiegl H, et al (2003) DNA methylation in serum of breast cancer patients: an independent prognostic marker. Cancer Res 63:7641–7645
91. Maruyama R, Toyooka S, Toyooka KO, et al (2001) Aberrant promoter methylation profile of bladder cancer and its relationship to clinicopathological features. Cancer Res 61:8659–8663
92. Bae SI, Lee HS, Kim SH, et al (2002) Inactivation of O6-methylguanine-DNA methyltransferase by promoter CpG island hypermethylation in gastric cancers. Br J Cancer 86:1888–1892
93. Yamamoto H, Perez-Piteira J, Yoshida T, et al (1999) Gastric cancers of the microsatellite mutator phenotype display characteristic genetic and clinical features. Gastroenterology 116:1348–1357
94. Simpson AJ, Caballero OL, Pena SD (2001) Microsatellite instability as a tool for the classification of gastric cancer. Trends Mol Med 7:76–80
95. Leon SA, Shapiro B, Sklaroff DM, et al (1977) Free DNA in the serum of cancer patients and the effect of therapy. Cancer Res 37:646–650
96. Stroun M, Anker P, Maurice P, et al (1989) Neoplastic characteristics of the DNA found in the plasma of cancer patients. Oncology 46:318–322
97. Kanyama Y, Hibi K, Nakayama H, et al (2003) Detection of p16 promoter hypermethylation in serum of gastric cancer patients. Cancer Sci 94:418–420
98. Ehrlich M, Gama-Sosa MA, Huang LH, et al (1982) Amount and distribution of 5-methylcytosine in human DNA from different types of tissues of cells. Nucleic Acids Res 10:2709–2721
99. Bird A (1999) DNA methylation de novo. Science 286:2287–2288
100. Robertson KD, Wolffe AP (2000) DNA methylation in health and disease. Nat Rev Genet 1:11–19
101. Kaneda A, Tsukamoto T, Takamura-Enya T, et al (2004) Frequent hypomethylation in multiple promoter CpG islands is associated with global hypomethylation, but not with frequent promoter hypermethylation. Cancer Sci 95:58–64
102. Chapman V, Forrester L, Sanford J, et al (1984) Cell lineage-specific undermethylation of mouse repetitive DNA. Nature (Lond) 307:284–286
103. Goelz SE, Vogelstein B, Hamilton SR, et al (1985) Hypomethylation of DNA from benign and malignant human colon neoplasms. Science 228:187–190
104. Narayan A, Ji W, Zhang XY, et al (1998) Hypomethylation of pericentromeric DNA in breast adenocarcinomas. Int J Cancer 77:833–838
105. Qu G, Dubeau L, Narayan A, et al (1999) Satellite DNA hypomethylation vs. overall genomic hypomethylation in ovarian epithelial tumors of different malignant potential. Mutat Res 423:91–101
106. Qu GZ, Grundy PE, Narayan A, et al (1999) Frequent hypomethylation in Wilms tumors of pericentromeric DNA in chromosomes 1 and 16. Cancer Genet Cytogenet 109:34–39
107. Alves G, Tatro A, Fanning T (1996) Differential methylation of human LINE-1 retrotransposons in malignant cells. Gene (Amst) 176:39–44
108. Yoder JA, Walsh CP, Bestor TH (1997) Cytosine methylation and the ecology of intragenomic parasites. Trends Genet 13:335–340
109. Rainier S, Johnson LA, Dobry CJ, et al (1993) Relaxation of imprinted genes in human cancer. Nature (Lond) 362:747–749
110. Falls JG, Pulford DJ, Wylie AA, et al (1999) Genomic imprinting: implications for human disease. Am J Pathol 154:635–647

Color Plates

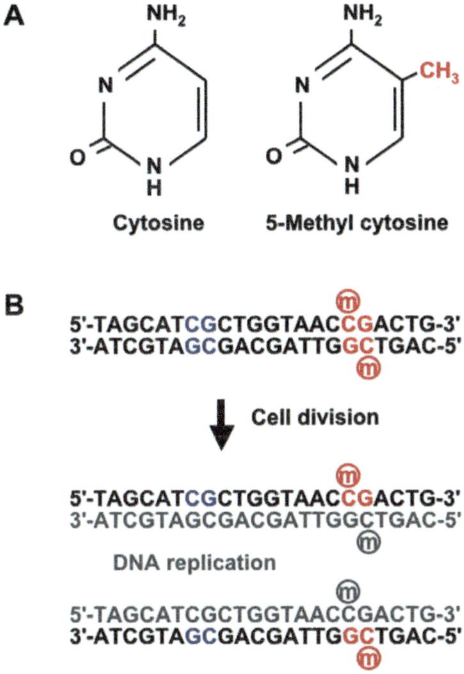

FIG. 1. **A** Cytosine methylation. DNA methylation is a covalent modification by a methyl group at C5 position of cytosine (*red*) at CpG dinucleotides. **B** Methylation at DNA replication. Hemi-methylated CpG sites are methylated by DNA methyltransferases into fully methylated CpG sites to inherit their methylated (*red*) and unmethylated (*blue*) status

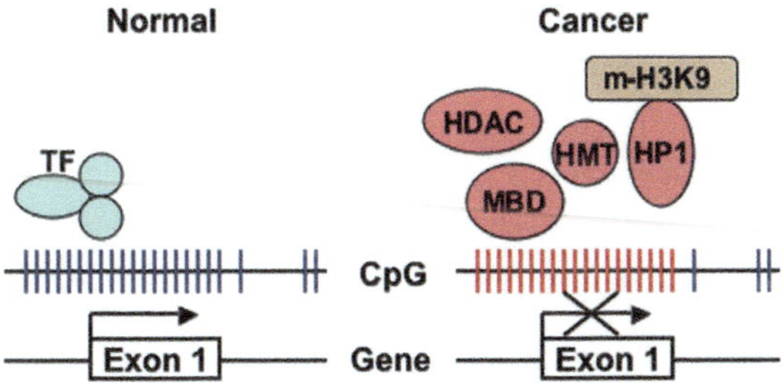

FIG. 2. Genes transcribed in normal cells, but silenced in cancer cells by aberrant methylation. *CpG*, distribution of CpG sites (*blue*, unmethylated; *red*, methylated); *TF*, transcription factor. Methyl-CpG binding domain containing protein (*MBD*) can be loaded onto methylated DNA through their interactions with histone deacetylase (*HDAC*) and histone methyltransferase (*HMT*). HMT can be recruited by the binding of the chromodomain protein HP1α (*HP1*) to methylated lysine 9 in histone H3 (*m-H3K9*) and maintains H3K9 methylations. HDAC deacetylates histone lysine residues, and the deacetylated histones are organized into tightly compacted nucleosomes, where transcriptionally silent DNA regions are packaged

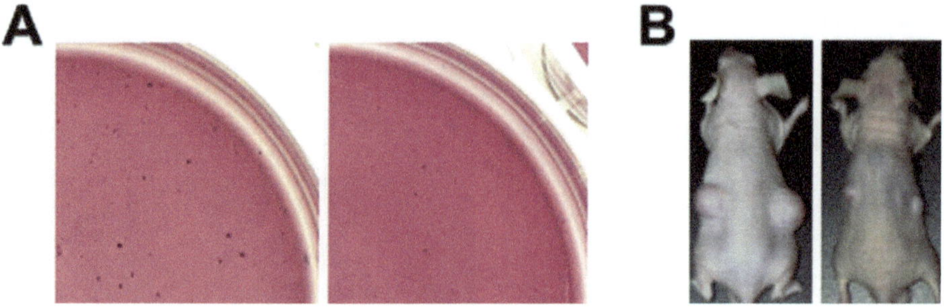

FIG. 3. Examination of tumor-suppressive function. After identification of genes silenced in cancer cells, their cDNA can be introduced in those cancer cells to confirm their tumor-suppressive functions by reduction of colony formation in soft agar (**A**) or reduction of subcutaneous tumor formation in nude mice (**B**) (Partly reproduced from [72] with permission from American Association for Cancer Research)

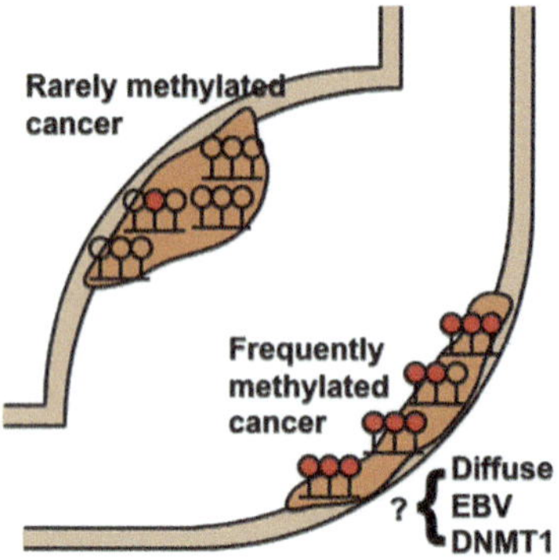

FIG. 4. Frequently methylated gastric cancers. When methylation statuses of multiple promoter CpG islands of genes are analyzed, a subset of gastric cancers with high frequency of aberrant promoter methylation is identified. This subset is reported to correlate with diffuse-type histology, EBV infection, and increased level of DNA methyltransferase 1

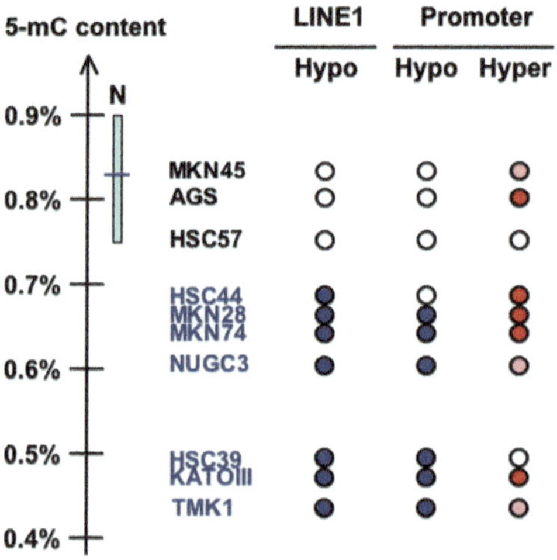

FIG. 5. Hypomethylation and hypermethylation in gastric cancer cell lines. *5-mC*, 5-methyl cytosine; *N*, 5-mC content in normal gastric epithelium shown by mean (*bar*) and SD (*box*). Lower level of 5-methyl cytosine, i.e., global hypomethylation, is detected in 7 of 10 gastric cancer cell lines (*blue*). Hypomethylation of LINE1 repetitive sequence is detected in 7 cell lines (*blue*). Hypomethylation of normally methylated promoters is detected frequently in 6 cell lines (*blue*), but not or rarely in 4 cell lines (*white*). These three aberrant hypomethylations correlate with each other, but do not correlate with aberrant promoter hypermethylations (*red*, frequent hyper-

pink

Distinction of High-Grade Intraepithelial Neoplasia and Tubular Gastric Adenocarcinoma

Michael Vieth[1] and Manfred Stolte[2]

Introduction

When searching the literature for the definition of intraepithelial neoplasia (formerly dysplasia), we found it has been described as structural change of surface epithelium [1] and atypical mucosa limited to the epithelium [2]. The first international classification by Morson et al. [3] did not add anything significant to these criteria, leaving room for subjective interpretation.

WHO Definition of High-Grade Intraepithelial Neoplasia

In 2000, the World Health Organization (WHO) recommended to no longer use the term "dysplasia" but rather "intraepithelial neoplasia" throughout the gastrointestinal tract. This change has been suggested because the term dysplasia has been overstressed in the past (Table 1) because of the weak descriptive nature of its definitions. Also, the term dysplasia was used in part for early carcinomas [4].

The WHO classification [5] describes high-grade intraepithelial neoplasia in the stomach as a lesion with "glandular crowding and prominent cellular atypia. Tubules can be irregular in shape, with frequent branching and folding: there is no stromal invasion." Mucin secretion is believed to be absent or minimized. Additionally, increased proliferative activity is present throughout the epithelium. According to the WHO classification, invasive adenocarcinoma is diagnosed whenever the tumor invades into the lamina propria or the submucosal layer. Also mentioned is that in bioptic diagnosis isolated tumor cells and glandlike and/or papillary projections are believed to help differentiate it from intraepithelial neoplasia.

[1] Institute of Pathology, University of Magdeburg, Leipziger Str. 44, 39120 Magdeburg, Germany
[2] Institute of Pathology, Klinikum Bayreuth, Preuschwitzer Str. 101, 95445 Bayreuth, Germany
e-mail: vieth.lkpathol@uni-bayreuth.de

TABLE 1. Use of the term "dysplasia" taken from a selection of histological diagnoses

Dysplasia I–III
Metaplastic dysplasia
"Proper gastric type" of dysplasia
Hyperplastic dysplasia
Intestinal dysplasia
Adenomatous dysplasia
Microglandular dysplasia
Anaplastic dysplasia
Regenerative dysplasia
Diffuse dysplasia
Globoid dysplasia
Strange dysplasia

Source: O. Stadelmann, personal communication

Are These Criteria Sufficient to Explain How to Make the Differential Diagnosis Between High-Grade Intraepithelial Neoplasia and Invasive Mucosal Carcinoma?

The WHO definition of high-grade intraepithelial neoplasia is mainly based on the descriptive terms "branching and folding" of the glands. These two descriptive terms especially leave a lot of room for subjective interpretation. On the other hand, infiltration of the submucosal layer by single neoplastic tubules is not described as "branching of glands" but as a clear carcinoma even without the presence of single tumor cells (Fig. 1).

Worldwide differences in the diagnostic criteria of mucosal carcinomas mostly apply to bioptic diagnoses but not to (endoscopic) resection specimens and are probably just a sign of uncertainty [6,7] rather than an expression of Japanese or Western points of view. Furthermore, some pathologists prefer the term high-grade intraepithelial neoplasia rather than adenocarcinoma for forensic reasons. Another reason seen by some pathologists is to avoid the patient's health insurance changing the contract as a result of carcinoma diagnosis. It should be noted that in addition to morphological criteria there are also forensic and social criteria that are applied by some pathologists. This practice is unacceptable because it prevents relating clinical outcomes worldwide [8].

When analyzing the literature for follow-up studies on high-grade intraepithelial neoplasia up to the development of invasive gastric adenocarcinoma (Table 2), it becomes apparent that all these studies showed that within a few months invasive carcinoma was present. Due to the very short time lag, this finding could be interpreted that these lesions were already carcinomas.

It is known that lesions designated as high-grade intraepithelial neoplasia do not differ much from invasive carcinoma concerning molecular and genetic changes. In our daily routine, the diagnosis of high-grade intraepithelial neoplasia is very rare. Most of these lesions are already invasive carcinomas.

TABLE 2. Results from follow-up studies of high-grade intraepithelial neoplasia up to invasive gastric adenocarcinoma

Author	Year	*n*	HGIEN → Ca in %	Months
Saraga et al. [15]	1987	21	81	4
Lansdown et al. [16]	1990	13	85	5
Rugge et al. [17]	1991	8	75	4
Fertitta et al. [18]	1993	31	81	5
Di Gregorio et al. [19]	1993	10	60	11
Rugge et al. [20]	1994	18	78	9
Kokkola et al. [21]	1996	3	67	18
Mean:			78%	8

HGIEN, high-grade intraepithelial neoplasia (formerly high-grade dysplasia); Ca, carcinoma

Differential Diagnosis

The differential diagnosis of intraepithelial neoplasia and early invasive carcinomas includes pseudoinvasions (cohesive type as in gastritis cystica profunda; diffuse type as in NHL-MALT-lymphoma with scattered remaining epithelial structures imitating invasive epithelial growth). Other differential diagnoses include neuroendocrine tumors and reactive changes as in chemical reactive gastritis (Fig. 2); especially, NSAID/ASA-induced lesions should be excluded. The endoscopic findings should be consistent with the neoplasia diagnosis and should be carefully reviewed. Sometimes criteria are difficult to interpret; therefore, a so-called matrix diagnostics with biopsies far from the questionable lesion from antrum and corpus (two each) should be taken to avoid overdiagnosis of a reactive lesion toward a neoplasia in case the patient is *Helicobacter pylori* negative, which would point more toward a reactive lesion.

How Can High-Grade Intraepithelial Neoplasia Be Reliably Distinguished from Invasive Adenocarcinoma?

Clinically, the distinction of gastric high-grade intraepithelial neoplasia and mucosal carcinoma does not play a role because both lesions after careful staging do require endoscopic resection [6], and most lesions should be already regarded as mucosal carcinomas rather than high-grade intraepithelial neoplasia.

An exact description of the term invasion is lacking in the European and American literature. In the WHO classification [5], invasion is defined through the presence of expansion of atypical cells through the basal membrane or even expansion through anatomical structures (e.g., muscularis mucosae in colorectal tumors). In Japan, pathologists use structural change of nuclei, hyperchromasia, anisonucleosis, etc., for the diagnosis of "malignancy" [6]. Precise descriptions of expansive growth of gastric neoplastic lesions are most available exclusively from Japanese authors [9–11] (Fig. 3).

In the European literature up until now, only one German author [12] ever tried to find an exact description of invasion that is in line with the criteria and findings from

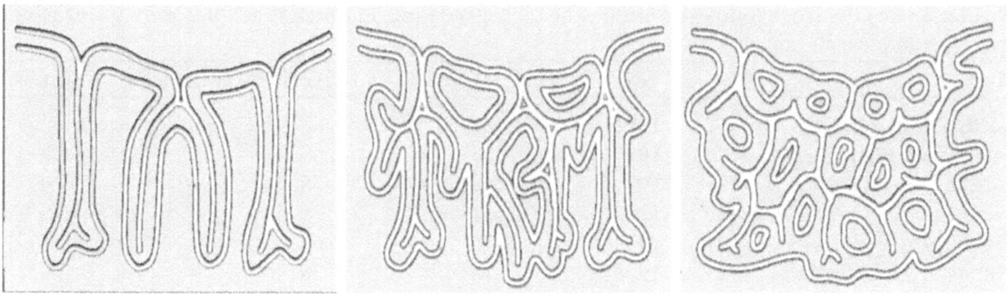

Fig. 3. Three-dimensional microstructure of normal gastric mucosa, adenoma, and well-differentiated (G1) gastric adenocarcinoma. (Modified after Refs. [10,11])

Table 3. Criteria of expansion in adenomas and early gastric carcinomas besides cytological criteria of malignancy

	Adenoma		Carcinoma	
Type of expansion	Tubular	Villous	Tubular	Diffuse
Septae	(+)	–	–	–
Intratubular expansion	+	++	–	–
Superficial lateral expansion	+	+	–	–
Luminal expansion	+	++	(+)	–
Intertubular vertical expansion	+	+	(+)	–
Intertubular lateral expansion	–	–	++	++
Undermining growth pattern	–	–	+	+
Compression and destruction	–	–	+	+
Loss of basal membrane	–	–	(–)+	++

Source: Modified from Refs. 12, 22

Japan (Tables 3, 4). According to Borchard, in carcinomas the expansion pattern is unique. The malignant epithelium shows a so-called primarily lateral intertubular expansion deriving from the proliferation zone within the mucosa (Figs. 4, 5). Expansion of atypical cells through the basal membrane, spreading of single tumor cells, and stromal fibrous reaction are criteria for more advanced lesions. The presence or absence of basal membranes correlates with the grading of the tumor. Well-differentiated adenocarcinomas are capable of generating basal membrane components by the tumor itself. Only poorly differentiated or diffuse carcinomas show a loss of basal membrane synthesis, mostly due to mutations of E-cadherin. Frequently this mutation can be detected in diffuse gastric carcinomas with loss of adhesion among the tumor cells. This complicates the diagnosis: is there a disruption of the basal membrane or a loss of the basal membrane? then the lesion shows definitively invasion but, as already pointed out, this criterion is not always present in well-differentiated adenocarcinomas.

TABLE 4. Cytological and structural criteria of high-grade intraepithelial neoplasia and invasive adenocarinoma

Criterion	High-grade intraepithelial neoplasia	Invasive carcinoma
Architecture	Irregular	Branching, anastomoses Rare: single tumor cells
Proliferation zone	Whole gland	Whole gland
Epithelial expansion	Surface epithelium	Also underneath surface epithelium
Epithelial differentiation	None	None
Foveolar epithelium	None	None
Nuclear layer in rows	2–5	Changing within one gland
Size of nucleus	Enlarged	Vesicular
Nucleoli	Some	Prominent, possible: >1

Source: Modified from Refs. [12, 22]

Fibrous stromal reactions around neoplastic tubules is an important criterion, but these are often detected in lesions that have already infiltrated the submucosal layer. This stromal fibrous reaction is most prominent in the submucosal and subserosal layer. Therefore, mucosal carcinomas almost never show such a fibrous reaction. Within the muscularis propria, the reaction is less dominant [13]. Fibroblasts of fibrous peritumoral reaction are less differentiated than peritubular fibroblasts [14]. Mucosal lesions of diffuse gastric carcinomas very rarely show a fibrous stromal reaction. The leading finding in well-differentiated mucosal carcinomas is, according to Borchard [12], the presence of a nonsuperficial lateral intertubular expansion that shows an abnormal branching of foveolae with tubular fissions; this results in a compression of the adjacent tissue (glands, capillaries), consecutive atrophy of neighboring glands, and stopping of regular cell movements during differentiation and proliferation. If stem cells of the gastric mucosa that are located very close to the surface (in the colorectum close to the base of the mucosa) are destroyed by the tumor, no further regeneration can be detected. Because of the lack of regeneration, subepithelial growth of cancerous tubules, and compression of capillaries, superficial destruction can occur in mucosal carcinomas. In adenomas with a regular vertical growth pattern, no erosion or superficial destruction can be observed.

Clinical Relevance

From a clinical point of view, the distinction of high-grade intraepithelial neoplasia and mucosal gastric carcinoma is without consequence because the diagnosis of high-grade intraepithelial neoplasia should always first lead to a (diagnostic) endoscopic resection. The final diagnosis could then be made on the basis of the resection specimen: high-grade intraepithelial neoplasia or mucosal adenocarcinoma. In routine practice, it should be noted that the diagnosis of high-grade intraepithelial neoplasia is very rare because most cases have already progressed to mucosal adenocarcinoma.

References

1. Oehlert W, Keller P, Henke M, Strauch M (1979) Gastric mucosal dysplasia: what is its clinical significance? Front Gastrointest Res 4:173–182
2. Grundmann E, Schlake W (1982) Histological classification of gastric cancer from initial to advanced stages. Pathol Res Pract 173:260–274
3. Morson BC, Sobin LH, Grundmann E, et al (1980) Precancerous conditions and epithelial dysplasia in the stomach. J Clin Pathol 33:711–721
4. Lewin KJ, Appelman HD (1995) Tumors of the esophagus and stomach. In: Atlas of Tumor Pathology, Third Series, Fascicle 18. Armed Forces Institute of Pathology, Washington, DC
5. Hamilton SR, Aaltonen LA (eds) (2000) WHO classification. Tumors of the digestive system. IARC Press, Lyon
6. Schlemper RJ, Riddell RH, Kato Y, et al (2000) The Vienna classification of gastrointestinal epithelial neoplasia. Gut 47:251–255
7. Stolte M (1999) Diagnosis of gastric carcinoma: Japanese fairy tales or Western deficiency? Virchows Arch 434:279–280
8. Stolte M (2003) The new Vienna classification of epithelial neoplasia of the gastrointestinal tract: advantages and disadvantages. Virchows Arch 442:99–106
9. Hattori T (1985) Histological and autoradiographic study on development of group III lesion (dysplasia grade III) in the stomach. Pathol Res Pract 180:36–44
10. Takahashi T, Iwama N (1984) Architectural pattern of gastric adenocarcinoma—a 3-dimensional study. Virchows Arch (Pathol Anat) 403:127–134
11. Takahashi T, Iwama N (1985) Three-dimensional microstructure of gastrointestinal tumors. Gland pattern and its diagnostic significance. Pathol Annu 20:419–440
12. Borchard F (2000) Forms and nomenclature of gastrointestinal epithelial expansion: what is invasion? Verh Dtsch Ges Pathol 84:50–61
13. Othani H, Sasano N (1983) Stromal cell changes in human colorectal adenomas and carcinomas. Virchows Arch Pathol Anat 401:209–299
14. Yao T, Tsuneyoshi M (1993) Significance of pericryptal fibroblasts in colorectal epithelial tumors: a special reference to the histologic features and growth patterns. Hum Pathol 24: 525–533
15. Saraga EP, Gardiol D, Costa J (1987) Gastric dysplasia. A histological follow-up study. Am J Surg Pathol 11:788–796
16. Lansdown M, Quirke P, Dixon MF, et al (1990) High-grade dysplasia of the gastric mucosa: a marker for gastric carcinoma. Gut 31:977–983
17. Rugge M, Farinati F, Di Mario F, et al (1991) Gastric epithelial dysplasia: a prospective multicenter follow-up study from the Interdisciplinary Group on Gastric Epithelial Dysplasia. Hum Pathol 22:1002–1008
18. Fertitta AM, Comin U, Terruzzi V, et al (1993) Clinical significance of gastric dysplasia: a multicenter follow-up study. Gastrointestinal Endoscopic Pathology Study Group. Endoscopy 25:265–268
19. Di Gregorio C, Morandi P, Fante R, et al (1993) Gastric dysplasia. A follow-up study. Am J Gastroenterol 88:1714–1719
20. Rugge M, Farinati F, Baffa R, et al (1994) Gastric epithelial dysplasia in the natural history of gastric cancer: a multicenter prospective follow-up study. Interdisciplinary Group on Gastric Epithelial Dysplasia. Gastroenterology 107:1288–1296
21. Kokkola A, Haapiainen R, Laxen F, et al (1996) Risk of gastric carcinoma in patients with mucosal dysplasia associated with atrophic gastritis: a follow up study. J Clin Pathol 49:979–984
22. Borchard F, Heilmann KL, Hermanek P, et al (1991) Definition und klinische Bedeutung der Dysplasie im Verdauungstrakt. Pathologe 12:50–56

Color Plates

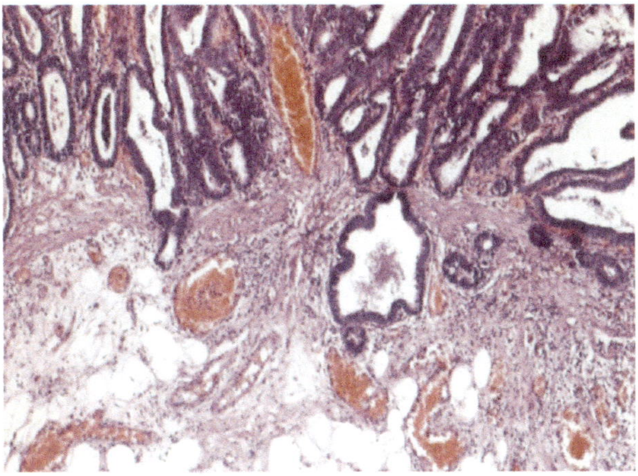

Fig. 1. Initial infiltration of the submucosal layer by a well-differentiated gastric adenocarci noma without presence of single tumor cells or branching or folding

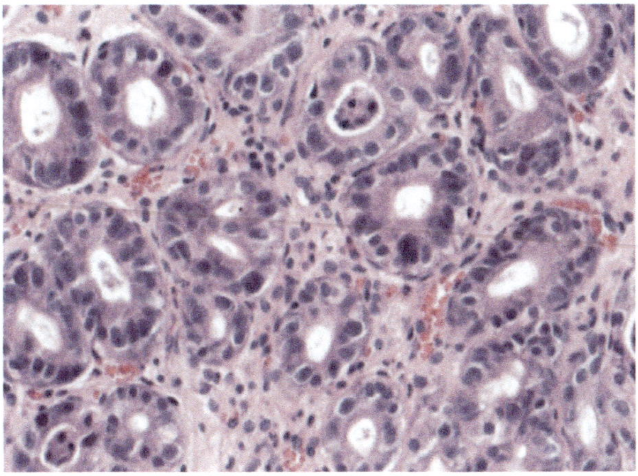

Fig. 2. Regenerative epithelium in chemical reactive gastritis of antrum mucosa with pleomorphic nuclei and even mitoses are seen; slight change of the architecture of the glands. Note basal orientation of nuclei. Hematoxylin and eosin. ×100

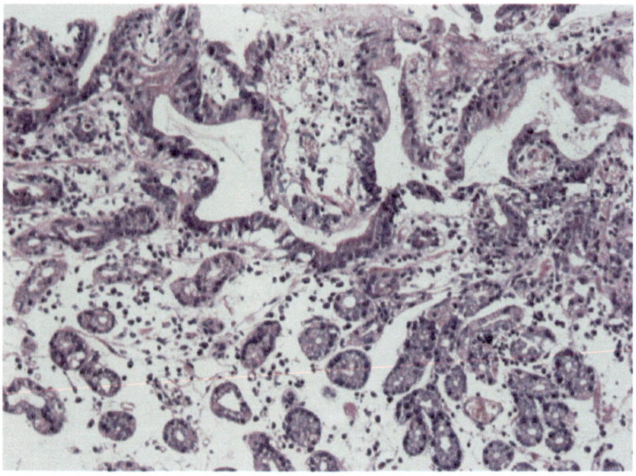

Fig. 4. Pattern of expansion in early mucosal carcinoma showing lateral intertubular expansion with initial discontinuing growth pattern with compression of neighboring glands and capillaries. Later destructions of the surface epithelium in the presence of erosions can be observed

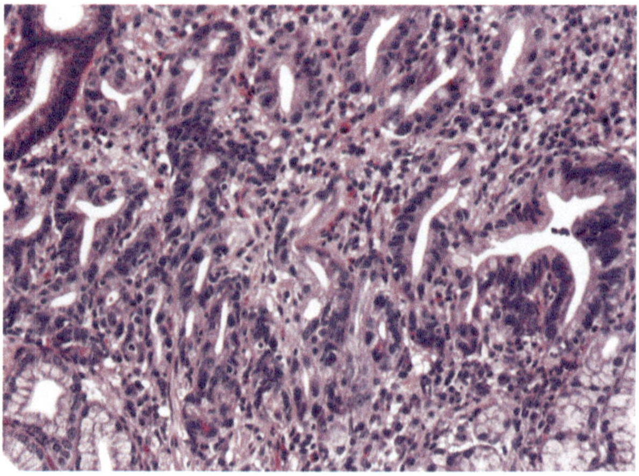

Fig. 5. Early well-differentiated gastric adenocarcinoma showing malignant single cells that expand downward through adjacent stromal tissue

Histological Diversity of Early Gastric Carcinoma

Yasuo Ohkura

Introduction

The histological types of gastric carcinoma (GC) vary in comparison with cancers in other parts of the gastrointestinal tract. The classification of the World Health Organization divides gastric adenocarcinomas into four main histological types: tubular, papillary, mucinous, and signet-ring cell carcinoma [1]. Also, GC often show mixed histological types in advanced stage. Lauren noted that tubular adenocarcinomas were accompanied by papillary fold formation or solid components, and glandular lumina were rarely seen in diffuse-type carcinoma [2]. Also, colloid carcinoma (mucinous adenocarcinoma) arose from carcinomas of intestinal as well as of diffuse type. When signet-ring cell carcinoma infiltrates the submucosa and deeper tissue, it is sometimes accompanied by poorly differentiated adenocarcinoma. Pathological diagnosis of GC is based on the predominant histological pattern according to the classification of the World Health Organization [1]. However, the predominant histological pattern may not show the true nature of mixed histological figures of GC.

Lauren divided GC into two groups from the general and cellular structure and in the mode of secretion [2], which was used world wide in much clinical and pathological research. However, 14% of tumors belong to carcinoma of intestinal and diffuse type. Ming mentioned a significant number of cancers could not be classified into these two types [3]. Tatematsu et al. suggest that Lauren confused intestinal phenotypic cancer cells with a diffuse structure and gastric phenotypic cells with the intestinal type [4]. We need to analyze a variety of histological types of gastric cancer.

Little is known about the histological diversity of GC. Thus, small early GCs, less than 2 cm in largest diameter, were collected and examined in this study. Because most large, advanced GCs are composed of several histological components, they are not suitable for this study. The results will help us to understand the nature of GC.

Department of Pathology, Kyorin University School of Medicine, 6-20-2 Shinkawa, Mitaka, Tokyo 181-8611, Japan
e-mail: ohkura@kyorin-u.ac.jp

Materials and Methods

Two hundred fifty cases of early GC with lesions less than 2 cm in largest diameter were examined. All materials were collected at Tokyo Metropolitan Cancer Detection Center, Tokyo, Japan, between 1990 and 1999. One hundred ninety cases were obtained by operation and 60 cases were endoscopic mucosal resection. Most of microcarcinomas less than 5 mm in largest diameter were multiple GC detectable only by pathological examination. Histological classification was made according to the Japanese Classification of Gastric Carcinoma [5]. Two hundred two cases were intramucosal and 48 cases demonstrated submucosal invasion.

All specimens were fixed in 15% (v/v) formalin. All specimens were cut into sections 5 mm wide and 3–4 cm long, parallel to the lesser curvature, and embedded in paraffin. The embedded sections were sliced into 2-μm-thick sections and examined after staining with hematoxylin and eosin (H&E); those with the greatest tumor diameters were sliced into 4-μm-thick sections for immunohistochemical investigation.

Immunohistochemical staining with mouse monoclonal antibodies against human gastric mucin (HGM) (45M1, 1:100; Novocastra, Newcastle upon Tyne, UK) [6], against MUC5AC (CLH2, 1:100; Novocastra) [7], against M-GGMC-1 (HIK1083, 1:50; Kanto Kagaku, Tokyo, Japan) [8], against MUC6 (CLH5, 1:100; Novocastra) [9], and against MUC2 (Ccp58, 1:100; Novocastra) [10] was performed for examining mucin expression in cancer cells. HGM and MUC5AC are expressed in the foveolar epithelial cells of the stomach, and M-GGMC-1 and MUC6 are expressed in the parietal cells of the fundic gland and pyloric gland cells. MUC2 is expressed in the goblet cells of intestinal gland. The results of each antibody staining were evaluated in terms of percentage of positively stained cancer cells, with more than 10% considered positive, as previously described [11,12]. The phenotypes of cancer cells were classified into four types according to the definition of Kawachi et al.: the gastric phenotype (G type), the intestinal phenotype (I type), the mixed gastric and intestinal phenotype (M type), and the null type (N type) [11].

Histological Features of Minute Gastric Carcinoma

Of 54 minute GC equal to or less than 5 mm in size, well-differentiated tubular adenocarcinoma (tub1) was 33 (60%), signet-ring cell carcinoma (sig) was 19 (35%), tub1 with moderately differentiated tubular adenocarcinoma (tub2) was 1 (2%), and sig with tub2 was 1 (2%) (Table 1). Minute GC less than 4 mm in size showed a monotonous histological figure. A mixed histological type was found that was more than 5 mm in size.

The histological figure of tub2 admixed with tub1 was irregularly shaped glands according to tumor dedifferentiation (Fig. 1a), and the component of tub2 with sig was microtubular adenocarcinoma with thin cytoplasm (Fig. 1b). Those lesions showed different morphological features. In spite of the mixed components of tub2, minute GCs were classified into two groups, tub1 and sig. The result was same as that of Nakamura et al. and Sugano et al. [12,13]; they classified GC as differentiated carcinoma (DCA) and undifferentiated carcinoma (UCA).

TABLE 1. Histological figure of minute gastric carcinoma

	1 mm	2 mm	3 mm	4 mm	5 mm	Total
sig	3	0	4	7	5	19
sig > tub2	0	0	0	0	1	1
tub1	2	9	15	5	2	33
tub1 > tub2	0	0	0	0	1	1
Total	5	9	19	12	9	54

Sig, signet-ring cell carcinoma; tub1, well-differentiated tubular carcinoma; tub2, tub1 with moderately differentiated tubular adenocarcinoma

a 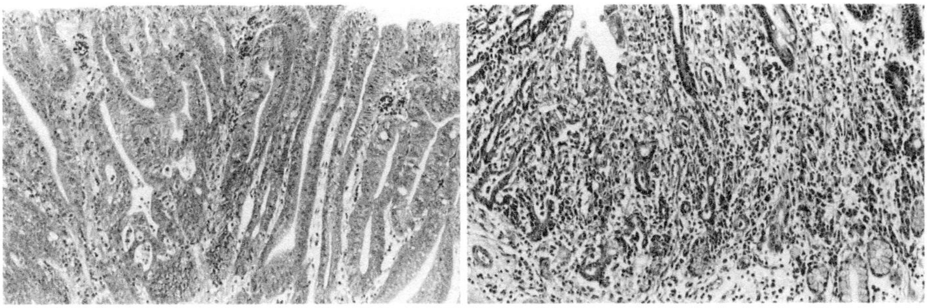 b

FIG. 1a,b. The components of well-differentiated tubular carcinoma (tub1) with moderately differentiated tubular adenocarcinoma (tub2) admixed with minute gastric carcinoma. **a** The components of tub2 admixed with tub1 showed irregularly shaped glands. Hematoxylin and eosin (H&E). ×400. **b** The components of tub2 admixed with signet-ring cell carcinoma (sig) showed microtubular glands. H&E. ×400

TABLE 2. The surrounding mucosa of minute gastric carcinoma

	P + IM	F + IM	F	C
sig	3	4	12	0
sig > tub2	1	0	0	0
tub1	29	3	0	1
tub1 > tub2	1	0	0	0

P + IM, pyloric gland mucosa with intestinal metaplasia; F + IM, fundic gland mucosa with intestinal metaplasia; F, fundic gland mucosa; C, cardiac gland mucosa

For the location of tub1, 29 (88%) were in the pyloric gland mucosa (P) with intestinal metaplasia (IM), 3 (9%) in the fundic gland mucosa (F) with IM, and 1 (3%) in the cardiac gland mucosa (C) without IM (Table 2); 1 case of tub1 with tub2 was in P with IM. All DCA were located almost in the gastric mucosa with IM. For the location of sig, 12 (63%) were in F without IM, 4 (21%) in F with IM, and 3 (16%) in P with IM; 1 case of sig with tub2 was located in P with IM. Most UCA was located in F without IM.

TABLE 3. Histological figure of small gastric carcinoma

	6mm	7mm	8mm	9mm	10mm	Total
sig	3	0	0	1	3	7
sig > tub2	0	0	0	1	1	2
tub1	6	10	4	7	9	36
tub2	0	0	0	1	0	1
pap	0	0	0	1	0	1
tub1 > tub2	1	2	4	2	0	9
tub2 > tub1	1	0	1	1	2	5
tub2 > por	0	0	1	1	1	3
tub2 > por > pap	0	0	1	0	0	1
Total	11	12	11	15	16	65

Pap, papillary adenocarcinoma; por, poorly differentiated adenocarcinoma

Immunohistochemically, all cases of sig showed G type, and 1 sig with tub2 showed G type. Of 33 cases of tub1, 14 (43%) were M type, 11 (33%) G type, 5 (15%) I type, and 3 (9%) N type; 1 tub1 with tub2 was M type. There was no relationship between phenotypes and IM of surrounding GC.

Histological Features of Small Gastric Carcinoma

Of 65 small early GC (6–10mm in size), 45 (69%) were simple in histological type (Table 3); these were 36 cases of tub1, 7 of sig, 1 of tub2, and 1 of papillary adenocarcinoma (pap). GC of mixed histological types comprised 20 cases (31%). Those mixed histological patterns were more various than minute GC. The mixed histological figures were classified into three types: (1) mixed tub1 and tub2, (2) tub2 admixed with poorly differentiated adenocarcinoma (por), and (3) sig admixed with tub2. The figure of tub2 was two different types, same as minute GC. The component of por showed a solid pattern or a scattered one, and both were derived from tubular adenocarcinoma. Thus, small GC was divided into DCA of 56 cases (86%) and UCA of 9 cases (14%).

All DCA were located in the gastric mucosa with IM; 48 DCA located in P with IM, 6 in F with IM, and 2 in C with IM. The location of UCA was various. Five cases of sig located in F without IM, two in F with IM, and two in P with IM. Two sig with tub2 were located in P with IM and F with IM (Table 4).

Concerning phenotypic expression of tub1, 22 cases (61%) were M type, 8 (22%) I type, 4 (11%) G type, and 2 (6%) N type. Both tub2 and pap showed M type. Nine (50%) mixed type of DCA were I type, seven (39%) M type, one (6%) G type, and one (6%) N type. All cases of sig expressed G type; two cases of sig with tub2 were I type and N type.

Histological Figures of Early Gastric Carcinoma

Early GCs from 11 to 20mm in size included 131 cases. As showed in Table 5, simple histological type was 57 cases (44%). Of 74 cases (56%) of mixed histological type, 66 showed two types and 8 showed three types. Those histological figures showed more

Table 4. The surrounding mucosa of small gastric carcinoma

	P + IM	F + IM	F	C + IM
sig	1	1	5	0
sig > tub2	1	1	0	0
tub1	31	3	0	2
tub2	1	0	0	0
pap	1	0	0	0
tub1 > tub2	9	0	0	0
tub2 > tub1	4	1	0	0
tub2 > por	1	2	0	0
tub2 > por > pap	1	0	0	0

P + IM, pyloric gland mucosa with intestinal metaplasia; F + IM, fundic gland mucosa with intestinal metaplasia; F, fundic gland mucosa; C + IM, cardiac gland mucosa with intestinal metaplasia

various patterns than small GC. However, early GC was classified in either DCA or UCA on the basis of histological features. As for DCA, variety was often noted in comparison with UCA.

Several glandular components were found in GC with sig. Those figures were microtubular adenocarcinoma, pyloric glandlike carcinoma, small gland carcinoma, and irregular shaped tubular adenocarcinoma with goblet cells (Fig 2). Microtubular adenocarcinoma and irregular shaped tubular adenocarcinoma with goblet cells were classified in tub2. Pyloric glandlike carcinoma was classified in sig and small gland carcinoma in sig or por.

All DCA was located almost in gastric mucosa with IM. Seventy-five (82%) DCA located in P with IM, 13 (14%) in F with IM, 3 (3%) in C with IM, and 1 (1%) in P without IM. Twenty-four (62%) UCA located in F without IM, 7 (18%) in F with IM, 7 (18%) in P with IM, and 1 (2%) in P without IM. There was no relationship between mixed histological pattern and location.

Forty (43%) DCA were M type, 32 (35%) I type, 11 (12%) G type, and 9 (10%) N type. Twenty (51%) UCA were M type, 15 (38%) G type, 3 (8%) I type, and 1 (3%) N type. There was no relationship between mixed histological pattern and phenotypic expression.

Histological Figures of Early Gastric Carcinoma with Submucosal Invasion

Early GC with submucosal invasion was 48 cases more than 6 mm in size. The histological figures are shown in Table 6. Mixed histological types were seen in 34 cases (71%); those showed various histological figures compared to mucosal GC. There was no relationship between histological type and location, and there was no relationship between histological type and phenotypic expression.

Table 5. Histological figure of early gastric carcinoma (11–20 mm in size)

	11 mm	12 mm	13 mm	14 mm	15 mm	16 mm	17 mm	18 mm	19 mm	20 mm	Total
sig	1	3	0	1	4	2	3	1	1	3	19
sig > por	0	0	0	0	0	0	0	1	1	0	2
por > sig	0	0	0	0	1	0	0	0	0	0	1
sig > tub2	0	0	2	1	0	0	0	2	0	0	5
tub2 > sig	0	0	1	4	1	0	1	1	0	0	8
sig > por > tub2	0	0	0	0	1	0	0	0	0	0	1
sig > tub2 > por	0	0	0	0	1	0	0	0	0	2	3
tub1	2	4	2	0	5	3	4	5	1	7	33
tub2	0	0	1	1	1	1	1	0	0	0	5
pap > tub1	1	0	0	0	0	0	0	0	0	0	1
tub1 > tub2	0	6	3	1	6	2	1	5	1	6	31
tub2 > tub1	1	2	1	2	2	0	2	1	0	0	11
tub2 > pap	0	0	0	0	0	0	0	0	1	0	1
pap > por	0	0	0	0	0	1	0	0	0	0	1
tub2 > por	1	0	0	0	0	0	0	0	0	1	2
tub2 > muc	0	0	0	0	1	0	0	0	0	0	1
por > tub2	0	0	0	0	1	0	0	0	0	1	2
tub1 > tub2 > pap	1	0	0	0	0	0	0	0	0	0	1
tub1 > tub2 > por	1	0	0	1	0	0	0	0	0	0	2
tub1 > tub2 > muc	0	1	0	0	0	0	0	0	0	0	1
Total	8	16	10	11	24	9	12	16	5	20	131

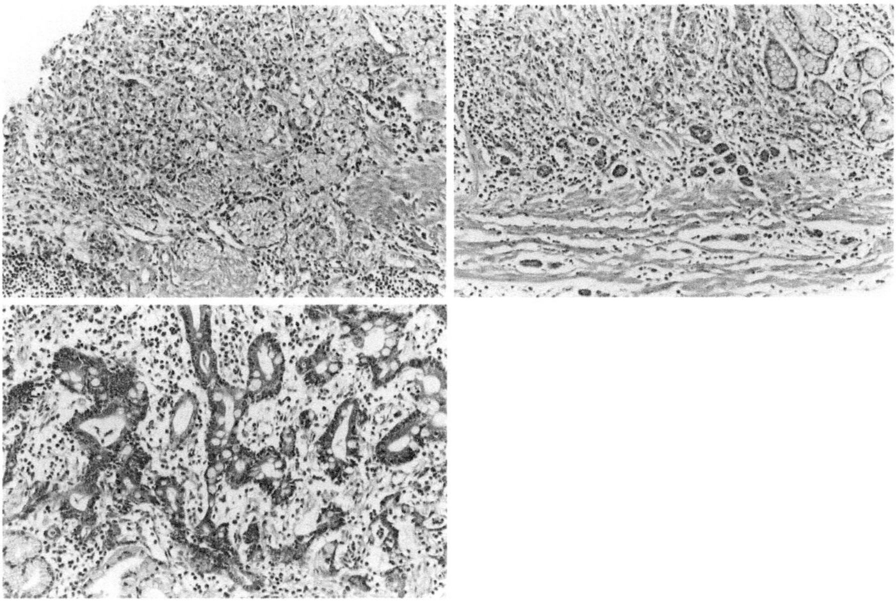

FIG. 2a–c. Glandular components admixed with sig of small gastric carcinoma, except microtubular glands. **a** Pyloric glandlike carcinoma. H&E. ×400. **b** Small gland carcinoma. H&E. ×400. **c** Irregularly shaped gland with goblet cells. H&E. ×400

TABLE 6. Histological figure of early gastric carcinoma with submucosa invasion

	6–10 mm	11–15 mm	16–20 mm	Total
sig	0	0	3	3
sig > por	0	0	2	2
sig > tub2	1	1	2	4
sig > por > tub2	0	1	0	1
sig > tub2 > por	0	1	1	2
tub1	3	3	2	8
tub2	0	1	2	3
tub1 > tub2	1	4	4	9
tub2 > tub1	1	5	2	8
tub2 > pap	0	0	1	1
pap > por	0	0	1	1
tub2 > por	0	1	1	2
por > tub2	0	0	1	1
tub1 > tub2 > pap	0	1	0	1
tub1 > tub2 > por	0	1	0	1
tub1 > tub2 > muc	0	1	0	1
Total	6	20	22	48

Histological Diversity of Small Early Gastric Carcinoma

It has been well known that GC shows various mixed histological patterns. However, very few examinations have been made of the histological diversity of GC. Nagayo et al. reported that mixed-type cancers comprised 42 cases (31%) of 137 early GC [14]. In this report, mixed type were 98 (39%) in 251 early GC equal to or less than 2 cm in size. The complexity of histological types appears in lesions more than 5 mm in size. The rate of mixed type was 4% in minute GC (1–5 mm), 31% in small early GC (6–10 mm), and 56% in early GC (11–20 mm). As tumor size is larger, histological complexity of GC increases. Most of them (95%) showed two histological types. Most GCs with submucosal invasion were of mixed histological type. Also, histological complexity increases according to submucosal invasion.

Minute GCs were morphologically homogeneous and showed two histological types, tub1 and sig. The result was the same as those of Nakamura et al. and Sugano et al. [12,13]. In this report, papillotubular type of Nakamura's classification was diagnosed as tub1 according to the criteria of the Japanese Research Society for Gastric Cancer [5]. In spite of increase of complexity, early GC was classified in DCA and UCA from morphological features.

The histological type of tub2 was found frequently in mixed-type GC. It is defined as a tumor that shows small or incomplete tubular structures with cubical or flat epithelium. However, histological figures of tub2 are various. The component of tub2 admixed with tub1 is an irregular gland according to dedifferentiation. On the other hand, the figures of tub2 admixed with sig are microtubular adenocarcinoma and irregular shaped tubular adenocarcinoma with goblet cells. Lauren noted the presence of miniature glandular elements admixed with sig [2], and this pattern is shown as poorly differentiated tubular adenocarcinoma in the AFIP Atlas of Tumor Pathology [15]. As for glandular components admixed with sig, pyloric glandlike carcinoma and small gland carcinoma were found. Ming noted pyloric glandlike carcinoma [3], and Fiocca et al. noted a microglandular pattern [16]. We have to consider histological findings to show those glandular formations to review the variety of gastric cancer.

Most DCA located in the gastric mucosa with IM and 62% UCA in the mucosa without IM. However, there was no relationship between histological figure and intestinal metaplasia of surrounding GC. Phenotypic expression of GC was various, and there was no relationship between histological figure and phenotypic expression except in minute GC. However, different results have been reported about phenotypic expression of minute DCA [11,17–19].

Histological complexity was found in lesions more than 5 mm in size, and histological diversity increases according to tumor size and invasion. Further study is needed for larger tumors to reveal the whole nature of GC.

Conclusions

1. Histological diversity of mixed figures is found in tumors more than 5 mm in size.
2. As size of GC becomes larger, histological diversity increases.
3. As GC invades the submucosa, histological diversity increases.

4. Both components of tub2 and por show various histological figures.
5. Despite diversity, early GC is classified into DCA and UCA.

References

1. Hamilton SR, Aalfonen LA (2000) World health organization classification of tumours, pathology and genetics of tumours of the digestive system. International Agency for Research on Cancer, Lyon, pp 43–46
2. Lauren P (1965) The two histological main types of gastric carcinoma: diffuse and so-called intestinal-type carcinoma: an attempt at a histo-chemical classification. Acta Pathol Microbiol Scand 64:31–49
3. Ming SC (1977) Gastric carcinoma: a pathological classification. Cancer (Phila) 39:2475–2485
4. Tatematsu M, Tsukamoto T, Inada K (2003) Stem cells and gastric cancer: role of gastric and intestinal mixed intestinal metaplasia. Cancer Sci 94:135–141
5. Japanese Research Society for Gastric Cancer (1995) Japanese classification of gastric carcinoma. Kanehara, Tokyo, pp 38–41
6. Bara J, Gautier R, Mouradian P, et al. (1991) Oncofetal mucin M1 epitope family: characterization and expression during colonic carcinogenesis. Int J Cancer 47:304–310
7. Reis CA, David L, Nielsen PA, et al. (1997) Immunohistochemical study of MUC5AC expression in human gastric carcinomas using a novel monocolonal antibody. Int J Cancer 74:112–121
8. Nakamura N, Ota H, Katsuyama T, et al. (1998) Histochemical reactivity of normal, metaplastic, and neoplastic tissues to α-like *N*-acetylglucosamine residue-specific monoclonal antibody HIK 1083. J Histochem Cytochem 46:793–801
9. Toribara NW, Robertson AM, Ho SB, et al. (1993) Human gastric mucin. Identification of a unique species by expression cloning. J Biol Chem 268:5879–5885
10. Xing P-X, Prenzoska J, Layton GT, et al. (1992) Second-generation monoclonal antibodies to intestinal MUC2 peptide reactive with colon cancer. J Natl Cancer Inst 84:699–703
11. Kawachi H, Takizawa T, Eishi Y, et al. (2003) Absence of either gastric or intestinal phenotype in microscopic differentiated gastric carcinomas. J Pathol 199:436–446
12. Nakamaura K, Sugano H, Takagi K (1968) Carcinoma of the stomach in incipient phase: its histogenesis and histological appearances. Gann 59:251–258
13. Sugano H, Nakamura K, Kato Y (1982) Pathological studies of human gastric cancer. Acta Pathol Jpn 32(suppl. 2):329–347
14. Nagayo T, Komagome T (1961) Histological studies of gastric mucosal cancer with special reference to relationship of histological pictures between the mucosal cancer and the cancer-bearing gastric mucosa. Gann 52:109–119
15. Lewin KJ, Appelman HD (1996) Tumors of the esophagus and stomach. In: Atlas of tumor pathology, 3rd series, fascicle 18. Armed Forces Institute of Pathology, Washington, DC, pp 267–321
16. Fiocca R, Villani L, Tenti P, et al. (1987) Characterization of four main cell types in gastric cancer: foveolar, mucopeptic, intestinal columnar and goblet cells: an histopathologic, histochemical and ultrastructural study of "early" and "advanced" tumours. Pathol Res Pract 182:308–325
17. Egashira Y, Shimoda T, Ikegami M (1999) Mucin histochemical analysis of minute gastric differentiated adenocarcinoma. Pathol Int 49:55–61
18. Sasaki I, Yao T, Nawata H, et al. (1999) Minute gastric carcinoma of differentiated type with special reference to the significance of intestinal metaplasia, proliferative zone and p53 protein during tumor development. Cancer (Phila) 85:1719–1729
19. Shiroshita H, Watanabe H, Ajioka Y, et al. (2004) Re-evaluation of mucin phenotypes of gastric minute well differentiated adenocarcinomas using a series of HGM, MUC5AC, MUC6, M-GGMC, MUC2 and CD10 stains. Pathol Int 54:311–321

Epstein–Barr Virus-Associated Gastric Carcinoma

Ja-Mun Chong, Hiroshi Uozaki, and Masashi Fukayama

Introduction

From the first report by MacCarty and Mahle in 1922 [1], gastric carcinoma with lymphoid stroma, characterized by a prominent lymphoid infiltration in the tumor stroma, has been recognized as associated with a favorable prognosis compared with the more common varieties of gastric carcinoma [1–3]. The suggestion was made that the infiltrating lymphocytes might play an important role in immune surveillance and protect against the invading carcinoma cells [4]. These investigations reveal that this specific type of gastric carcinoma might be a separate classification from ordinary gastric carcinoma. In the 1990s, several groups reported that virtually all gastric carcinomas with lymphoid stroma were associated with Epstein–Barr virus (EBV) [5–7]. Furthermore, EBV is also associated with some gastric carcinomas lacking a prominent lymphoid infiltrate [8]. EBV-associated gastric carcinoma (EBVaGC) occurs worldwide. Always a small minority of gastric cancers, the proportion of gastric cancers associated with EBV does not show the profound geographic variation that is characteristic of Burkitt's lymphoma [9]. EBVaGC shows characteristic features in many clinicopathological and genetic studies that differ from the features of gastric carcinoma without EBV, so EBVaGC is appropriately considered a distinct entity. However, in spite of many investigations, the pathogenesis of this tumor remains poorly understood. Advances in virology and molecular biology promise to shed light on this pathway. In this chapter, we review EBVaGC and associated epigenetic changes in the context of current therapy with an eye toward the possibility of targeted therapies in the future.

Department of Human Pathology, The University of Tokyo Graduate School of Medicine, 7-3-1 Hongo, Bunkyo-ku, Tokyo 113-0033, Japan
e-mail: jmchong-tky@umin.ac.jp

Background of EBV Infection

In 1964, Epstein and Barr reported the discovery of a human gamma herpes virus in cells cultured from endemic Burkitt's lymphoma in Africa [10]. Ultimately, the virus proven to be the ubiquitous EBV infection may be either lytic or latent [11]. Virions are only produced in lytic infection; these are icosahedral capsids that carry a large (172-kb) genome of linear double-strand DNA [12]. In latent infection, the viral DNA of EBV exists as an extrachromosomal circular molecule (episome) in the nucleus. More than 90% of the adults are seropositive for EBV. Infection is usually asymptomatic in childhood, but during adolescence frequently results in infectious mononucleosis (IM) [13,14]. Oropharyngeal infection results in infection of B cells and amplification of infection as the virus drives the proliferation of latently infected B cells [15]. Three types of latency have been described for lymphoid cell lines based on the variable expression of the latent gene products. A classification of EBV-associated neoplasms is shown in Table 1 [16–18]. Not only latent infection of circulation B cells in IM, but also opportunistic lymphoma and pyothorax-associated lymphoma, are characterized by the type III latency pattern [18,19], involving expression of six EBV nuclear antigens (EBNA 1, 2, LP, 3A, 3B, 3C), three latent membrane proteins (LMP1, LMP2A, and LMP2B), EBV-encoded small RNA (EBER)1 and EBER2, and the transcripts from the *Bam*H1A region. In type III latency, EBNA2 plays a central role in switching EBNA transcription from the *Bam*H1-W fragment of the genome W promoter (Wp) to C fragment (Cp), and the expression is driven from the Cp by alternative splicing from a primary transcript. In latency I, the antigen expression is restricted, such as EBNA1, which is driven by a promoter in the *Bam*H1-Q fragment of the genome (Qp). In latency type II, EBNA1 is also under the control of the Qp promoter, but there is also transcription of LMP1 and LMP2. EBNA1 is the virus genome maintenance protein, the remaining EBNAs are transcriptional regulators, and LMP1 is the major effecter of virus-induced cellular change.

A crucial mechanism involved in the silencing of Cp and LMP1 promoter in type I latency has been shown to be methylation of CpG dinucleotides [20–22]. Type III latency is associated with B-cell transformation (immortalization) [23]. However, EBV-specific cytotoxic T lymphocytes (CTL) can recognize all EBV-coded latent-phase proteins, except for EBNA1 [24]. Accordingly, the type III latency pattern is highly immunogenic, resulting in an expansion of EBV-specific CTL, which results in

TABLE 1. Latent infection phenotype in Epstein–Barr virus (EBV)-associated carcinoma

EBV-associated tumor	Latency	EBNA 1	EBNA 2,3s	EBNA LP	LMP1	EBER1
Gastric carcinoma	I	+	−	−	−	+
Burkitt's lymphoma	I	+	−	−	−	+
Nasopharyngeal carcinoma	II	+	−	−	+	+
Hodgkin's disease	II	+	−	−	+	+
Immortalized lymphocyte	III	+	+	+	+	+

EBNA, Epstein–Barr nuclear antigen; LMP, latent membrane protein; EBER, EBV-encoded small RNA

IM-like responses and regression of type III latently infected cells. A small proportion of infected B cells evade lysis by adopting and altering patterns of expression of latency proteins, type I or II, at different times. Then, EBV-infected B cells can escape the recognition of EBV-specific CTL. Although EBV-infected B cells with type III latency are never subsequently detected in the peripheral blood of healthy carriers, EBV infection persists for life in an incompletely defined cell–virus relationship [25]. Therefore, it is less likely that EBV is associated with carcinogenesis in latency type I malignancies. However, it has been shown in a Burkitt's lymphoma-derived cell line (Akata) that after cloning in soft agar, some clones will lose that viral episome [26]. EBV-positive clones can form colonies on soft agar and tumor masses in nude mice, but EBV-negative clones do not. EBV-reinfected clones exhibit restored capacity for growth on soft agar and tumorigenicity in mice [26,27]. Taken together, these results show that EBV relates carcinogenesis in latency type I malignancies.

EBV is associated with the genesis of Burkitt's lymphoma, Hodgkin's disease, undifferentiated nasopharyngeal carcinoma (NPC), and opportunistic lymphoma in immunocompromised hosts [9,28–30]. Recent studies demonstrate that EBV is also associated with gastric carcinoma and certain T-cell lymphomas [31,32]. All or a significant proportion of neoplastic cells of these tumors harbor EBV episomes and express a restricted number of latent viral proteins. Similar to many other EBV-associated malignancies, the malignant cell in EBVaGC is characterized by its unique viral phenotype [32,33]. Similar to Burkitt's lymphoma, EBVaGC tumor cells display a type I form of latency with latent gene expression limited to EBNA1, LMP2, EBER1, EBER2, and *Bam*HI-A transcripts.

Clinicopathological Features of EBVaGC

EBVaGC is reported to account for about 10% of GCs in various countries [8,34,35]. EBVaGC occurs more frequently in males [34,35]. The site of EBVaGC within the stomach is predominantly in the proximal stomach. EBVaGC is observed in gastric carcinomas at all depths of invasion (Fig. 1). A recent study in the Netherlands showed that there is no significant difference of tumor depth between EBVaGC and EBV-negative GC (T1 stage, 31.7% versus 26.1%) [36]. However, the proportion of EBVaGC in intramucosal carcinoma is relatively lower than that in invasive carcinomas in Japanese studies focused on the intramucosal stage [35,37]. The lower rate of EBVaGC in intramucosal carcinoma may reflect the presence of EBV-negative and less-aggressive neoplasms in intramucosal carcinoma in our series. This possibility has been pointed out in a comparative study of the criteria for gastric carcinoma used by Japanese and Western pathologists [38].

As for the histology of the carcinoma, gastric carcinomas with prominent lymphoid stroma are associated with EBV. The proportion of this particular type in EBVaGC varies considerably, from 0% to 80%, according to the strictness of the criteria. Nevertheless, EBVaGC with ordinary histology has certain characteristic morphological features: moderately differentiated tubular and poorly differentiated solid types are predominant, whereas papillary type or scirrhous type is extremely rare [37]. This finding suggests that EBVaGC may not have the same carcinogenic process as intestinal- or diffuse-type gastric carcinoma. It is also interesting that EBVaGC in its intramucosal stage is likely to exhibit a specific histological pattern: abortive

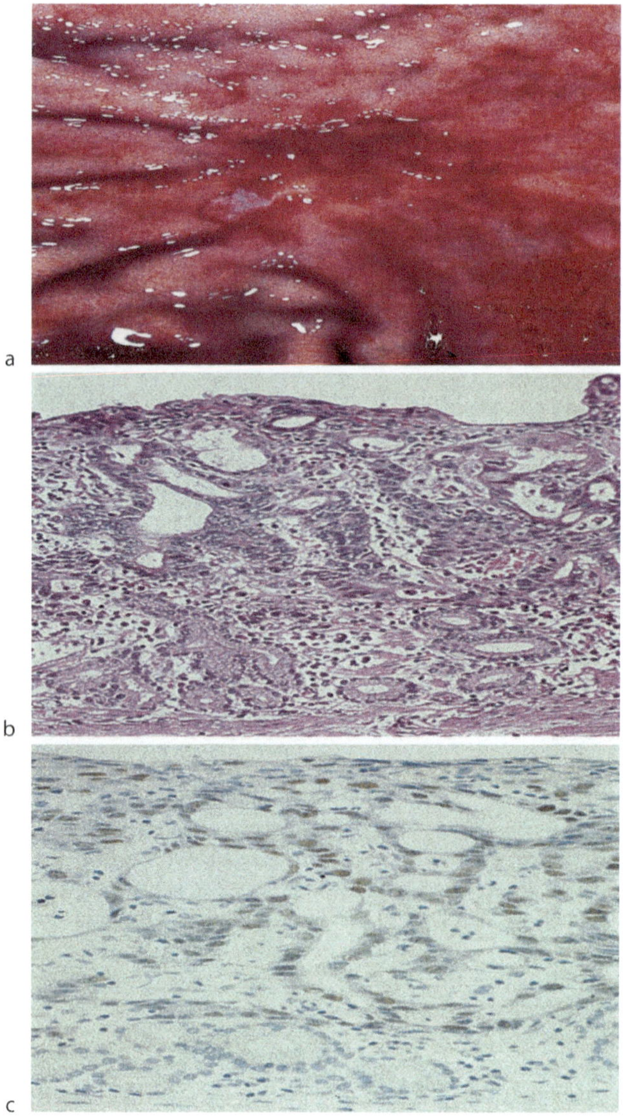

FIG. 1. An intramucosal case of Epstein–Barr virus (EBV)-associated gastric carcinoma. Gastric adenocarcinoma was limited to intramucosa with EBV infection. **a** Macroscopic finding of the carcinoma. **b** Microscopic finding with hematoxylin and eosin stain. **c** In situ hybridization finding using an EBV-encoded small RNA (EBER1) probe

tubular structures occupy the middle of the mucosa without destroying the mucosal architecture [39].

The prognosis of EBVaGC is controversial [36,40]. Nakamura et al. reported that the prognosis of patients with gastric carcinomas with prominent lymphoid stroma was not affected by whether the carcinoma was associated with EBV [40]. van Beek et al. showed that a better prognosis related to less lymph node involvement is significantly associated with EBV status [36]. Further study is needed, especially in determining whether the EBVaGC correlates with prominent lymphoid stroma.

Virological Features of EBVaGC

EBV-encoded small RNA (EBER)1 is detected in almost all carcinoma cells of the EBV-positive carcinomas [34]. Southern blot analysis for the terminal repeats in EBV-DNA demonstrated that the EBV genome is present in a monoclonal and episomal form in most EBV-positive gastric carcinomas. This finding suggests that EBV infects the gastric epithelial cell before or in the early stages of gastric carcinogenesis.

Transcriptional analyses demonstrated that EBERs, the putative *Bam*HI-A transcript (BARFs) and EBNA1, are expressed in the EBV-associated gastric carcinomas. However, none of the other EBNAs or LMPs except LMP2A is expressed in carcinoma tissues [32,33,41,42]. This is different from the pattern in nasopharyngeal carcinoma in which LMP1 is also expressed in carcinoma cells in up to approximately 65% of the patients [43].

zur Hausen et al. showed that in almost all cases of EBVaGC, BARF1 is expressed and can immortalize primary monkey epithelial kidney cells [44]. However, Iwakiri et al. reported that the EBER was responsible for insulin-like growth factor (IGF)-I expression, and the secreted IGF-I acts as an autocrine growth factor in transfection assays of individual EBV latent genes into NUGC-3 cells [45]. Thus, it is still controversial which latency gene is responsible for the carcinogenesis of EBVaGC.

EBVaGC Models

In vivo transplantation and in vitro cell culture of neoplastic cells, which retain the characteristics of the original tumor, are useful tools to further define the functional role of the EBV genes expressed and the biological or molecular alterations in carcinoma cells of EBVaGC. In vitro, EBV preferentially infects human B cells and transforms them into lymphoblastoid cell lines (LCLs). EBV initially enters B cells by binding the CD21, which is abundantly expressed on B cells. The abundance of CD21 explains why EBV infects B cells more efficiently than other types of cells [46,47]. In contrast, the lack of CD21 expression in epithelial cells, include stomach cells, has made establishing a stable cell line of EBVaGC difficult [48]. A stable cell line from NPC that carries the EBV genome in the nucleus is also difficult to establish, because the EBV genome tends to become lost during extensive in vitro passages [49]. We have attempted to transplant a human EBVaGC in severe combined immunodeficiency (SCID) mice. We succeeded in establishing a carcinoma line, designated KT, named after the patient from whom the tumor was derived [50]. The pattern of EBV latency gene expression in the KT line is the same in the original tumor: EBER1 was also found in tumor cell nuclei by in situ hybridization. Reverse transcription-polymerase chain reaction (PCR) analysis demonstrated Qp-driven EBNA1 expression, but not EBNA2- or LMP1 expression. Thus, the transplantable human EBVaGC retains the original EBV with the same latency gene expression as type I latency.

Several in vitro model systems have previously been established to study the role of EBV in gastric cancers [51–55]. These models are useful to investigate the behavior of the infected EBV in gastric carcinoma cells and allow comparison between the EBV-positive and EBV-negative epithelial cells. Also, they may be useful to study the EBV infection pathway of gastric cells, such as receptor-mediated infection [55].

However, these models are infected with an EBV strain derived from lymphoma cell lines and may not reflect the natural condition of EBV-associated gastric carcinoma, or are different from the majority of EBVaGC as they show EBV latency III and lytic replication. Recently, Oh et al. [56] found that a previously established gastric adenocarcinoma cell line, SNU-719, is infected with EBV. They confirmed EBV infection in the original carcinoma tissue of this cell line. This cell line reveals EBNA1 and LMP2A expression and the absence of LMP1 and EBNA2 expression. There are no lytic EBV proteins in this cell line. Interestingly, CD21 expression in the cell line is not found.

Presently, these spontaneous EBV-infected model cell lines, KT and SNU-719, are valuable tools. However, we need more cell lines for studying the functional role of EBV gene expression and the biological or molecular alteration in carcinoma cells of EBVaGC. These efforts may help progress toward a therapeutic approach.

Carcinogenic Pathway of EBVaGC

Recent molecular biological research shows that most tumors cause the alteration of its genome [57–60]. The alterations of various oncogenes and tumor suppressor genes are associated with carcinogenesis. There are many reports about the carcinogenic mechanism in gastric carcinomas [61–64]. One obvious question is whether the carcinogenic pathway of EBVaGC is the same as that of EBV-negative GC or is different. If it is different, what specific alterations occur in EBVaGC? Investigations of the molecular alterations in EBVaGC have remained few compared to the number of clinicopathological studies of EBVaGC. One of the first investigations of the genetic changes was performed by Chong et al. [65]. The study showed the deletion of 5q and/or 17p and microsatellite instability were found to be extremely rare in EBVaGC but were frequent in EBV-negative GC. Subsequent reports corroborated this result [66–68]. Although loss of chromosomes 4p, 11p, and 18q is found to be more frequent in EBVaGC than in EBV-negative GC by comparative genomic hybridization [69], there is no report that shows significant genetic changes such as a loss of heterozygosity, amplification, or point mutation in specific genes.

The EBV genome exists in episomal form in the nucleus of infected cells and does not integrate in the host cell genome. Accordingly, we hardly think that EBV directly affects the host cell DNA sequence, although some specific RNA and protein expressions in EBVaGC were found [70,71]. We found the carcinogenic pathway of EBVaGC is indeed different from that of EBV-negative GC. However, we must return to the second question in this section: What alterations occur in EBVaGC?

Recent investigations put light on this question. Kang et al. [72], Vo et al. [73], and our own group [74,75] demonstrated that promoter hypermethylation of various tumor-related genes occurs much more frequently in EBVaGC than in EBV-negative GC. Generally, promoter hypermethylation results in the reduction of the gene expressions [76]. In particular, the subsequent reduction of gene expression has been observed in p16 and E-cadherin [72–74,77]. When undergoing bisulfite sequencing to investigate the distribution and density of methylated CpG sites, EBVaGC exhibited concurrent methylation of $p14^{ARF}$ and $p16^{INK4A}$ promoters with extremely high density and distinctive methylation pattern in contrast to that for EBV-negative GC [78]. These findings suggest the presence of mechanisms of de novo and maintenance methylation specific to EBVaGC that might be associated with the EBV infection. We showed the possibility that EBV infects to a gastric epithelial cell before or in the early stage of gastric carcinogenesis. Now, we have newly arising questions. The first is how and when the promoter methylation in host cells occurs, whether before, with, or after EBV infection. In early gastric carcinomas infected with EBV with diameters less than 3 cm, frequent methylation is found in several tumor-related genes (our unpublished data). The second question is whether Cp methylation of EBV, which also occurs in EBVaGC [32], is related to this promoter methylation in host cells. To resolve these questions, we need to research the methylation status of cells and EBV DNA before and after infection. Thus, EBVaGC may be a good model to study the methylation mechanism and promoter methylation-targeted therapy.

With the foregoing investigations, some reports show therapeutic approaches for EBV-associated tumors. One therapeutic approach aims for the transition of EBV from latency to lytic cycle by inducing the products of immediate-early viral genes, BZLF1 and BRLF1 [79,80], or with chemotherapy [81]. This EBV-targeted therapy is plausible for EBVaGC, because almost all the carcinoma cells reveal EBV infection, and EBV infection of the surrounding noncancerous mucosa is quite rare [34]. The other therapeutic approach is to achieve demethylation with a DNA methyltransferase inhibitor, and gene reexpression [82]. This therapeutic approach based on epigenetic change of EBV genome also may adapt to the host cell gene reexpression suffering methylation in EBVaGC. Recent research showed that gene transcriptions were directly affected by RNA interference [83]. Therefore, we might be able to suppress EBV in carcinoma cells using RNA interference for EBNA1.

In summary, EBVaGC has characteristic features in clinicopathological study, and the carcinogenic pathway is different from that of EBV-negative GC. The promoter methylation may contribute to the carcinogenesis of EBVaGC. Although the carcinogenic mechanism including the promoter methylation must be clarified with further studies, EBV-targeted therapy is surely close to becoming reality.

Acknowledgment. The authors thank Dr. Richard F. Ambinder and Dr. Victor Lemas (Department of Oncology, Johns Hopkins University of Medicine, Baltimore, MD, USA) for reading our manuscript. Our own work as described in this chapter was supported by scientific research grants from the Ministry of Education, Science, Sports, and Culture of Japan.

References

1. MacCarty WC, Mahle AE (1922) Relation of differentiation and lymphocytic infiltration to postoperative longevity in gastric carcinoma. J Lab Clin Med 6:473–480
2. Watanabe H, Enjoji M, Imai T (1975) Gastric carcinoma with lymphoid stroma. Its morphologic characteristics and prognostic correlations. Cancer (Phila) 38:232–243
3. Ito H, Masuda H, Shimamoto F, et al (1990) Gastric carcinoma with lymphoid stroma: pathological and immunohistochemical analysis. Hiroshima J Med Sci 39:29–37
4. Minamoto T, Mai M, Watanabe K, et al (1990) Medullary carcinoma with lymphocytic infiltration of the stomach. Cancer (Phila) 66:945–952
5. Burke AP, Yen TSB, Shekitka KM, et al (1990) Lymphoepithelial carcinoma of the stomach with Epstein Barr virus demonstrated by polymerase chain reaction. Mod Pathol 3:377–380

6. Min KW, Holmquist S, Peiper SC, et al (1991) Poorly differentiated adenocarcinoma with lymphoid stroma (lymphoepithelioma-like carcinomas) of the stomach. Am J Clin Pathol 96:219–227
7. Shibata D, Tokunaga M, Uemura Y, et al (1991) Association of Epstein-Barr virus with undifferentiated gastric carcinomas with intense lymphoid infiltration. Am J Pathol 139:469–474
8. Shibata D, Weiss LM (1992) Epstein-Barr virus-associated gastric adenocarcinoma. Am J Pathol 140:769–774
9. Osato T (1998) Epstein-Barr virus infection and oncogenesis. In: Epstein-Barr virus and human cancer. Japan Scientific Societies Press, Tokyo, pp 3–16
10. Epstein A, Achong BG, Barr YM (1964) Virus particles in cultured lymphoblasts from Burkitt's lymphoma. Lancet 1:702–703
11. Kieff E (1996) Epstein-Barr virus and its replication. In: Fields virology, 3rd edn. Raven, Philadelphia, pp. 2343–2396
12. Baer R, Bankier AT, Biggin MD, et al (1984) DNA sequence and expression of the B95-8 Epstein-Barr virus genome. Nature (Lond) 310:207–211
13. Chan KH, Tam JS, Peiris JS, et al (2001) Epstein-Barr virus (EBV) infection in infancy. J Clin Virol 21:57–62
14. Evans AS (1972) Clinical syndromes associated with EB virus infection. Ann Intern Med 18:77–93
15. Sixby JW, Nedrud JG, Raab-Traub N, et al (1984) Epstein-Barr virus replication in oropharyngeal epithelial cells. N Engl J Med 310:1225–1230
16. Sbih-Lammali F, Djennaoui D, Belaoui D, et al (1996) Transcriptional expression of Epstein-Barr virus genes and proto-oncogenes in North African nasopharyngeal carcinomas. J Med Virol 49:7–14
17. Rowe M, Rowe D, Gregory C, et al (1987) Differences in B-cell growth phenotype reflect novel patterns of Epstein-Barr virus latent gene expression in Burkitt's lymphoma. EMBO J 6:2743–2751
18. Niedobitek G, Young LS, Herbst H (1997) Epstein-Barr virus infection and the pathogenesis of malignancy lymphomas. Cancer Surv 30:143–161
19. Fukayama M, Ibuka T, Hayashi, Y, et al (1993) Epstein-Barr virus in pyothorax-associated pleural lymphoma. Am J Pathol 143:1044–1049
20. Tao Q, Swinnen LJ, Yang J, et al (1999) Methylation status of the Epstein-Barr virus major latent promoter C in iatrogenic B cell lymphoproliferative disease: application of PCR-based analysis. Am J Pathol 155:619–625
21. Robertson KD, Ambinder RF (1997) Mapping promoter regions that are hypersensitive to methylaton-mediated inhibition of transcription: application of the methylation cassette assay to the Epstein-Barr virus major latency promoter. J Virol 71:6445–6454
22. Ernberg I, Falk K, Minarovits J, et al (1989) The role of methylation in the phenotype-dependent modulation of Epstein-Barr nuclear antigen 2 and latent membrane protein genes in cells latently infected with Epstein-Barr virus. J Gen Virol 70:2989–3002
23. Foss HD, Reusch R, Demel G, et al (1999) Frequent expression of the B-cell-specific activator protein in Reed-Sternberg cells of classical Hodgkin's disease provides further evidence for its B-cell origin. Blood 94:3108–3113
24. Rickinson AB, Moss DJ (1997) Human cytotoxic T lymphocyte responses to Epstein-Barr virus infection. Annu Rev Immunol 15:405–431
25. Miyashita EM, Yang B, Babcock GJ, et al (1997) Identification of the site of Epstein-Barr virus persistence in vivo as a resting B cell. J Virol 71:4882–4891
26. Shimizu N, Tanabe-Tochikura A, Kuroiwa Y, et al (1994) Isolation of Epstein-Barr virus (EBV)-negative cell clones from the EBV-positive Burkitt's lymphoma (B) line Akata: malignancy phenotypes of BL cells are dependent on EBV. J Virol 68:6069–6073
27. Komano J, Sugiura M, Takada K (1998) Epstein-Barr virus contributes to the malignant phenotype and to apoptosis resistance in Burkitt's lymphoma cell line Akata. J Virol 72: 9150–9156

28. Raab-Traub N (1992) Epstein-Barr virus and nasophryngeal carcinoma. Cancer Biol 3: 297–315
29. Borisch B, Finke J, Henning I, et al (1992) Distribution and localization of Epstein-Barr virus subtypes A and B in AIDS-related lymphomas and lymphatic tissue HIV-positive patients. J Pathol 168:229–236
30. Weiss LM, Strickler JG, Warnke RA, et al (1987) Epstein-Barr viral DNA in tissues of Hodgkin's disease. Am J Pathol 129:86–91
31. Korbjuhn P, Anagnostopoulos I, Hummel M, et al (1993) Frequent latent Epstein-Barr virus infection of neoplastic T cells and bystander B cells in human immunodeficiency virus-negative European peripheral pleomorphic T-cell lymphomas. Blood 82:217–223
32. Imai S, Koizumi S, Sugiura M, et al (1994) Gastric carcinoma: monoclonal epithelial malignant cells expressing Epstein-Barr virus latent infection protein. Proc Natl Acad Sci USA 91:9131–9135
33. Sugiura M, Imai S, Tokunaga M, et al (1996) Transcriptional analysis of Epstein-Barr virus gene expression in EBV-positive gastric carcinoma: unique viral latency in the tumor cells. Br J Cancer 74:625–631
34. Fukayama M, Hayashi Y, Iwasaki Y, et al (1994) Epstein-Barr virus-associated gastric carcinoma and Epstein-Barr virus infection of the stomach. Lab Invest 71:73–81
35. Tokunaga M, Land CE, Uemura Y, et al (1993) Epstein-Barr virus in gastric carcinoma. Am J Pathol 143:1250–1254
36. van Beek J, zur Hausen A, Kranenbarg EK, et al (2004) EBV-positive gastric adenocarcinomas: a distinct clinicopathologic entity with a low frequency of lymph node involvement. J Clin Oncol 22:664–670
37. Kaizaki Y, Sakurai S, Chong JM, et al (1999) Atrophic gastritis, Epstein-Barr virus infection, and Epstein-Barr virus-associated gastric carcinoma. Gastric Cancer 2:101–108.
38. Schlemper RJ, Itabashi M, Kato Y, et al (1997) Differences in diagnostic criteria for gastric carcinoma between Japanese and Western pathologists. Lancet 349:1725–1729
39. Arikawa J, Tokunaga M, Satoh E, et al (1997) Morphological characteristics of Epstein-Barr virus-related early gastric carcinoma: a case control study. Pathol Int 47:360–367
40. Nakamura S, Ueki T, Yao T, et al (1994) Epstein-Barr virus in gastric carcinoma with lymphoid stroma. Special reference to its detection by the polymerase chain reaction and in situ hybridization in 99 tumors, including a morphologic analysis. Cancer (Phila) 73:2239–2249
41. Rowlands DC, Ito M, Mangham DC, et al (1993) Epstein-Barr virus and carcinoma: rare association of the virus with gastric carcinomas. Br J Cancer 68:1014–1019
42. Ott G, Kirchner TH, Muller-Hermelink HK (1994) Monoclonal Epstein-Barr virus genomes but lack of EBV-related protein expression in different types of gastric carcinoma. Histopathology (Oxf) 25:323–329
43. Young LS, Dawson CW, Clark D, et al (1988) Epstein-Barr virus gene expression in nasopharyngeal carcinoma. J Gen Virol 69:1051–1065
44. zur Hauzen A, Brink AATP, Craanen ME, et al (2000) Unique transcription pattern of Epstein-Barr virus (EBV) in EBV-carrying gastric adenocarcinomas: expression of the transforming BARF1 gene. Cancer Res 60:2745–2748
45. Iwakiri D, Eizuru Y, Tokunaga M, et al (2003) Autocrine growth of Epstein-Barr virus-positive gastric carcinoma cells mediated by an Epstein-Barr virus-encoded small RNA. Cancer Res 63:7062–7067
46. Fingeroth JD, Weis JJ, Teddre TF, et al (1984) Epstein-Barr virus receptor of human B lymphocytes is the C3d receptor CR2. Proc Natl Acad Sci USA 81:4510–4514
47. Nemerow GR, Mold G, Schwend VK, et al (1987) Identification of gp350 as the viral glycoprotein mediating attachment of Epstein-Barr virus (EBV) to the EBV/C3d receptor of B cell: sequence homology of gp350 and C3 complement fragment C3d. J Virol 61:1416–1420
48. Shapiro IM, Volsky DJ (1983) Infection of normal human epithelial cells by Epstein-Barr virus. Science 219:1225–1228

49. Lin CT, Dee AN, Chen W, et al (1994) Association of Epstein-Barr virus, human papilloma virus, and cytomegalovirus with nine nasopharyngeal carcinoma cell lines. Lab Invest 71:731–736
50. Iwasaki Y, Chong JM, Hayashi Y, et al (1998) Establishment and characterization of a human Epstein-Barr virus-associated gastric carcinoma in SCID mice. J Virol 72:8321–8326
51. Yoshiyama H, Imai S, Shimizu N, et al (1997) Epstein-Barr virus infection of human gastric carcinoma cells: implication of the existence of a new virus receptor different from CD21. J Virol 71:5688–5691
52. Imai S, Nishikawa J, Takada K (1998) Cell-to-cell contact as an efficient mode of Epstein-Barr virus infection of diverse human epithelial cells. J Virol 72:4371–4378
53. Tajima M, Komuro M, Okinaga K (1998) Establishment of Epstein-Barr virus-positive human gastric epithelial cell lines. Jpn J Cancer Res 89:262–268
54. Takasaka N, Tajima M, Okinaga K, et al (1998) Productive infection of Epstein-Barr virus (EBV) in EBV-genome-positive epithelial cell lines (GT38 and GT39) derived from gastric tissues. Virology 247:152–159
55. Luo B, Murakami M, Fukuda M, et al (2004) Characterization of Epstein-Barr virus infection in a human signet ring cell gastric carcinoma cell line, HSC-39. Microbes Infect 6:429–439
56. Oh ST, Seo JS, Moon UY, et al (2004) A naturally derived gastric cancer cell line shows latency I Epstein-Barr virus infection closely resembling EBV-associated gastric cancer. Virology 320:330–336
57. Powell SM, Petersen GM, Krush AJ (1993) Molecular diagnosis of familial adenomatous polyposis. N Engl J Med 329:1982–1987
58. Iino H, Fukayama M, Maeda Y, et al (1994) Molecular genetics for clinical management of colorectal carcinoma. 17p, 18q, and 22q loss of heterozygosity and decreased DCC expression are correlated with the metastatic potential. Cancer (Phila) 73:1324–1331
59. Miyaki M, Nishio J, Konishi M, et al (1997) Drastic genetic instability of tumors and normal tissues in Turcot syndrome. Oncogene 15:2877–2881
60. Chong JM, Fukayama M, Hayashi Y, et al (1997) Microsatellite instability and loss of heterozygosity in gastric lymphoma. Lab Invest 77:639–645
61. Kushima R, Hattori T (1993) Histogenesis and characteristics of gastric-type adenocarcinomas in the stomach. J Cancer Res Clin Oncol 120:103–111
62. Tamura G, Sakata K, Maesawa C, et al (1995) Microsatellite alterations in adenoma and differentiated adenocarcinoma of the stomach. Cancer Res 55:1933–1936
63. Ooi A, Kobayashi M, Mai M, et al (1998) Amplification of c-erbB-2 in gastric cancer: detection in formalin-fixed, paraffin-embedded tissue by fluorescence in situ hybridization. Lab Invest 78:345–351
64. Tahara E (1993) Molecular mechanism of stomach carcinogenesis. Cancer Res Clin Oncol 119:265–272
65. Chong, JM, Fukayama M, Hayashi Y, et al (1994) Microsatellite instability in the progression of gastric carcinoma. Cancer Res 54:4595–4597
66. van Rees BP, Caspers E, zur Hausen A, et al (2002) Different pattern of allelic loss in Epstein-Barr virus-positive gastric cancer with emphasis on the p53 tumor suppressor pathway. Am J Pathol 161:1207–1213
67. Chang MS, Kim HS, Kim CW, et al (2002) Epstein-Barr virus, p53 protein, and microsatellite instability in the adenoma-carcinoma sequence of the stomach. Hum Pathol 33:415–420
68. Chang MS, Lee HS, Kim HS, et al (2003) Epstein-Barr virus and microsatellite instability in gastric carcinogenesis. J Pathol 199:447–452
69. zur Hausen A, van Grieken NC, Meijer GA, et al (2001) Distinct chromosomal aberrations in Epstein-Barr virus-carrying gastric carcinomas tested by comparative genomic hybridization. Gastroenterology 121:612–618
70. Chong JM, Fukayama M, Hayashi Y, et al (1997) Expression of CD44 variants in gastric carcinoma with or without Epstein-Barr virus. Int J Cancer 74:450–454

71. Chong JM, Sakuma K, Sudo M, et al (2002) Interleukin 1β expression in human gastric carcinoma with Epstein-Barr virus infection. J Virol 76:6825–6831
72. Kang GH, Lee S, Kim WH, et al (2002) Epstein-Barr virus-positive gastric carcinoma demonstrates frequent aberrant methylation of multiple genes and constitutes CpG island methylator phenotype-positive gastric carcinoma. Am J Pathol 160:787–794
73. Vo QN, Geradts J, Gulley ML, et al (2002) Epstein-Barr virus in gastric adenocarcinomas: association with ethnicity and CDKN2A promoter methylation. J Clin Pathol 55:669–675
74. Osawa T, Chong JM, Sudo M, et al (2002) Reduced expression and promoter methylation of p16 gene in Epstein-Barr virus-associated gastric carcinoma. Jpn J Cancer Res 93:1195–1200
75. Chong JM, Sakuma K, Sudo M, et al (2003) Global and non-random CpG-island methylation in gastric carcinoma associated with Epstein-Barr virus. Cancer Sci 94:76–80
76. Merlo A, Herman JG, Mao L, et al (1995) 5′-CpG island methylation is associated with transcriptional silencing of the tumor suppressor p16/CDKN2/MTS1 in human cancers. Nat Med 1:686–692
77. Sudo M, Chong JM, Sakuma K, et al (2004) Promoter hypermethylation of E-cadherin and its abnormal expression in Epstein-Barr virus-associated gastric carcinoma. Int J Cancer 109:194–199
78. Sakuma K, Chong JM, Sudo M, et al (2004) High-density methylation of $p14^{ARF}$ and $p16^{INK4A}$ in Epstein-Barr virus-associated gastric carcinoma. Int J Cancer 112:273–278
79. Ragoczy T, Heston L, Miller G (1998) The Epstein-Barr virus Rta protein activates lytic cycle genes and can disrupt latency in B lymphocytes. J Virol 72:7978–7984
80. Feng WH, Westphal E, Mauser A, et al (2002) Use of adenovirus vectors expressing Epstein-Barr virus (EBV) immediate-early protein BZLF1 or BRLF1 to treat EBV-positive tumors. J Virol 76:10951–10959
81. Feng WH, Israel B, Raab-Traub N, et al (2002) Chemotherapy induces lytic EBV replication and confers ganciclovir susceptibility to EBV-positive epithelial cell tumors. Cancer Res 62:1920–1926
82. Chan ATC, Tao Q, Robertson KD, et al (2004) Azacitidine induces demethylation of the Epstein-Barr virus genome in tumors. J Clin Oncol 22:1373–1381
83. Elbashir SM, Harborth J, Lendeckel W, et al (2001) Duplexes of 21-nucleotide RNAs mediate RNA interference in cultured mammalian cells. Nature (Lond) 411:494–498

Hepatoid Adenocarcinoma of the Stomach: Biological Significance of Hepatic Transdifferentiation in Adenocarcinoma Cells

Hiroshi Ishikura[1], Yana Supriatna[1], Kazuhiro Kojima[1,2], Shigeyuki Kamata[1,2], Hiroki Nakaya[3], and Takashi Kishimoto[1]

Clinicopathology of Hepatoid Adenocarcinoma of the Stomach

Hepatoid adenocarcinoma was first described in the stomach as a subtype of alpha-fetoprotein (AFP)-producing gastric cancers with distinct clinicopathological properties [1,2]. Hepatoid adenocarcinoma of the stomach is defined as a primary gastric carcinoma with areas of functionally and structurally distinctive foci of hepatocellular differentiation. It usually arises as a circumscribed mass in the antrum to body of the stomach in middle-aged to elderly persons (Fig. 1).

Tumor cells in a certain type of AFP-producing gastric carcinomas were once regarded as poorly differentiated or undifferentiated due to the sheetlike arrangement of tumor cells with abundant, eosinophilic cytoplasm. However, after the recognition of a liverlike trabecular arrangement, as well as production of a set of liver-specific proteins [2,3], the sheetlike proliferation of AFP-producing gastric carcinoma has now come to be regarded as a morphological mimicry of the liver structure (Figs. 2–5).

Most importantly, hepatoid adenocarcinomas exhibit hepatocellular differentiation, usually in association with well-differentiated tubular or papillary adenocarcinoma [2,4]. Adenocarcinoma cells are either of intestinal epithelial type with production of mucin, or of clear cell type with a primitive appearance. Adenocarcinoma cells usually can be found in the mucosal layer of the gastric wall (Fig. 6), which strongly indicates the emergence of hepatoid cells from adenocarcinoma through neometaplasia or transdifferentiation. Rare cases of hepatoid adenocarcinoma, however, have no obvious adenocarcinoma components; in such cases, de novo development has not been excluded. Transition between adenocarcinoma and hepatoid cells is gradual in some cases (Fig. 7) and abrupt in others.

[1] Department of Molecular Pathology, [2] Department of General Surgery, Chiba University Graduate School of Medicine, 1-8-1 Inohana, Chuo-ku, Chiba, Japan
[3] Department of Gastroenterology and Hematology, Hokkaido University Graduate School of Medicine, Sapporo, Japan
e-mail: hishik@med.m.chiba-u.ac.jp

Hepatocellular differentiation in a hepatoid adenocarcinoma includes structural mimicry of liver tissue, for example, trabecular arrangement with sinusoid-like vasculature and formation of bile (Fig. 8), glycogen, and bile canaliculus-like structures (Fig. 9), and production of liver-specific proteins such as AFP [1,2], albumin [3,5], transferrin [2], PIVKA-II [6], and Hep-par 1 [7,8] antigens. Periodic acid-Schiff (PAS) staining-positive hyaline globules are numerous in some cases (Fig. 10). The hepatocellular phenotype in a hepatoid adenocarcinoma is determined by a collective consideration of the afore-mentioned factors; the mere presence or absence of AFP production does not necessarily characterize phenotype. Thus, not all AFP-producing gastric carcinomas are hepatoid adenocarcinoma, whereas there are many hepatoid adenocarcinomas that do not produce AFP (Fig. 11) [4]. The nonhepatoid, AFP-producing tumors include enteroblastic gastric tumors [9], medullar tumors with gastrointestinal tract-specific AFP [10], and yolk sac tumors [11]. The biological behavior of hepatoid adenocarcinomas is definitively worse than that of other types of AFP-producing gastric cancers, both clinically [4] and experimentally [12].

A striking feature exhibited by hepatoid adenocarcinoma is its invasion of vessels, usually extending to veins. This invasion can readily be seen by light microscopy as expanded veins in the gastric wall that are filled with tumor cells (Fig. 12). In addition, intravenously invading tumor cells can even be seen grossly as tumor thrombi from the serosal surface in occasional hepatoid adenocarcinoma cases (Fig. 13). Hepatoid adenocarcinoma of the stomach, therefore, is characterized by almost inevitable blood-borne metastasis to the liver, which results in an extremely poor prognosis of patients with hepatoid adenocarcinoma [4]. In a study with a limited number of cases, hepatoid adenocarcinoma metastasizes to the liver even if its invasion is limited to the submucosal layer of the gastric wall [13,14].

In rare circumstances, tumor thrombi were in direct continuity with those in the portal vein. Considering that morphology of liver metastatic foci also resembles that of hepatocellular carcinoma, the presence of portal vein thrombi that are contiguous to gastric veins causes a diagnostic problem; it is difficult to differentiate between hepatocellular carcinoma metastatic to the stomach and hepatoid adenocarcinoma metastatic to the liver [15]. Our previous study revealed that the absence of liver cirrhosis and the presence of intramucosal adenocarcinoma favor the origin of the stomach, that is, hepatoid adenocarcinoma metastatic to the liver [15]. In contrast, hepatocellular carcinoma metastatic to the stomach is characterized by the gross appearance of a gastric submucosal tumor in association with liver cirrhosis or hepatitis virus-associated hepatitis. Before the introduction of hepatoid adenocarcinoma, several case studies had concluded the former cases were rare examples of hepatocellular carcinoma metastatic to the stomach [15].

Hepatoid Adenocarcinoma as a Ubiquitously Occurring Carcinoma with Hepatocellular Transdifferentiation

Hepatoid adenocarcinoma was first described in the stomach, followed by reports of it in a variety of other organs, with gastric primaries being most common [16–19]. Extragastric hepatoid adenocarcinoma has been found in the digestive organs, including the esophagus [20,21], duodenum [22], large intestine [23], gallbladder [24], and pancreas [25]. It has also been found in the lung [26,27]. In addition, the genitourinary organs are one of the most common sites of origin; it has been described in the renal pelvis [28], urinary bladder [29], uterus [30–32], fallopian tube [33], and ovary [34–37]. In all these organs except the ovary, hepatoid adenocarcinomas almost always arise from the mucosa. Hepatoid carcinoma of the ovary was classified into the miscellaneous tumor category in the WHO classification in 2003, but the proposal that it belongs in the common epithelial category has been made by several investigators [37–39].

Hepatoid Adenocarcinoma as a Model for Transdifferentiation in Adenocarcinoma

Phenotypic microheterogeneities are well known in a variety of human and animal tumors. For example, the occurrence of argentaffin/argyrophil cells in otherwise common-type gastric adenocarcinoma cells has been shown [40]. This finding may be due to maturation or transdifferentiation of adenocarcinoma cells with a questionable clinicopathological impact; the occurrence has not clearly been related to an altered prognosis. In contrast, the emergence of transdifferentiated oat cell-type neuroendocrine tumor cells in gastric adenocarcinoma may profoundly alter the clinicopathology [41]. Similarly, the emergence of transdifferentiated hepatocellular tumor tissues in gastric adenocarcinoma has a great impact on the biology of gastric adenocarcinoma through frequent blood-borne metastases to the liver [2,4]. This biological modification seen in hepatocellular transdifferentiation in hepatoid adenocarcinoma warrants intensive study of its genesis and regulation.

Several cell lines of AFP-producing gastric cancers have been cultured [42–44]. These lines provide an opportunity to study phenotypic regulation of gastric carcinoma at the molecular level. Currently, some of them have been shown to represent hepatocellular transdifferentiation based on the production of a set of liver-specific proteins (Supriatna et al. 2005, manuscript in preparation).

Liver-Enriched Nuclear Factors, Hepatogenesis, and Hepatic Transdifferentiation in Carcinoma Cells

We showed that FU97 cells, an AFP-producing gastric adenocarcinoma cell line, produced a set of liver-specific proteins (Supriatna et al. 2005, manuscript in preparation). In addition, transcriptional factors positively regulate transcription of the AFP gene in FU97 cells, which is indicated by the fact that FU97 cells expressed the herpes simplex tymidine kinase (HSVtk) gene through the function of the AFP promoter/enhancer sequence [45]. It is probable that other genes for liver-specific proteins may also be expressed by a mechanism identical or similar to it.

Cooperative expressions of multiple master transcriptional factors have been shown in multiple organogenesis sites such as the lung [46]. In hepatogenesis, several important transcriptional factors, collectively called liver-enriched nuclear factors, exert their role on structural and functional development of the liver [47,48]. Based on the fact that transdifferentiation of adenocarcinoma toward the hepatocellular phenotype might be homologous to liver bud emergence in the primitive digestive tract at the duodenum, some of the liver-enriched nuclear factors might well be involved in the genesis of hepatoid adenocarcinoma, as suggested by the HSVtk autocidal experiment [45].

Our previous data indicated that HNF-4α mRNA is expressed in the gastric hepatoid adenocarcinoma tissues [3]. However, gastric adenocarcinoma tissues without distinctive hepatocellular transdifferentiation also expressed similar amounts of HNF-4α mRNA, indicating that this liver-enriched nuclear factor may not be the sole factor responsible for hepatic transdifferentiation in gastric carcinomas [3]. With regard to the lung, upregulation of HNF-4α mRNA was specifically seen in hepatoid adenocarcinoma but not in the normal lung and conventional lung carcinoma tissues. Furthermore, HNF-4α was specifically stained in the nuclei in the transdifferentiated but not in the conventional areas of the hepatoid adenocarcinoma of the lung, indicating an organ-specific role of liver-enriched nuclear factors in the genesis of hepatoid adenocarcinoma (Kishimito et al. 2005, manuscript in preparation).

Hepatic transdifferentiation has been shown in neoplastic and nonneoplastic rodent pancreas cells [49]. In rodent models, regenerated pancreas contained liver cells [50,51]. A recent experiment demonstrated a C/EBP-β-rendered transdifferentiation of rat pancreatic carcinoma cells into tumor cells with a hepatocellular phenotype [52]. This observation exemplifies that a single, or a few, master transcriptional protein(s) indeed have the potential to transdifferentiate tumor cells into another phenotype, in this case, into a hepatocellular phenotype. The transcriptional regulatory region of the mdr-1/p-glycoprotein gene contains a C/EBP-β site [53]. This finding adds to the possible importance of liver-enriched nuclear factors in the treatment of transdifferentiated tumor cells.

Conclusions

Hepatoid adenocarcinoma is an extrahepatic carcinoma with functionally and structurally distinctive foci of hepatocellular differentiation. The usual presence of adenocarcinoma indicates the emergence of hepatocellular transdifferentiation from adenocarcinoma cells. Hepatoid adenocarcinoma most commonly occurs in the stomach, but other gastrointestinal and genitourinary organs are also common sites of origin. Master transcriptional regulators, particularly liver-enriched nuclear factors, might be involved in the transdifferentiation process, as well as in the biology of hepatoid adenocarcinoma tissues.

References

1. Ishikura H, Fukasawa Y, Ogasawara K, et al (1985) An AFP-producing gastric carcinoma with features of hepatic differentiation. A case report. Cancer (Phila) 56:840–848
2. Ishikura H, Kirimoto K, Shamoto M, et al (1986) Hepatoid adenocarcinoma of the stomach: an analysis of seven cases. Cancer (Phila) 58:119–126
3. Yano T, Kishimoto T, Tomaru U, et al (2003) Further evidence of hepatic transdifferentiation in hepatoid adenocarcinomas of the stomach: quantitative analysis of mRNA for albumin and hepatocyte nuclear factor-4α. Pathology 35:75–78

4. Nagai E, Ueyama T, Yao T, et al (1993) Hepatoid adenocarcinoma of the stomach. A clinicopathologic and immunohistochemical analysis. Cancer (Phila) 72:1827–1835
5. Foschini MP, Baccarini P, Dal Monte PR, et al (1998) Albumin gene expression in adenocarcinomas with hepatoid differentiation. Virchows Arch 433:537–541
6. Kudo M, Takamine Y, Nakamura K, et al (1992) Des-γ-carboxy prothrombin (PIVKA-II) and α-fetoprotein-producing IIc-type early gastric cancer. Am J Gastroenterol 87:1859–1862
7. Maitra A, Murakata LA, Albores-Saavedra J (2001) Immunoreactivity for hepatocyte paraffin 1 antibody in hepatoid adenocarcinoma of the gastrointestinal tract. Am J Clin Pathol 115:689–694
8. Villari D, Caruso R, Grosso M, et al (2002) Hep Par 1 in gastric and bowel carcinomas: an immunohistochemical study. Pathology 34:423–426
9. Matsunou H, Konishi F, Jalal REA, et al (1994) Alpha-fetoprotein-producing gastric carcinoma with enteroblastic differentiation. Cancer (Phila) 73:534–540
10. Ooi A, Nakanishi I, Sakamoto N, et al (1990) Alpha-fetoprotein (AFP)-producing gastric carcinoma: is it hepatoid differentiation? Cancer (Phila) 65:1741–1747
11. Motoyama T, Aizawa K, Watanabe H, et al (1993) α-Fetoprotein producing gastric carcinomas: a comparative study of three different subtypes. Acta Pathol Jpn 43:654–661
12. Aizawa K, Motoyama T, Suzuki T, et al (1994) Different characteristics of hepatoid and nonhepatoid α-fetoprotein-producing gastric carcinomas: an experimental study using xenografted tumors. Int J Cancer 58:430–435
13. Aoyagi K, Koufuji K, Yano S, et al (2003) Alpha-fetoprotein-producing early gastric cancer: report of two cases. Kurume Med J 50:63–66
14. Tsurumachi T, Yamamoto H, Watanabe K, et al (1997) Resection of liver metastasis from alpha-fetoprotein-producing early gastric cancer: report of a case. Surg Today 27:563–566
15. Ishikura H, Kishimoto T, Andachi H, et al (1997) Gastrointestinal hepatoid adenocarcinoma: venous permeation and mimicry of hepatocellular carcinoma: a report of four cases. Histopathology (Oxf) 31:47–54
16. Kang GH, Kim YI (1998) α-Fetoprotein-producing gastric carcinoma presenting focal hepatoid differentiation in metastatic lymph nodes. Virchows Arch 432:85–87
17. Ihling C, Shaefer HE, Baumgartner U, et al (1995) Hepatoid adenocarcinoma of the stomach: a case report. Gen Diagn Pathol 141:61–65
18. Roberts CC, Colby TV, Batts KP (1997) Carcinoma of the stomach with hepatocyte differentiation (hepatoid adenocarcinoma). Mayo Clin Proc 72:1154–1160
19. Morinaga S, Takahashi Y (1996) Primary hepatocellular carcinoma and hepatoid adenocarcinoma of the stomach with liver metastasis: an unusual association. Jpn J Clin Oncol 26:258–263
20. Motoyama T, Higuchi M, Taguchi J (1995) Combined choriocarcinoma, hepatoid adenocarcinoma, small cell carcinoma and tubular adenocarcinoma in the oesophagus. Virchows Arch 427:451–454
21. Tanigawa H, Kida Y, Kuwao S, et al (2002) Hepatoid adenocarcinoma in Barrett's esophagus associated with achalasia: first case report. Pathol Int 52:141–146
22. Gardiner GW, Lajoie G, Keith R (1992) Hepatoid adenocarcinoma of the papilla of Vater. Histopathology (Oxf) 20:541–544
23. Hocking GR, Shembrey M, Hay D, et al (1995) Alpha-fetoprotein-producing adenocarcinoma of the sigmoid colon with possible hepatoid differentiation. Pathology 27:277–279
24. Nakashima H, Nagafuchi K, Satoh H, et al (2000) Hepatoid adenocarcinoma of the gallbladder. J Hepatobiliary Pancreat Surg 7:226–230
25. Yano T, Ishikura H, Wada T, et al (1999) Hepatoid adenocarcinoma of the pancreas. Histopathology (Oxf) 35:90–92
26. Ishikura H, Kanda M, Ito M, et al (1990) Hepatoid adenocarcinoma: a distinctive histological subtype of alpha-fetoprotein-producing lung carcinoma. Virchows Arch A Pathol Anat Histopathol 417:73–80

27. Arnould L, Drouot F, Fargeot P, et al (1997) Hepatoid adenocarcinoma of the lung: report of a case of an unusual α-fetoprotein-producing lung tumor. Am J Surg Pathol 21:1113–1118
28. Ishikura H, Ishiguro T, Enatsu C, et al (1991) Hepatoid adenocarcinoma of the renal pelvis producing alpha-fetoprotein of hepatic type and bile pigment. Cancer (Phila) 67:3051–3056
29. Sinard J, Macleay L Jr, Melamed J (1994) Hepatoid adenocarcinoma in the urinary bladder. Unusual localization of a newly recognized tumor type. Cancer (Phila) 73:1919–1925
30. Hoshida Y, Nagakawa T, Mano S, et al (1996) Hepatoid adenocarcinoma of the endometrium associated with alpha-fetoprotein production. Int J Gynecol Pathol 15:266–269
31. Takahashi Y, Inoue T (2003) Hepatoid carcinoma of the uterus that collided with carcinosarcoma. Pathol Int 53:323–326
32. Yoyoda H, Hirai T, Ishii E (2000) Alpha-fetoprotein producing uterine corpus carcinoma: a hepatoid adenocarcinoma of the endometrium. Pathol Int 50:847–852
33. Aoyama T, Mizuno T, Andoh K, et al (1996) α-Fetoprotein-producing (hepatoid) carcinoma of the fallopian tube. Gynecol Oncol 63:261–266
34. Ishikura H, Scully RE (1987) Hepatoid carcinoma of the ovary. A newly described tumor. Cancer (Phila) 60:2775–2784
35. Senzaki H, Kiyozuka Y, Mizuoka H, et al (1999) An autopsy case of hepatoid carcinoma of the ovary with PIVKA-II production: immunohistochemical study and literature review. Pathol Int 49:164–169
36. Badreddine J, Rabouille Y, Heron JF, et al (1993) Ovarian tumor with hepatoid differentiation. Discussion and review of the literature. Report of a case. Ann Pathol 13:37–39
37. Scurry JP, Brown RW, Jobling T (1996) Combined ovarian serous papillary and hepatoid carcinoma. Gynecol Oncol 63:138–142
38. Matsuta M, Ishikura H, Murakami K, et al (1991) Hepatoid carcinoma of the ovary: a case report. Int J Gynecol Pathol 10:302–310
39. Tochigi N, Kishimoto T, Supriatna Y, et al (2003) Hepatoid carcinoma of the ovary: a report of three cases admixed with a common surface epithelial carcinoma. Int J Gynecol Pathol 22:266–271
40. Proks C, Feit V (1982) Gastric carcinoma with argyrophil and argentaffin cells. Virchows Arch A Pathol Anat Histol 395:201–206
41. Lechago J (1994) Gastrointestinal neuroendocrine cell proliferations. Hum Pathol 25: 1114–1122
42. Nozue M, Nishida M, Todoroki T, et al (1991) Establishment and characterization of a human scirrhous type gastric cancer cell line, GCIY, producing CA19-9 (in Japanese). Hum Cell 4: 71–75
43. Matsuda M, Watanabe A, Sawada H, et al (1999) Establishment of an α-fetoprotein-producing cell line derived from gastric cancer. In Vitro Cell Dev Biol Anim 35:555–557
44. Sekiguchi M, Fujii Y, Saito A, et al (1995) Alpha-fetoprotein-producing gastric carcinoma: biological properties of a cultured cell line. J Gastroenterol 30:589–598
45. Nakaya H, Ishizu A, Ikeda H, et al (2003) In vitro model of suicide gene therapy for alpha-fetoprotein-producing gastric cancer. Anticancer Res 23:3795–3800
46. Warburton D, Wuenschell C, Flores-Delgado G, et al (1998) Commitment and differentiation of lung cell lineages. Biochem Cell Biol 76:971–995
47. Schrem H, Klempnauer J, Borlak J (2002) Liver-enriched transcription factors in liver function and development. Part I: The hepatocyte nuclear factor network and liver-specific gene expression. Pharmacol Rev 54:129–158
48. Schrem H, Klempnauer J, Borlak J (2004) Liver-enriched transcription factors in liver function and development. Part II: The C/EBPs and D site-binding protein in cell cycle control, carcinogenesis, circadian gene regulation, liver regeneration, apoptosis, and liver-specific gene regulation. Pharmacol Rev 56:291–330
49. Liu Y, Rao MS (2003) Transdifferentiation: fact or artifact. J Cell Biochem 88:29–40
50. Scarpelli DG, Rao MS (1981) Differentiation of regenerating pancreatic cells into hepatocyte-like cells. Proc Natl Acad Sci USA 78:2577–2581

51. Rao MS, Subbarao V, Scarpelli DG (1988) Development of hepatocytes in the pancreas of hamsters treated with 2,3,7,8-tetrachlorodibenzo-*p*-dioxin. J Toxicol Environ Health 25: 201–205
52. Shen CN, Horb ME, Slack JM, et al (2003) Transdifferentiation of pancreas to liver. Mech Dev 120:107–116
53. Combates NJ, Rzepka RW, Chen YN, et al (1994) NF-IL6, a member of the C/EBP family of transcription factors, binds and trans-activates the human MDR1 gene. J Biol Chem 269: 29715–29719

Color Plates

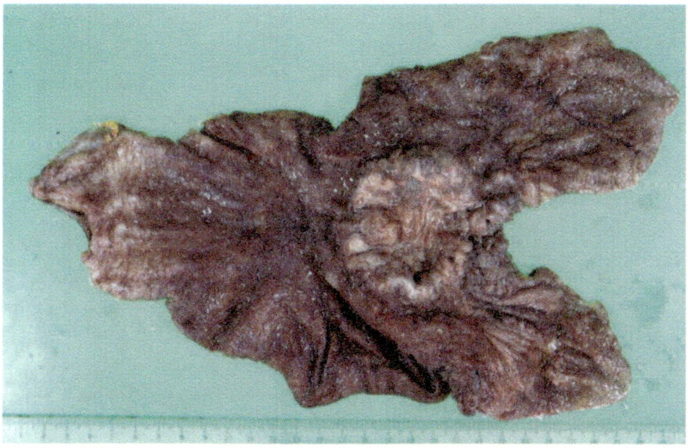

FIG. 1. Hepatoid adenocarcinoma of the stomach. A 5 × 8 cm, circumscribed mass with ulceration is seen in the body of the stomach in a 76-year-old man. Serum alpha-fetoprotein (AFP) was 7600 ng/ml

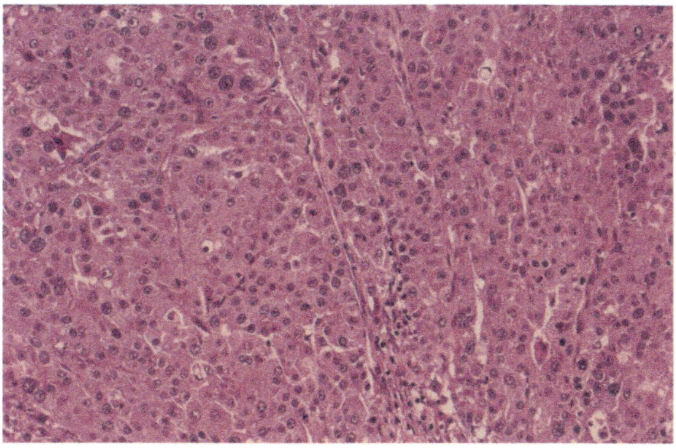

FIG. 2. Sheetlike proliferation of polygonal carcinoma cells with abundant, eosinophilic cytoplasm in a hepatoid adenocarcinoma. This pattern was once regarded as "patternless," resulting in the designation of this area as poorly differentiated or undifferentiated carcinoma. Thin networks of microvessels give an appearance of vague thick trabeculae

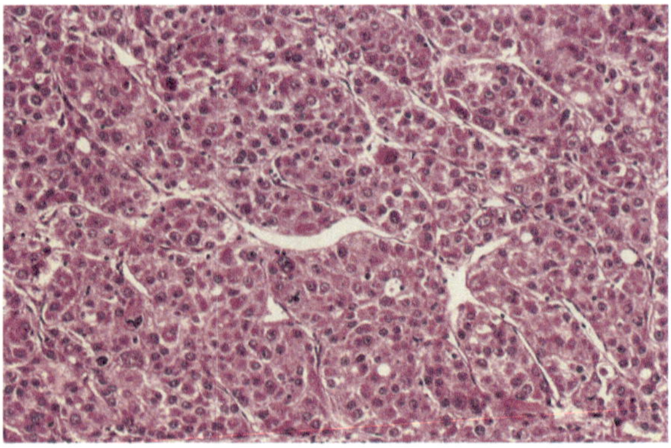

FIG. 3. Sheetlike proliferation of polygonal carcinoma cells with abundant, eosinophilic cytoplasm in a hepatoid adenocarcinoma. Anastomosing networks of capillaries are dilated in several areas, giving the appearance of a distinct middle trabecular pattern

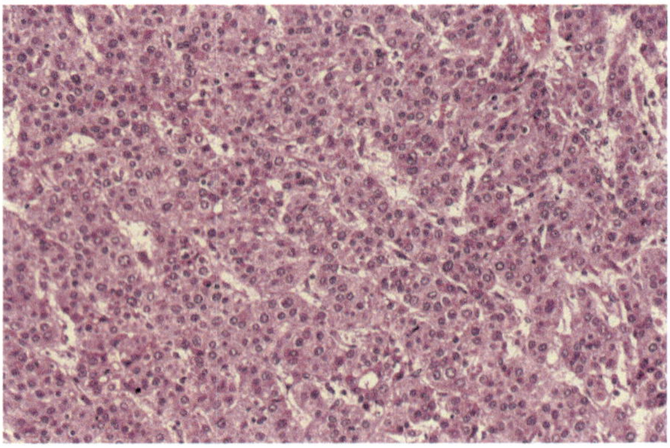

FIG. 4. Sheetlike proliferation of polygonal carcinoma cells with abundant, eosinophilic cytoplasm in a hepatoid adenocarcinoma. Capillary networks are incomplete. Middle-to-thin trabeculae are conspicuous

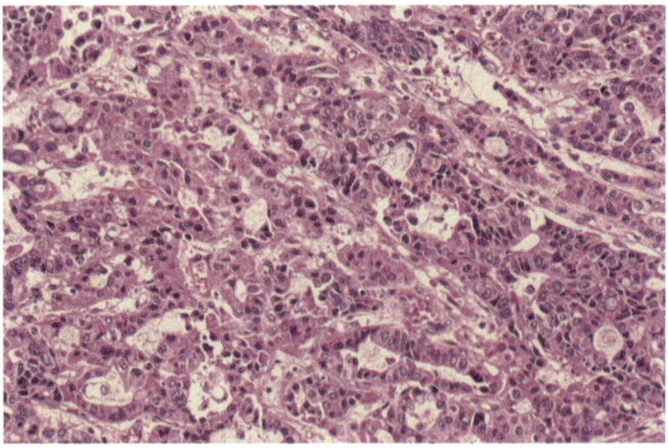

FIG. 5. Cords and sheets of hyperchromatic carcinoma cells in a hepatoid adenocarcinoma. Glandlike spaces are filled with mucin. Cytoplasm of these tumor cells is abundant and eosinophilic, giving the appearance of hepatoid cells

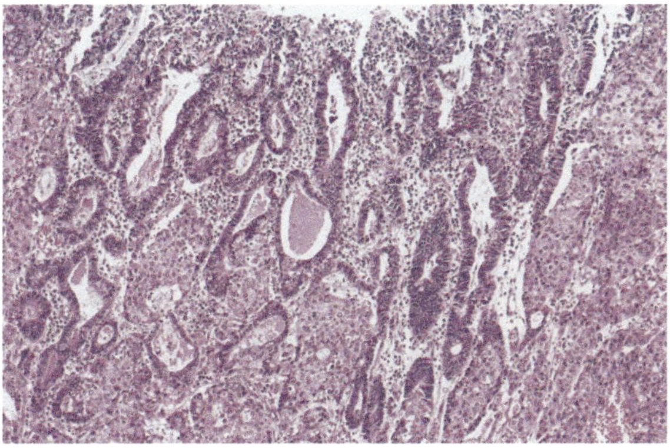

FIG. 6. Adenocarcinoma seen in the mucosal layer of a hepatoid adenocarcinoma of the stomach. Note the transition of tall, columnar, mucin-producing adenocarcinoma cells to hepatoid cells with large eosinophilic cytoplasm

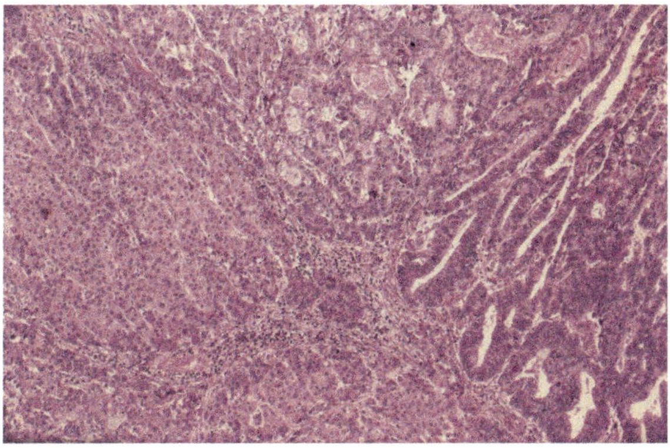

FIG. 7. Close apposition of adenocarcinoma (*right*) and hepatoid cells (*left*). There is a transition between these areas at the *middle upper portion* of the figure

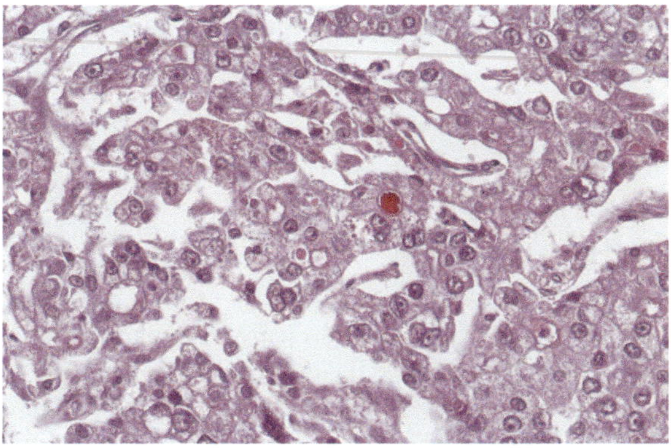

FIG. 8. Production of bile pigment in a hepatoid adenocarcinoma. Only a limited number of cases show bile production, but this finding demonstrates a clear-cut hepatocellular differentiation

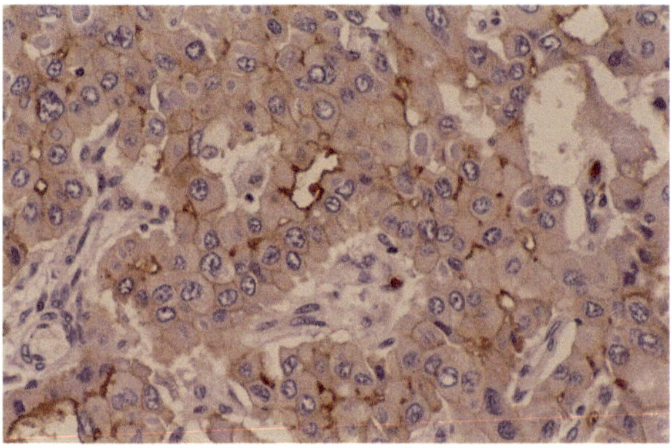

Fig. 9. Canalicular structures in a hepatoid adenocarcinoma. These structures are intermingled in the hepatoid portion, and positive for polyclonal anticarcinoembryonic antigen antibodies. Given that these antibodies cross-react with biliary glycoprotein, the morphological finding in combination with this immunohistochemical finding suggests a development of bile canaliculi in hepatoid adenocarcinoma cells, even in the absence of visible bile pigment

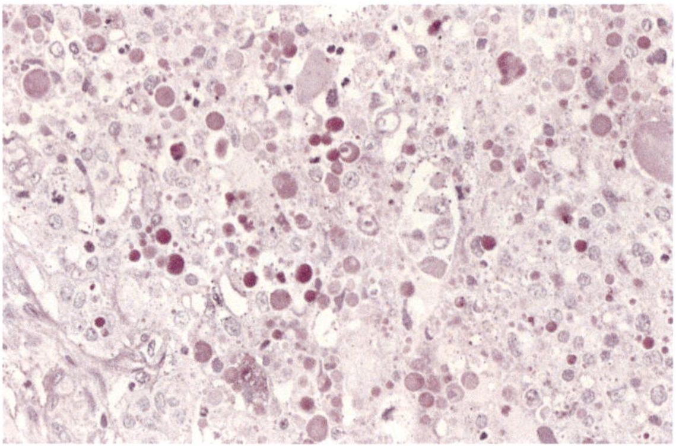

Fig. 10. Periodic acid-Schiff (PAS)-positive hyaline globules in a hepatoid adenocarcinoma

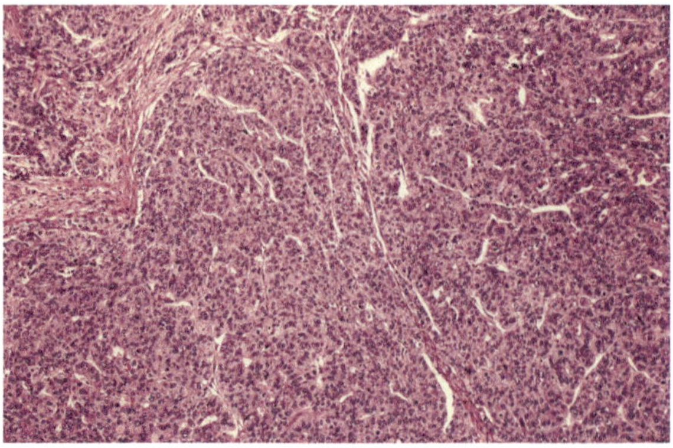

Fig. 11. Hepatoid adenocarcinoma with no obvious AFP production. There was no elevation in the patient's serum AFP level. Immunostaining for AFP was negative. Vascular permeation was extensive, and multiple liver metastases were seen. The histopathological pattern indicated a hepatoid adenocarcinoma

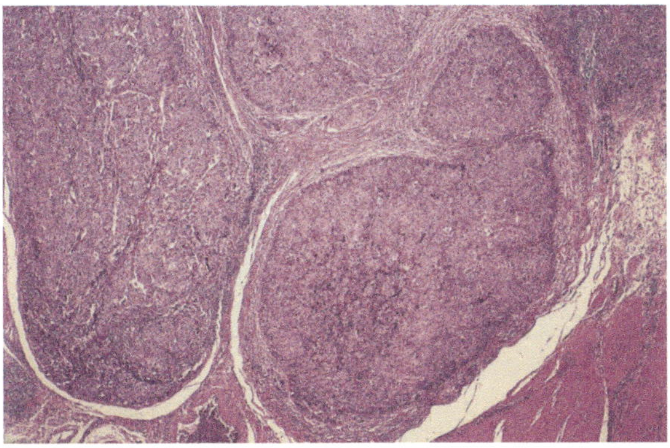

FIG. 12. Extensive vascular involvement seen in the primary gastric wall in a hepatoid adenocarcinoma

a

b

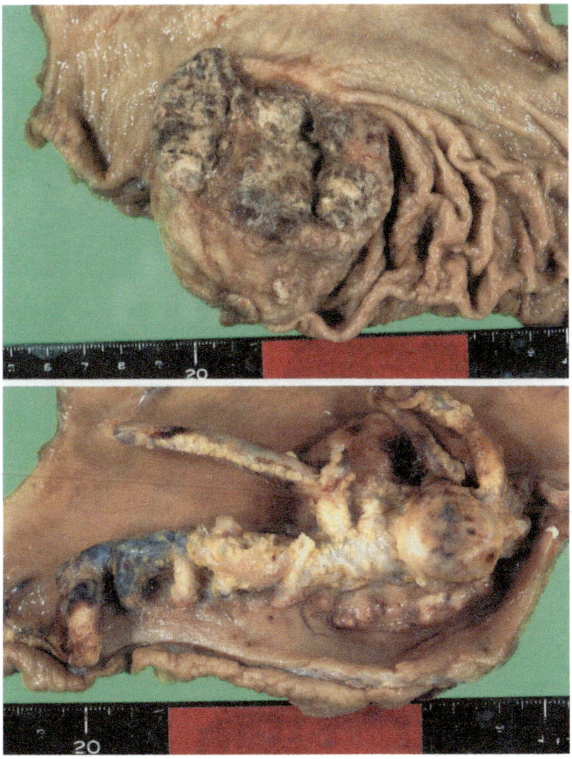

FIG. 13a,b. Gross appearance of hepatoid adenocarcinoma with wormlike tumor thrombi within veins in the gastric serosa. **a** A mucosal view of the primary gastric hepatoid adenocarcinoma. **b** A serosal view. Adipose tissues surrounding the veins were removed. Note the expanded, wormlike veins radiating from the primary site

Oncocytic Adenocarcinoma of the Stomach: Comparison with Parietal Cell Carcinoma

Kaiyo Takubo[1] and Tomio Arai[2]

Introduction

Primary adenocarcinomas of the stomach are usually divided histologically into diffuse and intestinal types [1]. However, a number of rare histologic variants have been reported, including choriocarcinoma, hepatoid carcinoma, carcinoma with lymphoid stroma (Epstein–Barr virus-related carcinoma), Paneth cell carcinoma [2], neuroendocrine carcinoma, small cell carcinoma, gastric carcinoma with rhabdoid features [3], and parietal cell carcinoma [4]. Among them, hepatoid carcinoma and carcinoma with lymphoid stroma are described elsewhere in this volume (see the chapters by H. Ishikura and J.-M. Chong). Some of these variants have been reported to have a better or worse prognoses than the usual type of adenocarcinoma.

Parietal cell carcinoma of the stomach is very rare, with only 16 cases reported to date [5–11], and is suggested to have a better prognosis than the usual type of gastric adenocarcinoma. It consists of cells with abundant eosinophilic cytoplasm that, on ultrastructural examination, have numerous mitochondria, intracytoplasmic secretory canaliculi, and cytoplasmic tubulovesicles. These histologic and ultrastructural features are considered to be very similar to those of parietal cells in the normal gastric fundic mucosa [7]. The carcinomas in the 16 reported cases showed solid sheets of rather uniform or fusiform cells with only focal glandular structures [5–11]. We have reported a category different from parietal cell carcinoma, although the morphologic features are similar.

We have described 10 well- to moderately differentiated papillotubular adenocarcinomas of the stomach with oncocytic features and compared them with the features of the 16 reported cases of parietal cell carcinoma [12]. Over the last few years we have found 4 more papillotubular adenocarcinomas with oncocytic differentiation; these differed histologically from gastric parietal cell carcinoma cells but were ultrastructurally similar to them and also to normal gastric parietal cells. However, all 14 adenocarcinomas were negative on immunostaining with four different antibodies against H^+-K^+-ATPase.

---

[1] Human Tissue Research Group, Tokyo Metropolitan Institute of Gerontology, 35-2 Sakaecho, Itabashi-ku, Tokyo 173-0015, Japan
[2] Tokyo Metropolitan Geriatric Medical Center, Tokyo, Japan
e-mail: takubo@tmig.or.jp

Incidence of Oncocytic Adenocarcinoma Among Gastric Carcinomas in Terms of Patient Age and Sex

In a previous article [12], we described 10 patients (9 male, 1 female) with well- to moderately differentiated tubular or papillotubular adenocarcinoma in which the carcinoma cells had eosinophilic, finely granular cytoplasm. These cases were encountered over an 8-year period (1993–2000) at the Department of Clinical Pathology, Tokyo Metropolitan Geriatric Medical Center, and accounted for 1.8% of a total of 554 gastric carcinomas encountered over this period. In the 2 years (2001–2002) since then, we have newly encountered 4 (2.5%) patients (all male) with gastric oncocytic carcinoma among 162 patients with gastric malignancy, making the overall incidence 14 (2.0%) of 716 patients.

The 14 patients ranged in age from 58 to 84 years (mean, 70.2 years). Four were in their eighties, 5 in their seventies, 4 in their sixties, and 1 in his fifties. Nine of the patients were treated by gastrectomy and the remaining 5, who were considered on the basis of endoscopy and endoscopic ultrasonography to have mucosal carcinomas without metastasis, were treated by laser ablation or endoscopic resection. On the basis of WHO staging, 10 patients (including the 5 treated by laser ablation or endoscopic resection) were in stage IA, 2 were in stage IB, and 2 were in stage IIIA. The 10 stage IA carcinomas were macroscopically type 0-IIa, superficial elevated type (Fig. 1) [13].

Histopathologic Findings

The intramucosal and deeply invasive portions of the 14 carcinomas were always well- to moderately differentiated tubular or papillotubular adenocarcinoma without poorly differentiated or undifferentiated areas (Fig. 2). The carcinoma cells in the mucosal components and superficially invasive portions had finely granular eosinophilic cytoplasm and round nuclei. However, in the deeply invasive portions, the carcinoma cells contained less eosinophilic cytoplasm. The carcinoma cell cytoplasm was relatively abundant. In the mucosa, the cell nuclei occasionally had very prominent nucleoli and intranuclear invaginations of cytoplasm. Cells with irregular, large nuclei with prominent nucleoli were also frequent, especially in the area near the lamina muscularis mucosae (Fig. 3). In the invasive portions, the nuclei had relatively small nucleoli. Therefore, oncocytic features were typically present in the mucosal components with invasive carcinoma or intramucosal carcinoma. Oncocytes have been described as cells with abundant, finely granular eosinophilic cytoplasm that are normally found in the salivary glands [14] and parathyroid glands [14]. Benign oncocytic tumors may arise in the salivary glands, gastrointestinal tract [15], lung, kidney, and other sites. Papotti et al. [15] have suggested the existence of a gastric neoplasm that is rich in mitochondria.

Malignant oncocytomas, although rare, are known to occur occasionally in the salivary glands, thorax, breast, pancreas, and other sites. Both neoplastic and nonneoplastic oncocytes exhibit solid and papillary-tubular architectural patterns and have oxyphilic granular cytoplasm because of the presence of numerous mitochondria in their cytoplasm. These histologic and ultrastructural features are similar to those of the carcinomas in the present study. Our carcinomas can therefore be termed oncocytic carcinomas, or carcinomas showing oncocytic differentiation.

Mucin and Lectin Histochemistry and Immunohistochemistry

A few cells in some of the carcinomas showed cytoplasmic periodic acid-Schiff (PAS) and/or alcian blue positivity but were negative for lectin by the concavalin A (Con A) method. The cells were generally also negative for Muc-2, with only a few cells in the mucosal layer staining positive, and were negative for HGM .

The normal parietal cells and the carcinoma cells near the lamina muscularis mucosae showed the most strongly positive staining with the antimitochondrial antibody MAB 1273. Chief cells and metaplastic absorptive cells were less strongly positive than carcinoma cells, whereas the gastric surface epithelium, pyloric glands and goblet cells showed much weaker staining (Fig. 4).

The normal gastric parietal cells showed strongly positive staining with all four antiparietal cell antibodies. The gastric pyloric glands, the metaplastic mucosa, and the carcinoma cells did not stain with any of the four antibodies. A micrograph of a section stained using anti-H^+-K^+-ATPase-subunit (N-terminal sequence) is shown in Fig. 5.

Ultrastructural Study

The present carcinoma cells formed tubules with microvilli on their luminal surfaces, and there were junctional complexes and desmosomes between cells. Intracytoplasmic and intercellular lumina, with many microvilli, were also seen occasionally. The nuclei had prominent and irregular nucleoli. The cytoplasm contained numerous mitochondria near the lamina muscularis mucosae (Fig. 6), while fewer mitochondria were observed in the cells in or near the mucosal surface (Fig. 7). This result was consistent with the findings of immunohistochemical mitochondrial staining.

Normal gastric parietal cells have H^+-K^+-ATPase as a proton pump. It is located mainly near free cellular membranes and the membranes of intracytoplasmic canaliculi. The normal gastric parietal cells were stained very strongly positive with four different antiparietal cell antibodies, whereas the carcinoma cells were negative. If the presence of H^+-K^+-ATPase is one of the most important features of parietal cells, then our carcinomas cannot be said to have shown parietal cell differentiation, and therefore cannot be diagnosed as parietal cell carcinomas. Amorphous secretory material was present in some intracytoplasmic canaliculi (Fig. 8), but well-developed tubulovesicles were rarely observed. If present, tubulovesicles were adjacent to cell-surface membranes.

It has been reported that intracytoplasmic canaliculi are ultrastructural markers of glandular tissue and adenocarcinoma, including gastric adenocarcinoma of the usual

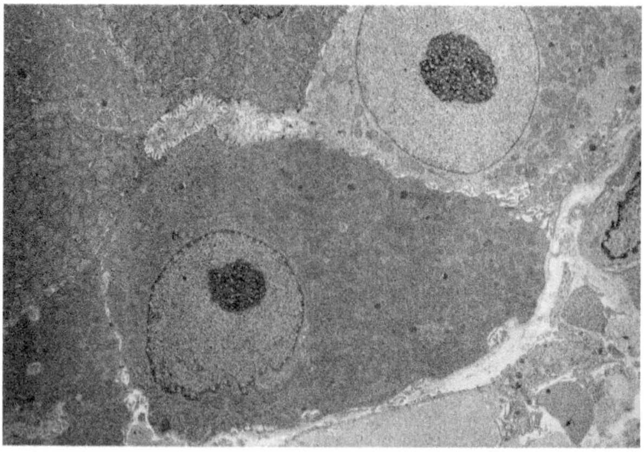

FIG. 6. Carcinoma cells near the lamina muscularis mucosae. The tumor cells have microvilli at their luminal surfaces, and there are junctional complexes with desmosomes between cells. The cells have numerous mitochondria. The nucleus has prominent and irregular nucleoli. An intercellular lumen is seen and is associated with microvilli (*left top*). There is amorphous secretory material in the lumen. ×4800

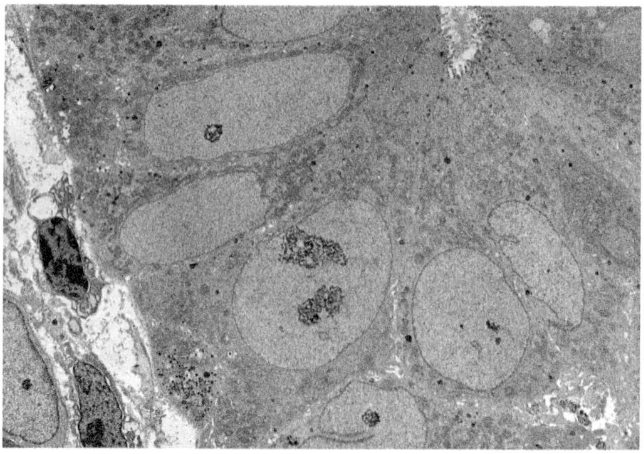

FIG. 7. The carcinoma cells in the mucosal surface layer. The tumor cells have fewer mitochondria than those near the lamina muscularis mucosae. The nucleus also has irregular nucleoli. An intercellular lumen is seen and is associated with microvilli (*right top*). There is amorphous secretory material in the lumen. ×3600

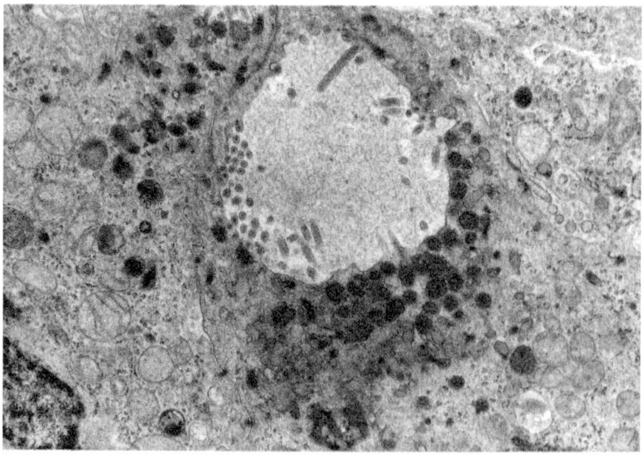

FIG. 8. An intracytoplasmic lumen is seen and is associated with long microvilli. There is amorphous secretory material in the lumen. Tubulovesicles are not observed around the intracytoplasmic lumen. ×19 000

type, but they are rare in adenomas and normal secretory cells [16]. However, the intracytoplasmic lumina seen in parietal cell carcinomas differ from those seen in gastric adenocarcinomas of the usual type and carcinomas arising at other sites [16]. The intracytoplasmic canaliculi of usual-type gastric adenocarcinomas contain electron-dense homogeneous granular material, and there is no communication between the canaliculi and the extracellular space [16]. In the carcinomas we studied, it was difficult to determine whether communication existed between the canaliculi and the extracellular space. The presence of intracytoplasmic canaliculi with microvilli, many mitochondria, and tubulovesicles, but with an absence of mucin secretory granules, is a characteristic feature of parietal cell differentiation [7,16].

Differences between Parietal Cell Carcinoma and Oncocytic Adenocarcinoma

It has been said that parietal cell carcinoma of the stomach is very rare, and indeed only 16 cases have been reported previously; however, our findings suggest that our variant may not be so rare in Japan. Previously reported cases of gastric parietal cell carcinoma were diagnosed on the basis of staining using hematoxylin and eosin (H&E), phosphotungstic acid-hematoxylin (PTAH), and Klüver–Barrera Luxol Fast Blue, and also by electron microscopy [5–11]. The PTAH and Luxol Fast Blue methods are known to stain parietal cells and other cells rich in mitochondria, including oncocytes [7].

The previously reported carcinomas diagnosed as gastric parietal cell carcinoma have been variously described as showing a diffuse, poorly differentiated, or solid pattern with a rare tubular pattern [5–8,10], a leiomyosarcoma- or leiomyoblastoma-like pattern [9,11], or spindle [11] cells. Therefore, on the basis of histology, our carcinomas may be in a different category from these parietal cell carcinomas. Parietal cell carcinoma has been reported to be generally negative on PAS and alcian blue staining, and electron microscopy has not revealed cytoplasmic mucin granules [5,6,10,11]. We observed no Con A- or HGM-positive cells in our carcinomas, and Muc-2-positive cells were very infrequent. Thus, our carcinomas did not show the mucin phenotype of normal gastric mucosa, and the intestinal mucin phenotype was observed in only a few of the cells.

The carcinomas reported previously as parietal cell carcinomas often had intracytoplasmic canaliculi and multiple mitochondria, but tubulovesicles were said to be either absent or infrequent. Capella et al. [7] described a discrete number of tubulovesicles, intermingled with mitochondria, in a small group of gastric parietal cell carcinomas.

Intracytoplasmic lumina were occasionally observed in our carcinomas, but tubulovesicles were infrequent. Intracytoplasmic lumina have been observed in oncocytic neoplasms of the pancreas. Therefore, as with the immunohistochemical findings, the ultrastructural findings of our study do not allow a diagnosis of parietal cell carcinoma or carcinoma with parietal cell differentiation, but only one of oncocytic adenocarcinoma or carcinoma with oncocytic differentiation.

We believe that the diagnosis of parietal cell carcinoma of the stomach should be based not only on histologic and ultrastructural findings but also on immunohistochemical staining using antiparietal cell antibodies. The previously reported parietal cell carcinomas could not be tested with these antibodies; they showed wide variations in their histological and ultrastructural features, and it seems doubtful that all of them showed true parietal differentiation.

Prognosis of Parietal Cell Carcinoma and Oncocytic Adenocarcinoma

All 16 parietal cell carcinomas reported to date were said to have a favorable outcome [7]. Our present 14 carcinomas were at mainly very early stages and it was thus difficult to determine whether their prognosis would have been significantly different from that of gastric adenocarcinoma of the usual type. Further investigation of the prognosis of this group of carcinomas is needed.

Conclusion

The carcinomas we have described here may constitute a different category from those reported previously as parietal cell carcinoma, but it would be of interest to stain the latter carcinomas using antiparietal cell antibodies, now that such antibodies have become available. Similar to parietal cell carcinoma, oncocytic adenocarcinoma of the stomach is an uncommon variant of gastric cancer that occurs particularly in older patients, and most cases were detected in the early stages. More needs to be learned about the clinicopathologic features of this subtype, and especially the prognosis.

References

1. Laurén P (1965) The two histological main types of gastric carcinoma: diffuse and so-called intestinal-type carcinoma. Acta Pathol Microbiol Scand 64:31–49
2. Ooi A, Nakanishi I, Itoh T, et al (1991) Predominant Paneth cell differentiation in an intestinal type gastric cancer. Pathol Res Pract 187:220–225
3. Ueyama T, Nagai E, Yao T, et al (1993) Vimentin-positive gastric carcinomas with rhabdoid features. Am J Surg Pathol 17:813–819
4. Lewin KJ, Appelmen HD (1996) Morphological variants of gastric adenocarcinoma. In: Tumors of the esophagus and stomach. Armed Forces Institute of Pathology, Washington, DC, pp 313–317
5. Barbosa AJA, Nogueira AMMF, Leite VHR, et al (1987) Parietal cell carcinoma of the stomach and Menetrier's disease. Arch Gastroenterol (Sao Paulo) 24:36–40
6. Byrne D, Holley MP, Cuschieri A (1988) Parietal cell carcinoma of the stomach: association with long-term survival after curative resection. Br J Cancer 58:85–87
7. Capella C, Frigerio B, Cornaggia M, et al (1984) Gastric parietal cell carcinoma. A newly recognized entity: light microscopic and ultrastructural features. Histopathology (Oxf) 8:813–824
8. Gaffney EF (1987) Favourable prognosis in gastric carcinoma with parietal cell differentiation. Histopathology (Oxf) 11:217–218
9. Hedenbro JL, Hägerstand I, Rychterova V (1990) Parietal cell carcinoma. A new differential diagnosis for submucosal gastric tumors. Endoscopy 22:47–48

10. Robey-Cafferty SS, Ro JY, McKee EG (1989) Gastric parietal cell carcinoma with an unusual, lymphoma-like histologic appearance: report of a case. Mod Pathol 2:536–540
11. Rychterova V, Hägerstrand I (1991) Parietal cell carcinoma of the stomach. APMIS 99:1008–1012
12. Takubo K, Honma N, Sawabe M, et al (2002) Oncocytic adenocarcinoma of the stomach: parietal cell carcinoma. Am J Surg Pathol 26:458–465
13. Japanese Research Society for Gastric Cancer (1995) Japanese classification of gastric carcinoma. Kanehara, Tokyo
14. Hamperl H (1962) Onkocyten und Onkocytome (in German with English abstract). Virchows Arch Path Anat 335:452–483
15. Papotti M, Cassoni P, Taraglio S, et al (1999) Oncocytic and oncocytoid tumors of the exocrine pancreas, liver, and gastrointestinal tract. Semin Diagn Pathol 16:126–134
16. Ghadially FN (1985) Intracellular or intracytoplasmic lumina. In: Diagnostic electron microscopy of tumours, 2nd edn. Butterworths, London, pp 92–94

Color Plates

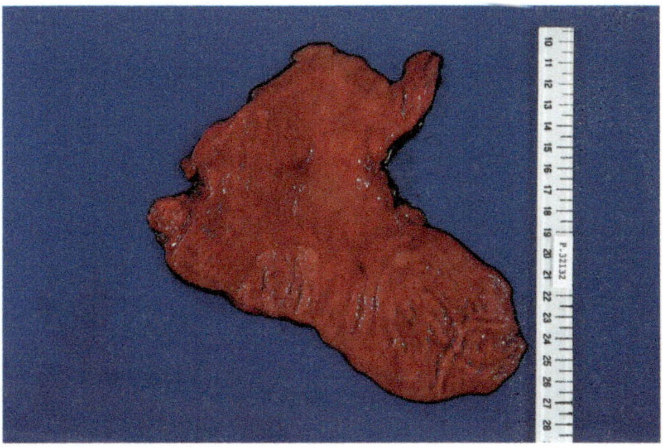

Fig. 1. Macroscopic features of an early-stage oncocytic adenocarcinoma. A slightly elevated intramucosal tumor is evident in the posterior wall of the stomach, and shows only a small focus of submucosal invasion

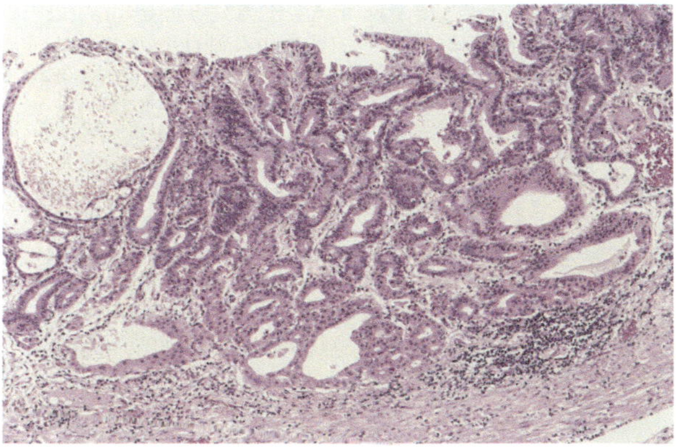

Fig. 2. Intramucosal components of oncocytic adenocarcinoma of the stomach. The carcinoma shows a tubular pattern and the cells have markedly eosinophilic cytoplasm. ×100

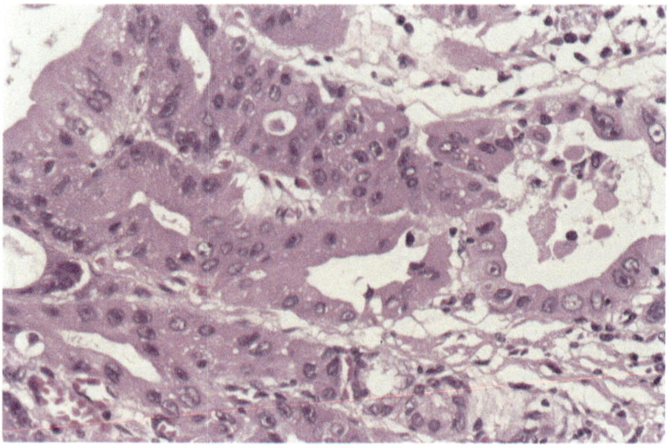

FIG. 3. Intramucosal oncocytic adenocarcinoma near the lamina muscularis mucosae. The carcinoma cells have prominently eosinophilic, finely granular cytoplasm and atypical nuclei with very prominent nucleoli. ×400

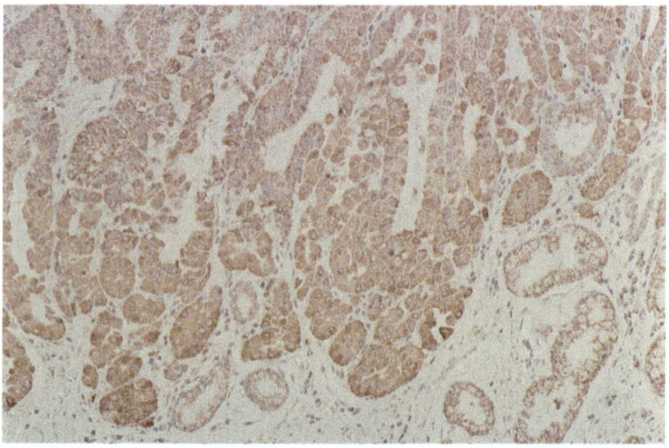

FIG. 4. The carcinoma cells near the lamina muscularis mucosae are stained strongly positive with antimitochondrial antibody MAB 1273, but the pyloric glands (*right bottom*) react much more weakly. ×200

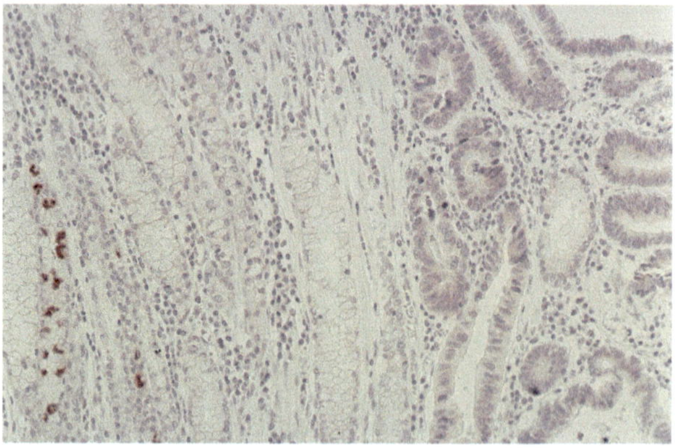

FIG. 5. Nonneoplastic parietal cells stain positively with anti-H^+-K^+-ATPase-subunit (N-terminal sequence) antibody (*right*); carcinoma cells are negative (*left*). Normal gastric parietal cells were stained strongly positive with all four different anti-H^+-K^+-ATPase-subunit (N-terminal and C-terminal) polyclonal antibodies used, whereas carcinoma cells were unstained with any of the antibodies. ×100

Gastric Carcinoma in the Elderly

Tomio Arai

Introduction

Gastric cancer is currently the second major cause of death in Japan from malignancy [1]. As such, it affects a wide range of the Japanese population, from young adults to those older than 100 years of age. Despite the diversity of ages affected, this malignancy has come to be recognized as a disease of the aged. Peak incidence of gastric cancer death occurs in men between the ages of 75 and 79 and in women between 85 and 89 years of age [1]. Moreover, elderly patients eventually make up the greatest proportion of the victims of this disease: 75.2% of the men and 78% of the women who die of gastric cancer are older than 65 years of age [1].

As the geriatric population increases in Japan, an increasing number of elderly patients are presenting with gastric cancer. This rise in patient numbers highlights the need to elucidate the characteristics of this disease particular to the elderly population. Although it is generally believed that malignancies in the elderly tend to be well differentiated with slower growth rates and less metastatic potential, there are those tumors that exhibit aggressive biological behavior and which are resistant to therapy. Analyses limited to surgical gastrectomy specimens can be misleading. The elderly are susceptible to many other sources of morbidity, such as heart failure, arteriosclerosis, cerebral infarction, and dementia. These comorbid disease states render many elderly patients, even those with early-stage cancers, poor operative candidates. Thus, when performing an analysis of clinicopathologic characteristics, unresectable and autopsy cases should be included in studies of the elderly.

In this chapter, I elaborate on the clinicopathologic features of gastric cancer among the elderly (Table 1), as well as the natural history, associated prognoses, and molecular aspects of this tumor in this age group.

Department of Pathology, Tokyo Metropolitan Geriatric Medical Center, 35-2 Sakaecho, Itabashi-ku, Tokyo 173-0015, Japan
e-mail: arai@tmig.or.jp

TABLE 1. Characteristics of gastric cancer in the elderly and the young

	Elderly	Young
Location	Predilection for lower third	Predilection for middle third
Gross features		
Early cancers	Protruding type predominant (50%)	Superficial depressed predominant (90%)
Advanced cancers	Type 2 & 3 predominant (70%)	Infiltrating type predominant (50%)
Histology		
Early cancers	Differentiated type[a] >> undifferentiated type[b]	Undifferentiated type >> differentiated type
Advanced cancers	Differentiated type ≧ undifferentiated type	Undifferentiated type >> differentiated type
Patterns of metastases	Relatively low rate of metastasis Liver metastases	Peritoneal metastases Lymph node metastases
Synchronous tumors	8%–15%	3%

[a] Differentiated-type carcinoma includes tubular adenocarcinoma and papillary adenocarcinoma

[b] Undifferentiated-type carcinoma includes poorly differentiated adenocarcinoma and signet-ring cell carcinoma

Metaplasia of Gastric Mucosa

It has been widely believed that the gastric mucosa atrophies with age, thus giving rise to the increased incidence of intestinal metaplasia among the aged. This belief has been based upon pathologic analyses of post-operative gastrectomy specimens. However, when a broader range of specimens are analyzed, the findings are markedly different. Examination of autopsy specimens reveals that intestinal metaplasia and fundic gland atrophy occur in only 40% to 50% of patients between the ages of 65 and 69 years. This percentage increases with advancing age, reaching 50% to 60% in those who are 90 years of age or older [2]. The gastric mucosa is thus well preserved in approximately half the elderly population, and the rate of intestinal metaplasia does not appear to occur on an incremental basis with aging. Atrophy and intestinal metaplasia of the gastric mucosa appear then to be pathologic phenomena unrelated to the physiological process of aging.

Anatomic Location

Gastric cancers in the elderly are localized predominantly in the lower third of the stomach [3–12]. In those patients who are 60 years of age and older, 42% to 63% of gastric carcinomas occur in the lower third of the stomach, whereas in patients less than 40 years old, only 31% to 44% of these tumors are thus located [3–14]. The predisposition of this tumor for the lower third of the stomach is even more striking in those patients 85 years and older (Fig. 1). Given these findings, the risk of carcinoma developing in this particular region of the stomach appears to increase with advancing age, particularly after patients reach the age of 85.

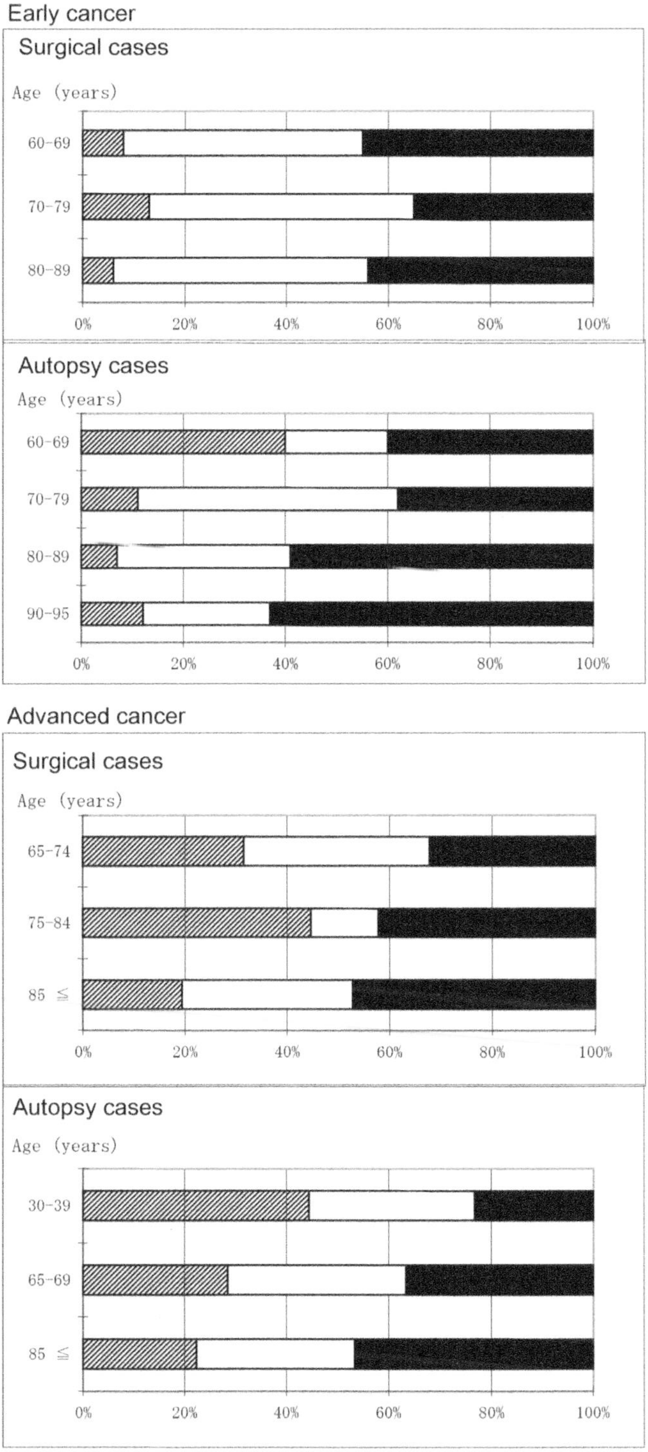

FIG. 1. Distribution of gastric carcinomas in surgical and autopsy cases. Carcinomas in the lower third of the stomach increase with advancing age. Locations within the stomach are as follows: *open rectangles with oblique lines*, upper third; *open rectangles*, middle third; *closed rectangles*, lower third. (Data from Esaki et al. [3] and Inoshita et al. [6])

Conversely, there is no clear risk pattern for gastric carcinomas involving the upper third of the stomach. Some investigators have reported that these upper third stomach cancers are more common in younger patients whereas others have found no such significant differences.

Macroscopic Appearance

The macroscopic appearance of gastric carcinoma tumors varies according to age. In the elderly patient population, the incidence of tumors of the polypoid type or superficial elevated type increases with advancing age, whereas the incidence of infiltrating type or superficial depressed type tumors decreases [6,15]. This trend is observed not only in surgical specimens but also in autopsy cases [16].

In patients younger than 40 years of age with early gastric cancers, approximately 90% have tumors of the superficial depressed type. In patients older than 65 years of age, this superficial depressed type of macroscopic appearance accounts for only 46% of gastric cancers whereas the polypoid and superficial elevated type makes up 43% of the gastric tumors in this age group [6].

In elderly patients with advanced cancers, the fungating type or ulcerative-invasive type account for 70% of tumors. Although the infiltrating type of cancer makes up a small proportion of these advanced cases among the elderly, it is by no means a rarity. In the elderly with advanced-stage tumors, up to 17.6% of surgical specimens [6], 16.6% of autopsy specimens [17], and 11.4% of unresectable cases [16] reveal tumors of the infiltrating type. Additionally, among those patients older than 85 years of age, polypoid tumors constitute 10% of the advanced cancers.

Although macroscopic appearance generally reflects a tumor's histology, there are some age-related differences. In those young patients where superficial depressed-type tumors account for the overwhelming majority of early-stage cancers, many of these tumors are signet-ring cell carcinomas or poorly differentiated adenocarcinomas [5]. However, in the elderly with early cancers, those patients with the same type of tumor often have histologically well or moderately differentiated adenocarcinomas [6].

Histology

Tumor differentiation has long been believed to be related to age, with younger patients having predominantly poorer and elderly patients having better differentiated cancers [18]. Such observations appear to hold true in early cancers. In young patients, up to 90% of early gastric cancers are poorly differentiated adenocarcinomas whereas 90% of those found in elderly patients are well differentiated [6,15].

These age-related differences are less striking in advanced cancers. Although most young patients continue to have poorly differentiated adenocarcinomas, 40% to 50% of advanced tumors among the elderly also demonstrate these more aggressive characteristics [6,15,19]. This change in distribution of histologic patterns among the elderly suggests that gastric carcinoma in this age group may develop principally as a well-differentiated tumor that then progresses to a more poorly differentiated one over time (Table 2).

TABLE 2. Histopathologic patterns of early and advanced gastric carcinomas in young and elderly patients

	Early cancer		Advanced cancer
Young patients	Well-differentiated adenocarcinoma	→	Well-differentiated adenocarcinoma
	Poorly differentiated adenocarcinoma[a]	→	Poorly differentiated adenocarcinoma
Elderly patients	Well-differentiated adenocarcinoma[b]	→ ↘	Well-differentiated adenocarcinoma
	(Poorly differentiated adenocarcinoma)[c]	→	Poorly differentiated adenocarcinoma

[a] Most young patients with gastric carcinoma have tumors that are poorly differentiated adenocarcinomas exclusive of stage

[b] Gastric cancer in the elderly may occur as a well-differentiated adenocarcinoma that progresses to a more poorly differentiated histology; these well-differentiated adenocarcinomas show increasing histological diversity with tumor growth

[c] It is postulated that poorly differentiated adenocarcinomas in the early-stage gastric cancers of the elderly are missed because of rapid tumor growth

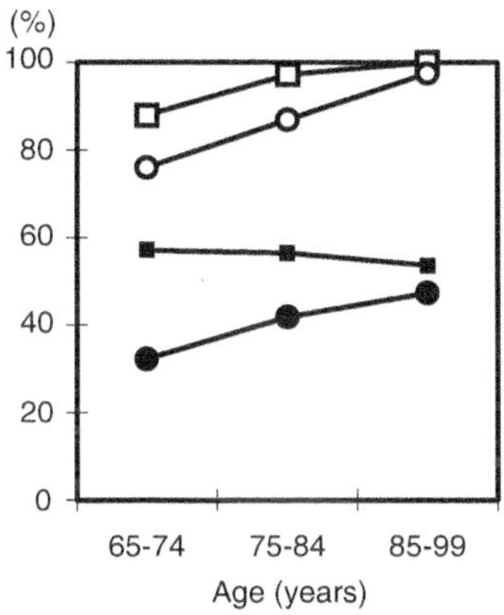

FIG. 2. Proportions of differentiated-type carcinoma of the stomach in the elderly. Note the increased proportion of differentiated-type carcinomas with advancing age in early and advanced cancers, with the exception of male advanced cancer. *Open squares*, male early cancer; *open circles*, female early cancer; *closed squares*, male advanced cancer; *closed circles*, female advanced cancer. (From Arai et al. [15], with permission)

There are two hypotheses for this progression [6]. One theorizes that gastric cancer in the elderly may initially develop as a well-differentiated type of tumor and then progress to a less well differentiated type. The other hypothesis is that early-stage, poorly differentiated types of cancers are never identified because of their rapid growth in older patients. In all cases, however, histopathologic diversity appears to increase with tumor growth in the elderly.

In both early- and advanced-stage cancers, male elderly patients have a higher proportion of differentiated-type carcinomas compared to female elderly patients (Fig. 2). The proportion of differentiated-type carcinoma increases with age, except in cases of male advanced cancers [15].

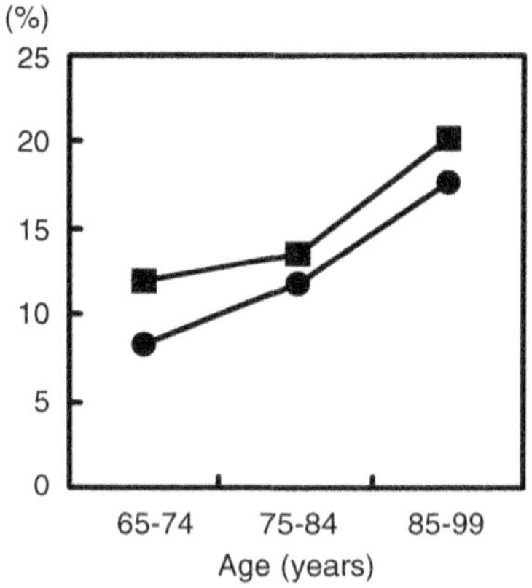

Fig. 3. Multiplicity of gastric cancers. The rate of multiple gastric cancers increases with advancing age in both sexes. *Closed squares*, males; *closed circles*, females. (From Arai et al. [15], with permission)

Multiplicity of Gastric Cancers

Across all tumor histologies, synchronous tumors tend to be more prevalent among elderly patients compared to younger patient populations. Although certain types of tumors, such as colorectal cancers, in the elderly show no predilection for increasing multiplicity with age [15,20,21], the incidence of multiple gastric cancers does increase with advancing age [9,15,22–24], particularly among the elderly population (Fig. 3). In gastric cancer, synchronous tumors occur in 8% to 15% of patients older than 65 years of age [9,15,18,22,23], whereas patients less than 40 years old have significantly fewer such tumors (2.9%) [9].

Given this propensity for synchronous lesions, clinicians and pathologists should examine the stomach carefully, taking into consideration the possibility of multiple neoplasms when searching for foci of gastric cancer in elderly patients.

Metastatic Disease

In general, differentiated-type gastric carcinomas tend to metastasize to the liver whereas undifferentiated-type tumors tend to develop peritoneal implants and lymph node metastases. Among the elderly, metastases present more often in the liver (11%–32% of metastatic cases), compared to younger patients in whom peritoneal dissemination is more frequent and liver lesions make up only 4% to 10% of metastases [9,12,13]. Interestingly enough, most reports show no significant difference in the rate of lymph node metastases between younger and elderly patients [8–10,13–15]. In those patients with end-stage gastric cancer, younger patients will more often have evidence of peritoneal and lymph node disease, and both younger and older patients have developed hepatic metastases at the same rate [25].

Unresectable Gastric Cancer

Generally, gastric cancers deemed unresectable are those tumors that have grown beyond the stomach wall and have metastasized, through hematogenous or lymphatic means or by direct extension, to other organs. In elderly patients, gastric cancer metastasizes most frequently to the liver (54%). Additionally, although peritoneal implants are less frequently found in those patients 85 years of age or older [16,25], direct invasion into the esophagus or pancreas and distant metastases to the lung or skin tend to occur more frequently with advancing age [16].

In the elderly population, however, factors other than metastatic disease may preclude surgical extirpation. Comorbidity is an important issue in this population, and many pathologically resectable cases are deemed otherwise because of diseases such as pneumonia, arteriosclerosis, cerebrovascular disease, myocardial infarction, dementia, and even other malignancies. Among patients aged 70 or older, 12% have an additional malignant neoplasms. Elderly patients may eventually succumb to these metachronous lesions even if the gastric cancer could have otherwise been cured.

Psychological and social factors also may preclude surgical therapy. Refusal by patients or their families accounts for 10% to 30% of cases where surgery was not performed, even though these patients were deemed good operative candidates. Moreover, the rate of refusal tends to increase with advancing age [16]. These psychological and social considerations may be quite important in this patient population. Although the survival rate for gastric cancer patients improves with aggressive treatment without any relation to age, there can be an unexpected decrease in the ability to perform activities of daily living (ADLs) after surgery in the elderly [16]. Consequently, the decision to proceed with gastrectomy or surgical therapy should be considered carefully in elderly patients.

Prognosis

Prognosis for elderly patients with gastric cancer is uniformly dismal. In those patients with unresectable tumors, two-thirds will survive less than a month after diagnosis, and 80% of these patients eventually die of the cancer within 2 years [16]. Even with early-stage cancers, prognosis is poor. One-year and 2-year survival rates for elderly patients are 51% and 16% to 36%, respectively [16]. Eighty percent of these elderly patients with early cancers eventually die of other causes, and 20% succumb to their tumor [16].

When compared to young and middle-aged patients, elderly patients with gastric carcinoma have poorer long-term prognoses [5,11,12,18]. The overall 5-year survival rate, inclusive of all stages of tumor, is lower in the elderly (44.6%–53.2%) compared to that in younger patients (57.1%–82.0%) [5,11,12,18]. In early gastric cancer treated with curative resection, however, survival rates do not differ between young and elderly patients [8]. Even comparing those patients who undergo curative resection, survival rates among the elderly stage for stage are poorer than those rates for their clinically equivalent younger counterparts [5,14,18]. While it is unclear what might account for the elderly patients' poorer prognoses, one possible explanation is their generally weaker host-defense status.

Molecular Aspects of Gastric Cancer in the Elderly

Several molecular alterations may play important roles in the development of gastric cancer in the elderly. Promoter methylation, for example, has been found to be present not only in tumors but also in normal tissues as an age-related and tissue-specific phenomenon that can precede the development of neoplasms [26,27]. In gastric cancers, the frequency of absent hMLH1 expression and hypermethylation increases with age [26]. In addition, gastric carcinomas with microsatellite instability tend to present as poorly differentiated adenocarcinomas in the antrum of elderly patients. These tumors display abundant T-cell infiltration and carry a relatively good prognosis [28]; they are considered to be a kind of gastric cancer counterpart of colorectal medullary-type poorly differentiated adenocarcinomas [29].

References

1. Minister's Secretariat, Statistics and Information Department (2002) Vital statistics of Japan, Vol. 3. Ministry of Health, Labour and Welfare of Japan, Tokyo, pp 384–385
2. Esaki Y, Sawabe M, Arai T, et al (1997) Autopsy findings of gastric mucosa from elderly people without gastric disease (in Japanese with English abstract). Jpn J Geriatr (Nippon Ronen Igakkai Zasshi) 34:114–119
3. Esaki Y, Yamashiro M (1981) Gastric carcinoma in the aged population (in Japanese with English abstract). Stomach Intest (I to Cho) 16:27–33
4. Ishigami S, Natsugoe S, Saihara T, et al (1997) Clinical and pathologic features of early gastric cancer in elderly patients. Hepatogastroenterology 44:1164–1168
5. Hanazaki K, Wakabayashi M, Sodeyama H, et al (1998) Surgery for gastric cancer in patients older than 80 years of age. Hepatogastroenterology 45:268–275
6. Inoshita N, Yanagisawa A, Arai T, et al (1998) Pathological characteristics of gastric carcinomas in the very old. Jpn J Cancer Res 89:1087–1092
7. Medina-Franco H, Heslin MJ, Cortes-Gonzalez R (2000) Clinicopathological characteristics of gastric carcinoma in young and elderly patients: a comparative study. Ann Surg Oncol 7:515–519
8. Fujimoto S, Takahashi M, Ohkubo H, et al (1994) Comparative clinicopathologic features of early gastric cancer in young and older patients. Surgery (St Louis) 115:516–520
9. Maehara Y, Emi Y, Tomisaki S, et al (1996) Age-related characteristics of gastric carcinoma in young and elderly patients. Cancer (Phila) 77:1774–1780
10. Wang JY, Hsieh JS, Huang CJ, et al (1996) Clinicopathologic study of advanced gastric cancer without serosal invasion in young and old patients. J Surg Oncol 63:36–40
11. Kubota H, Kotoh T, Dhar DK, et al (2000) Gastric resection in the aged (> or = 80 years) with gastric carcinoma: a multivariate analysis of prognostic factors. Aust N Z J Surg 70:254–257
12. Okuno K, Shigeoka H, Tanaka A, et al (2000) Clinicopathological evaluation of T2-gastric cancer among age groups. Hepatogastroenterology 47:1180–1182
13. Wu CW, Lo SS, Shen KH, et al (2000) Surgical mortality, survival, and quality of life after resection for gastric cancer in the elderly. World J Surg 24:465–472
14. Habu H, Endo M (1989) Gastric cancer in elderly patients: results of surgical treatment. Hepatogastroenterology 36:71–74
15. Arai T, Esaki Y, Inoshita N, et al (2004) Pathologic characteristics of gastric cancer in the elderly: a retrospective study of 994 surgical cases. Gastric Cancer 7:154–159
16. Hashimoto H, Takahashi T, Kino K, et al (1996) Clinical and pathological study of gastric cancer treated without surgery in elderly patients (in Japanese with English abstract). Jpn J Geriatr (Nippon Ronen Igakkai Zasshi) 33:518–523
17. Hashimoto H, Esaki Y, Kino K, et al (1997) Gastric cancer in the elderly—relationship between macroscopic appearance and histological type in autopsy specimens (in Japanese with English abstract). Jpn J Geriatr (Nippon Ronen Igakkai Zasshi) 34:499–504
18. Kitamura K, Yamaguchi T, Taniguchi H, et al (1996) Clinicopathological characteristics of gastric cancer in the elderly. Br J Cancer 73:798–802

19. Hermanek P, Wittekind C (1993) Histological typing and grading of gastric carcinomas. In: Nishi M, Ichikawa H, Nakajima T, et al (eds) Gastric cancer. Springer-Verlag, Tokyo, pp 40–52
20. Kimura T, Iwagaki H, Fuchimoto S, et al (1994) Synchronous colorectal carcinomas. Hepatogastroenterology 41:409–412
21. Arai T, Sawabe M, Takubo K, et al (2001) Multiple colorectal cancers in the elderly: a retrospective study of both surgical and autopsy cases. J Gastroenterol 36:748–752
22. Esaki Y, Hirokawa K, Yamashiro M (1987) Multiple gastric cancers in the aged with special reference to intramucosal cancers. Cancer (Phila) 59:560–565
23. Mitsudomi T, Watanabe A, Matsusaka T, et al (1989) A clinicopathological study of synchronous multiple gastric cancer. Br J Surg 76:237–240
24. Kitamura K, Yamaguchi T, Okamoto K, et al (1997) Clinicopathologic features of synchronous multifocal early gastric cancers. Anticancer Res 17:643–646
25. Esaki Y, Hirayama R, Hirokawa K (1990) A comparison of patterns of metastasis in gastric cancer by histologic type and age. Cancer (Phila) 65:2086–2090
26. Nakajima T, Akiyama Y, Shiraishi J, et al (2001) Age-related hypermethylation of the hMLH1 promoter in gastric cancers. Int J Cancer 94:208–211
27. Waki T, Tamura G, Tsuchiya T, et al (2002) Promoter methylation status of E-cadherin, hMLH1, and p16 genes in nonneoplastic gastric epithelia. Am J Pathol 161:399–403
28. Seruca R, Santos NR, David L, et al (1995) Sporadic gastric carcinomas with microsatellite instability display a particular clinicopathologic profile. Int J Cancer 64:32–36
29. Arai T, Esaki Y, Sawabe M, et al (2004) Hypermethylation of the hMLH1 promoter with absent hMLH1 expression in medullary-type poorly differentiated colorectal adenocarcinoma in the elderly. Mod Pathol 17:172–179

Adenocarcinoma with Gastric Mucin Phenotype

Hiroshi Yokozaki, Tadateru Hasuo, Dong Li, and Shuho Semba

Introduction

Gastric cancer is the most common cancer in many countries. The highest incidence is still observed in Japan because of the remarkable increase in the aged population over 60 years old. A comparison between Japan and other countries of the survival rates for gastric cancer patients in terms of cancer registries has revealed that survival rates in Japan are significantly higher than those in other countries because of two factors: (1) an increase in the number of early-stage patients, and (2) an increase in the number of patients who received curative resection during the first course of treatment for cancer [1].

In contrast to colorectal carcinoma, which almost always produces a relatively uniform histological picture of highly differentiated tubular adenocarcinoma, gastric carcinoma takes several histological forms, even in its early stage, and this variability in its histology increases in accordance with the advancement of intramural growth. The histological classification by Japanese Gastric Cancer Association (JGCA) [2], subdividing gastric cancer mainly into papillary, tubular, and poorly differentiated adenocarcinoma, is widely accepted in Japan. Papillary and tubular adenocarcinoma correspond to "so-called intestinal type" and poorly differentiated adenocarcinoma to "diffuse type" carcinoma according to Lauren's classification (1965), which is commonly used in the Western world [3]. Lauren's classification roughly corresponds to that of Nakamura et al. (1968) from analysis of the incipient phase of stomach cancer, in which "differentiated type" and "undifferentiated type" are equivalent to "so-called intestinal type" and "diffuse type," respectively [4]. According to the observations by Nakamura et al. as well as those by Ming (1977), it has been accepted that the "so-called intestinal type" developed on the bases of intestinal metaplasia and related intestinalized gastric mucosa, whereas "diffuse type" stomach cancer arose from proper gastric mucosa [4,5].

Division of Surgical Pathology, Department of Biomedical Informatics, Kobe University Graduate School of Medicine, 7-5-1 Kusunoki-cho, Chuo-ku, Kobe 650-0017, Japan
e-mail: hyoko@med.kobe-u.ac.jp

Parts of differentiated-type stomach cancers that developed from nonintestinalized background gastric mucosa have also been reported. Recently, efforts to classify gastric cancers according to the mucin phenotype into gastric type and intestinal type and to clarify its clinicopathological significance have been conducted mainly by Japanese researchers. Although the recent classification of World Health Organization mentions this briefly [6], the significance of this phenotypical difference, especially of the gastric type, is not well recognized in the Western world. In this chapter, historical background, definition, morphological features, and biological behavior as well as gene abnormalities of adenocarcinomas of the stomach with gastric-type mucin phenotype are introduced and overviewed.

Historical Background

According to the mucin phenotypes of gastric cancer, Tatematsu et al. have conducted extensive studies on the rat *N*-methyl-*N'*-nitro-*N*-nitrosoguanidine (MNNG) or 4-nitroquinoline 1-oxide (4-NQO) carcinogenesis model [7]. Using the paradoxical concanvalin A staining [8] and high-iron diamine-alcian blue (pH 2.5) staining for the differentiation of gastrointestinal mucin phenotypes, they demonstrated that well-differentiated adenocarcinomas consisted of a mixture of four types of cancer cells as follows: (1) surface mucous cells with sulfated and/or sialated class II mucins, (2) pyloric gland cells with sialated and/or sulfated class III mucins, (3) goblet cells with sulfated class II mucins, and (4) intestinal absorptive cells with a striated cell border. They also described that signet ring cell carcinomas, mucinous adenocarcinomas, and poorly differentiated adenocarcinomas also consisted of cells containing sulfated and/or sialated class II mucins (surface mucous cell type) or sialated and/or sulfated class III mucins (pyloric gland type). These initial findings have been further confirmed using newly developed histochemical techniques [the modified method with labeled peanut lectin, the galactose oxidase-Schiff (GOS) reaction for surface mucous cells, and the sialidase-GOS reaction for goblet cells] and immunohistochemistry for pepsinogen isozyme 1 (Pg 1) for mucous neck cells and pyloric gland cells [9]. Observations on the rat stomach carcinogenesis model have been demonstrated to be also applicable to human gastric adenocarcinomas [10,11].

The entity of gastric or foveolar type adenocarcinoma of the stomach was first proposed by Hattori (1985) from the morphological analysis of hyperplastic polyp and carcinoma arising in hyperplastic polyp of the stomach [12]. The original report described that cancer cells were tall columnar cells with periodic acid-Schiff (PAS) reaction-positive neutral mucin, resembling the normal foveolar epithelial cells, in 2 of 3 differentiated-type adenocarcinomas arising in hyperplastic polyps of the stomach. Kushima and Hattori extended their study using a significant number of endoscopically removed hyperplastic polyps and intramucosal cancers found in surgically resected stomachs [13]. Fourteen (3.3%) differentiated-type adenocarcinomas were found in 421 hyperplastic polyps. Eleven (78.6%) of 14 carcinomas in hyperplastic polyps demonstrated gastric phenotype with positive reaction to GOS and/or class III paradoxical concanavalin A staining. Among 43 intramucosal differentiated-type adenocarcinomas in surgically resected stomachs, 10 (23.2%) exhibited the gastric mucin phenotype.

Ishiguro (1987) described the histochemical and clinicopathological similarities between foveolar-type tubular adenocarcinoma and signet ring cell carcinoma of the stomach from the histological review of 377 lesions of small gastric carcinoma less than 20 mm in diameter using mucin histochemistry and suggested that the two types of carcinoma arose from common ancestral cells [14].

Definition

Markers for Gastric and Intestinal Epithelia

As mentioned previously, several specific markers have been identified and used to differentiate the gastric or intestinal epithelial phenotypes (Table 1). Among them, monoclonal antibodies to MUC5AC (clone CLH2, Novocastra Lab., Newcastle upon Tyne, UK), MUC6 (clone CLH6, Novocastra), MUC2 (Ccp58, Novocastra), and CD10 (clone 56C6, Novocastra) [15] are commonly used for the immunohistochemical differentiation of foveolar epithelium, pyloric/cardiac gland epithelium, goblet cell, and brush border of intestinal absorptive epithelium, respectively, with conventional formalin-fixed and paraffin-embedded histological specimens.

A monoclonal antibody M-GGMC-1 (clone HIK 1083, Kanto Kagaku, Tokyo, Japan) binds alpha-linked *N*-acetylglucosamine (alpha-GlcNAc), whose reaction is equivalent to that of class III paradoxical concanavalin A staining [16]. The core antigen of M-GGMC-1-reactive mucin is detected by antibody to MUC5AC [17]. The reaction of a monoclonal antibody to HGM (human gastric mucin; clone 45M1; Novocastra) [18]

TABLE 1. Markers for gastric and intestinal epithelia

Cancer type	Cell type	Marker
Gastric type	Foveolar epithelium	MUC5AC
		HGM
		GOS
	Pyloric gland epithelium	MUC6
		M-GGMC-1
		Class III paradoxical concanvalin A staining
		Pepsinogen
Intestinal type	Absorptive cell	CD10
		Sucrase
		Villin
		CAI (colon)
	Goblet cell	MUC2
		Sialidase GOS
		TKH-2
		91.1 (colon)
	Paneth cell	Lysozyme
		Defensin 5, 6

HGM, human gastric mucin; GOS, galactose oxidase Schiff; M-GGMC-1, mucin monoclonal antibody-recognizing gastric gland mucous cells; CAI, carbonic anhydrase I

is similar to that of GOS, and MUC6 is a core antigen of HGM-reactive mucin [19]. MUC2 is a core peptide of intestinal goblet cell mucin [20]. CD10, originally identified as common acute lymphoblastic leukemia antigen (CALLA), is a 100-kDa surface neutral endopeptidase that is expressed abundantly at the brush border of enterocytes and renal tubular epithelia as well as lymphoid precursor cells [21].

Subclassification of Gastric Adenocarcinomas According to the Epithelial Phenotypes

Combinations of immunoreactivities of cancer cells to the aforementioned markers are employed for the epithelial phenotyping of adenocarcinomas of the stomach. Japanese investigators have proposed the following criteria for the assessment of the results; however, the consensus criteria for the evaluation is still under discussion.

Tajima et al. subclassified gastric cancers as gastric or intestinal phenotype if more than 10% of cancer cells exhibited gastric (HGM and/or MUC6) or intestinal (CD10 and/or MUC2) marker(s), respectively [22]. Tumors were classified as gastric and intestinal mixed when more than 10% of neoplastic cells showed both gastric and intestinal markers.

On the other hand, Tsukashita et al. proposed a scoring system of MUC2, MUC5AC, MUC6, and CD10 immunoreactivity for the subclassification of the epithelial phenotype of gastric adenocarcinomas. The extent of positivity of each marker is scored according to the percentage of neoplastic cells stained; score 0, <5%; score 1, 30%–60%; score 2, 30%–60%; score 3, >60% of cancer cells show positive immunoreaction [23]. According to the sum of scores of gastric (MAC5AC and MAC6) and intestinal (MUC2 and CD10) epithelial markers, each case is phenotypically classified as either a complete intestinal phenotype, MAC5AC + MUC6 = 0 and MUC2 + CD10 ≥ 1; mixed phenotype (intestinal predominant), MAC5AC + MUC6 < MUC2 + CD10; mixed phenotype (gastric = intestinal), MAC5AC + MUC6 = MUC2 + CD10; mixed phenotype (gastric predominant), MAC5AC + MUC6 > MUC2 + CD10; completely gastric phenotype, MAC5AC + MUC6 ≥ 1 and MUC2 + CD10 = 0; nonclassified phenotype, MAC5AC + MUC6 = 0 and MUC2 + CD10 = 0. Takahasi et al. [24] used sialosyl-Tn [25] as a marker of small intestinal mucin antigen instead of MUC2.

Watanabe et al. [26] emphasized distinguishing CD10-positive intestinal-type gastric carcinomas as "small intestinal type" from MUC2-positive ones because CD10 positive colorectal cancers have been reported to show a high grade of malignancy [27].

The reported incidence of adenocarcinomas with gastric phenotype in early gastric carcinomas ranged from 24.6% to 85% depending on the criteria for the subtyping of phenotypes [13,23,26,28,29].

Morphological Characteristics

Macroscopic Features

From the review of 168 well-differentiated type early gastric carcinomas resected endoscopically, Oda et al. analyzed the epithelial phenotype using HGM, type III paradoxical concanavalin A staining, MUC2, and CD10 and reported the macroscopic features of adenocarcinomas of the stomach with gastric phenotype [30]. On endoscopic examination, tumors with gastric phenotype frequently show superficial depressed (type 0-IIc) macroscopic type (23/45, 51.1%); in addition, superficial elevated and depressed-type (type 0-IIa + IIc) tumors were found more frequently in gastric- (14/45, 31.1%) than in the gastrointestinal- (12/90, 13.3%) or intestinal-phenotype (3/33, 9.1%) cancers. Importantly, a significant number of the gastric-phenotype adenocarcinomas showed an unclear margin (55.6%) and normal mucosal color (53.3%) in contrast to the gastrointestinal- (21.1%, 21.1%) and intestinal-phenotype (9.1%, 18.2%) tumors. These findings were compatible with those reported previously [13,14,28]. From these descriptions, it is emphasized that any slight abnormality in the gastric area, abnormal barium adhesion, and granular mucosa at the margin of the lesions should be checked at the time of X-ray or endoscopic examination for the accurate diagnosis of gastric-type adenocarcinomas.

According to distribution in the stomach, Ishiguro et al. demonstrated that gastric-type adenocarcinoma had a tendency to localize at the middle portion and the anterior wall of the lower portion of the stomach in comparison with intestinal-type tumors [28]. On the other hand, Oda et al. reported that no significant difference was observed in the localization between gastric- and intestinal-type cancers [30]. Gastric-type adenocarcinomas arising in hyperplastic polyps were shown to localize preferentially at the cardia [13].

Microscopic Features

In general, gastric-type adenocarcinomas were composed of columnar cells with clear to slightly basophilic cytoplasm and well-polarized nuclei microscopically [13]. In spite of mild cellular atypia, structural atypism such as villous or papillary proliferation and retelike undefined tubular structure has been described as the histological character of gastric-type carcinomas of the stomach [13,14] (Fig. 1). In addition, Ishiguro emphasized that gastric-type adenocarcinomas change into undifferentiated-type carcinomas including signet ring cell and poorly differentiated adenocarcinomas on the basis of his observation that the frequency of undifferentiated-type carcinomas was significantly lower in the lesions of 10 mm less than those of 11 mm or more in the greatest dimension, and that gastric-type adenocarcinomas were included in all undifferentiated-type carcinomas mixed with other histological types [14]. Watanabe et al. also reported lesions morphologically identical to poorly differentiated adenocarcinoma and signet ring cell carcinoma in the lower part of minute gastric-type adenocarcinomas [31].

In terms of the histogenesis of these lesions, Tsukashita et al. reported from observation of gland-forming intramucosal neoplastic lesions of the stomach that the majority of low-grade adenoma/dysplasia strongly expressed intestinal markers in which proliferating cell zones were formed, but generally expressed no gastric markers, whereas more than 50% of high-grade adenoma/dysplasia and intramucosal carcinoma expressed gastric markers, indicating that adenocarcinomas arise de novo [23]. Moreover, Kawachi et al. examined the phenotype of minute differentiated gastric adenocarcinomas of the stomach and found that more than half the lesions less than 1.4 mm in diameter demonstrated neither gastric (HGM or M-GGMC-1) nor intestinal (CD10 or MUC2) phenotype; they concluded that differentiated-type

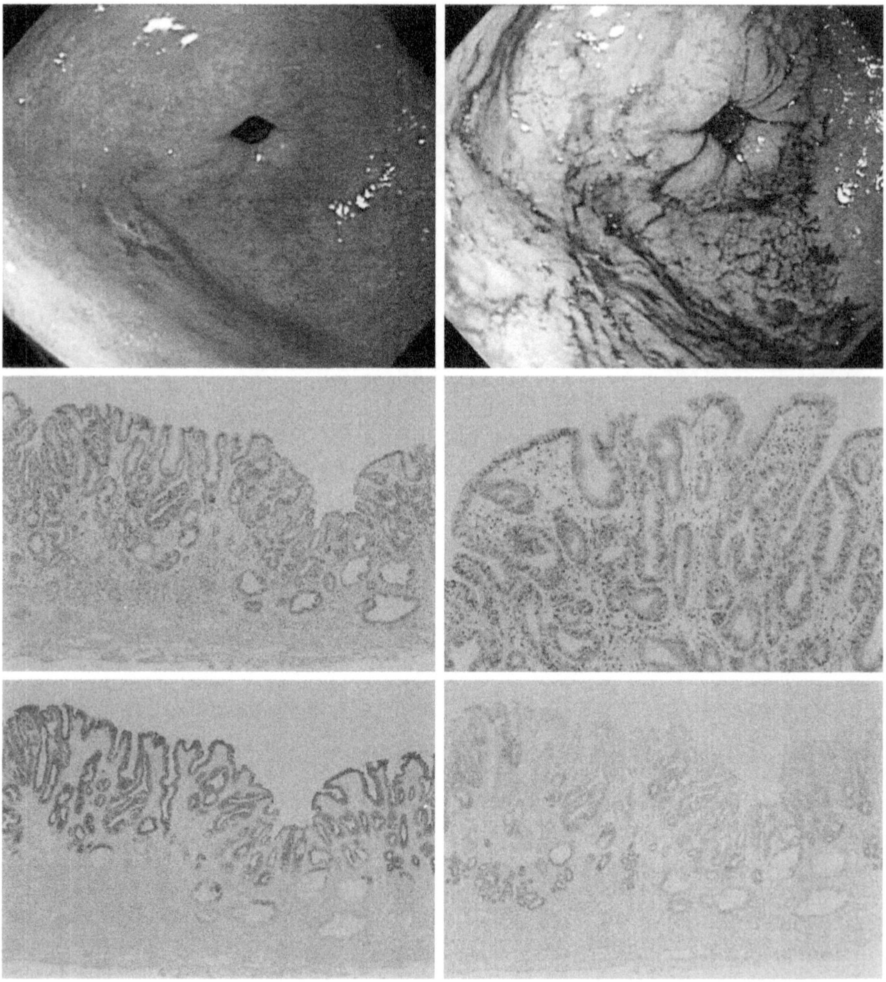

a b c d e f

Fig. 1a–f. A case of adenocarcinoma of the stomach with gastric mucin phenotype. **a** Endoscopic picture demonstrates an irregularly shaped, elevated- and depressed-type (0-IIa + IIc) lesion on the anterior wall of the antrum. This lesion has a rather normal colored surface and unclear margin. **b** Endoscopic view of the same lesion under dye spray. **c** Histological features of the lesion removed by endoscopic mucosal resection reveal a slightly elevated and depressed lesion composed of the growth of irregularly shaped atypical tubular structures in the mucosa. Hematoxylin and eosin (H&E) stain, lower magnification. **d** The tubular structures are composed of columnar epithelia with pale stained cytoplasm and rather hyperchromatic nuclei. H&E stain, higher magnification. **e** Immunohistochemical staining of MUC5AC reveals diffuse as well as strong immunoreactions in cancer cells. **f** Parts of cancer cells also show MUC6 immunoreactivity

adenocarcinomas of the stomach might arise from gastric mucosa affected by intestinal metaplasia or not, without having either gastric or intestinal phenotype [32].

The aforementioned histological characteristics of gastric-type adenocarcinomas have been mainly described on the analysis of small intramucosal carcinomas of the stomach. Tatematsu et al. [33] investigated the mucin phenotype of early and advanced adenocarcinomas of the stomach and reported that of 122 papillary and tubular adenocarcinomas, the proportion consisting mainly of intestinal-type cells increased with progression from 22.9% (early) to 41.9% (advanced). Similarly, intestinal features increased with progression from 8.3% (early) to 25.4% (advanced) in the 107 poorly differentiated adenocarcinomas, signet ring cell carcinomas, and mucinous adenocarcinomas. Moreover, the expression of sialosyl-Tn, a carbohydrate marker for intestinal epithelia, was manifested more extensively in advanced-stage gastric carcinomas [34]. A similar phenomenon was also observed in intramucosal differentiated-type adenocarcinomas of the stomach as the extension of tumor growth [29]. Therefore, it must be noted that a phenotypic shift from gastric- to intestinal-type expression occurs with progression of gastric cancer regardless of the histological type [35].

Clinicopathological Significance and Biological Behavior

Ishiguro et al. [28] summarized the clinicopathological significance of gastric-type adenocarcinomas after extensive analysis of significant number of cases as follows. (1) There is a possibility of histopathological underdiagnosis because of their cellular atypia, especially at routine biopsy interpretation. (2) They sometimes invade deeply into the gastric wall in spite of their low grade of atypism. (3) On the other hand, substantial parts of superficially spreading type gastric cancers are composed of adenocarcinomas with gastric phenotype. (4) A significant number of gastric-type tumors show unclear margin and normal mucosal color at endoscopic or macroscopic examination, making precise detection and diagnosis difficult.

To elucidate the biological behavior of gastric-type adenocarcinomas of the stomach, Ito and Takizawa subclassified 117 differentiated-type gastric adenocarcinomas with submucosal invasion Aimmunohistochemically using gastric-type (MUC5AC, MUC6) and intestinal-type (MUC2, CD10) markers into simplified gastric phenotype (sG-type, gastric phenotype > intestinal phenotype), simplified intestinal phenotype (sI-type, intestinal phenotype > gastric phenotype), and null phenotype (N-type, lacking gastric and intestinal phenotype) and investigated their relationship with histology and clinicopathological factors [36]. When these tumors were subdivided histologically into papillary and tubular adenocarcinomas, the frequency of lymph node metastasis was significantly higher in papillary adenocarcinomas (44%) than in tubular adenocarcinomas (6%). Among papillary adenocarcinomas, the frequency of lymph node metastasis was 56% and 30% in sG type and sI type, respectively. Moreover, all the sG-type papillary adenocarcinomas demonstrated lymphatic or venous invasion. Therefore, part of papillary adenocarcinoma with gastric phenotype is high-grade malignancy.

Takahashi et al. examined mucin phenotypes of 63 surgically resected carcinomas from 25 patients with early multiple gastric cancers and 39 early solitary gastric cancers [24]. A significant difference in the incidence of gastric-type cancers was found between multiple gastric cancers (59%) and solitary tumors (23%). Therefore, special clinical attention should be paid to the possibility of multiple cancers when gastric-type early carcinoma is detected.

Genetic and Epigenetic Alterations

In general, genetic and epigenetic alterations of multiple cancer-related genes and molecules are implicated in the development and progression of human gastric carcinomas [37,38]. Reactivation of telomerase, inactivation of *p53* tumor suppressor gene, overexpression of cyclin E, and reduced expression of $p27^{KIP1}$ by disorganized degradation in the proteasome are common events of both differentiated- and undifferentiated-type gastric adenocarcinomas. Inactivation of *hMLH1* mismatch repair gene by CpG hypermethylation resulting in microsatellite instability, amplification of c-*erb*B2 oncogene, inactivation of *APC* tumor suppressor gene, and K-*ras* mutations are preferentially associated with differentiated-type gastric cancer. Conversely, reduction or loss of E-cadherin and catenins by both mutation and CpG hypermethylation, K-*sam*, and c-*met* oncogene amplification are necessary for the development and progression of undifferentiated-type gastric carcinomas.

As already mentioned, K-*ras*, whose gene product p21 transduces mitogenic signals of receptor tyrosine kinases, is activated by point mutation reported to be detected in 18% (3/17) of differentiated-type gastric adenocarcinomas [39]. Kushima and Hattori investigated point mutations at codon 12 of the K-*ras* gene in 9 gastric-type, 10 intestinal-type, 10 mixed-type, and 15 undifferentiated mucosal carcinomas as well as in 10 gastric-type adenocarcinomas in hyperplastic polyps of the stomach using the dot blot hybridization technique [13]. Among them, point mutations were detected in 1 gastric-type adenocarcinoma (11%) and in 2 intestinal-type adenocarcinomas (20%), suggesting occurrence through a common genetic abnormality.

Gene *p73*, which encodes a product sharing considerable protein sequence homology with p53, has been cloned [40]. This gene maps to the subtelomeric region of chromosome 1 (1p36.33), where frequent deletions have been reported in neuroblastoma. Although p73 has a physiological function similar to that of p53 when overexpressed [41], the inactivation mechanism is somehow different from that of well-known tumor suppressor in neuroblastoma as well as other cancer cell lines. To establish the possible involvement of *p73* in human stomach carcinogenesis, Yokozaki et al. investigated the allelic status, allele-specific expression, and mutations of the gene in 95 cases of gastric adenocarcinomas [42]. Of these, 32 exhibited the heterozygous *p73* allele for the *Sty*I restriction site in exon 2. Among them, the cancer DNA of 12 revealed loss of heterozygosity (LOH) of *p73*. Interestingly, all the cancers with *p73* LOH demonstrated phenotypes of foveolar epithelium of the stomach showing positive pS2 (a stomach-specific trefoil factor [43,44]) immunoreactivity (Fig. 2). Reverse transcription-polymerase chain reaction (RT-PCR) single-strand conformation polymorphism (SSCP) analysis of *p73* heterozygous cases demonstrated not only biallelic expression of the gene but also relatively reduced expression of the affected allele in six of eight tumors with *p73* LOH. No gene mutation was detected in the remaining allele of *p73* LOH-positive cancers. These findings suggested that alterations of *p73*, including LOH and abnormal expression, might play roles in the genesis of gastric-type adenocarci-

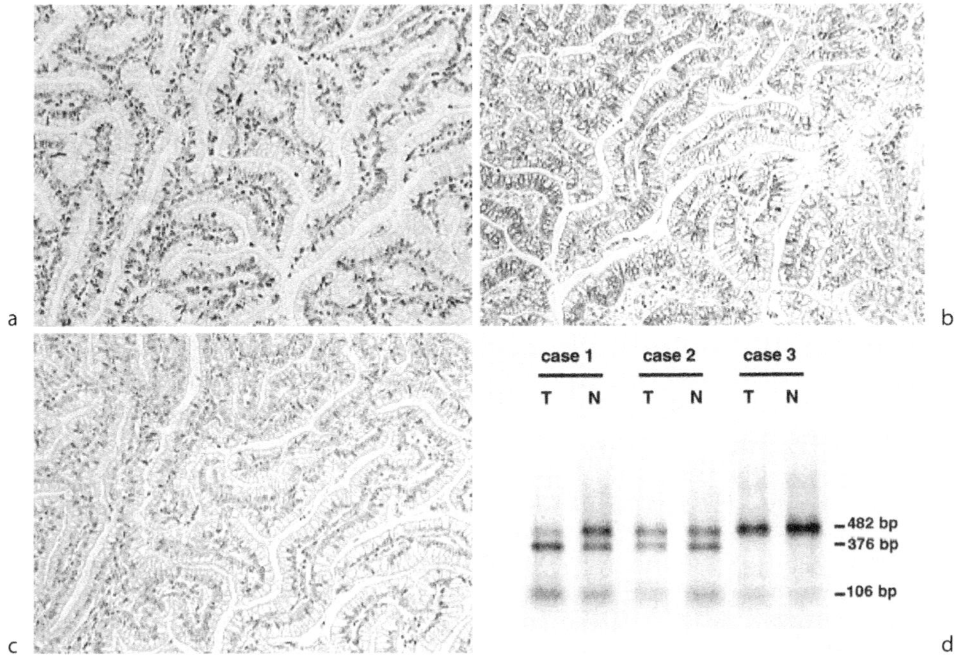

FIG. 2a–d. Gastric adenocarcinoma with *p73* loss of heterozygosity (LOH). **a** Representative histology of gastric adenocarcinoma with *p73* LOH (*case 1* in **d**). Papillary adenocarcinoma composed of cancer cells closely resembling that of foveolar epithelium of the stomach. H&E stain. **b** Immunohistochemical staining of pS2 gastric-specific trefoil factor. Strong membrane and cytoplasmic pS2 immunoreactivity is observed in cancer cells. **c** Immunohistochemical staining of p53 tumor suppressor gene product. Abnormal accumulation of p53 was not observed in cancer cells. **d** Representative polymerase chain reaction-restriction fragment length polymorphism (PCR-RFLP) analyses of *p73* G/C and A/T alleles in human gastric carcinomas. Electrophoresis of genomic PCR products including *p73* exon 2 on 1.5% agarose gel yields a 482-bp fragment. PCR products derived from A/T alleles are digested by *Sty*I and yield 376-bp and 106-bp fragments as in cases 1 and 2, whereas the amplicons from G/C alleles remain uncut as in all the cases presented. *T*, gastric carcinoma tissues; *N*, nonneoplastic mucosae. *Case 1* is *p73* heterozygous and shows LOH with the reduction of 482-bp fragments that stand for G/C alleles in cancer DNAs. *Case 2* is heterozygous with preserved alleles. *Case 3* reveals only G/C allele and was regarded as a noninformative case

nomas of the stomach, although this is not in line with the classic Knudson's "two-hit" model.

During the normal course of DNA replication, single base mismatches may result from misincorporation by polymerase and larger mismatches may result from strand slippage. The resulting mismatch is recognized by mutS homologues. In humans, optimal mismatch recognition is thought to require at lease two mutS homologues, hMSH2 and hMSH6 or hMSH2 and hMSH3. MutL homologues, hMLH1 and PMS, are then recruited to the complex and the mismatch is repaired by a process that in bacteria involves an exonuclease, helicase II, DNA polymerase III, single-strand binding protein, and DNA ligase. Mutations of the gene(s) involved in this mismatch repair (MMR) system, for example, *hMSH2* and *hMLH1*, have been found in germline DNA of patients with hereditary non-polyposis colorectal cancer (HNPCC) and in DNA from their tumors [45–48]. Microsatellites are short repeated sequences that are found interspersed throughout the genome. The repeating unit comprising a microsatellite can be as short as one or two nucleotides. These regions of the genome tend to be polymorphic or variable between different individuals. Altered length of microsatellites, called replication error (RER) or microsatellite instability (MSI), has been reported in DNA from the tumors of HNPCC patients as a consequence of the defect in the MMR system [49–51]. Mutations in the four major MMR genes, that is, *hMSH2*, *hMLH1*, *hPMS1*, and *hPMS2*, have been reported to be a quite rare event in gastric cancers with MSI. Recently, hypermethylation of *hMLH1* and loss of its expression was reported as the main mechanism of MMR deficiency in sporadic gastric carcinomas with high-frequency MSI [52–54]. Endoh et al. investigated the relationship between genetic alterations and cellular phenotypes in differentiated-type adenocarcinomas and precancerous lesions of the stomach [55]. MSI occurred in 45% of tumors with an extremely well preserved gastric foveolar phenotype (foveolar type) detected by GOS mucin staining or HGM immunoreactivity, whereas tumors with an extremely well preserved complete-type intestinal metaplastic phenotype (CIM type) having predominant sialomucin, MUC2-positive cells, and a brush border did not exhibit MSI. On the other hand, alterations of *p53* tumor suppressor gene were significantly frequent in CIM type (31%) in comparison with foveolar type (5%). From these observations the mutator pathway, characterized by MSI, is suggested to play an important role in the tumorigenesis of the foveolar type, whereas the suppressor pathway, represented by *p53* alteration, could participate in the tumorigenesis of CIM-type gastric adenocarcinomas. To clarify the significance of hMLH1 promoter hypermethylation in the development of foveolar-type well-differentiated adenocarcinomas of the stomach, Endoh et al. conducted methylation-specific PCR for the *hMLH1* promoter region [56]. Hypermethylation of *hMLH1* promoter, well correlated with the reduction of *hMLH1* immunoreactivity, was detected in 74% of the foveolar-type, 33% of the intestinal-type, and 83% of the combined-type adenocarcnomas of the stomach.

Kushima et al. examined chromosomal abnormalities in 13 cases of early well-differentiated gastric adenocarcinomas with the completely gastric phenotype using laser capture microdissection and comparative genomic hybridization [57]. Gains of 1p36-pter, 9q34-qter, 17p12-ter, 20pq, and 22q, losses of 6q and 18q, and amplification of 15q26 were frequently and commonly identified. Although most of the cancer cells showed low-grade nuclear atypia, gastric-type adenocarcinomas, even in the early stage, harbored considerable chromosomal abnormalities, as has been previously reported in advanced gastric carcinomas and cancer cell lines.

Concluding Remarks

In this section, we overviewed the present condition of the studies on adenocarcinomas of the stomach with gastric mucin phenotype. Accumulating clinical as well as pathological findings suggest that both tubular and papillary differentiated-type adenocarcinomas with gastric mucin phenotype show distinct clinicopathological behavior in contrast to those with intestinal phenotype and should be considered as a distinct pathological entity. Although differentiated-type adenocarcinomas in hyperplastic polyp also frequently show the gastric mucin phenotype, they should be separated from those that arose de novo from the point of view of biological behavior. Several investigators have tried to elucidate the genetic and epigenetic background of these carcinomas. However, the precise molecular pathway(s) of the carcinogenesis of adenocarcinomas with gastric mucin phenotype remains to be further clarified.

To make this type of gastric adenocarcinoma an internationally recognized clinicopathological entity, efforts should be spared to build a consensus criteria for the evaluation of each epithelial marker and phenotypical subclassification of adenocarcinomas of the stomach.

References

1. Hanai A, Tsukuma H, Hiyama T, et al (1997) Survival of patients with stomach cancer: results from population-based cancer registrations. In: Sugimura T, Sasako M (eds) Gastric cancer. Oxford University Press, New York, pp 22–30
2. Japanese Gastric Cancer Association (1998) Japanese Classification of Gastric Carcinoma, 2nd English edn. Gastric Cancer 1:10–24
3. Lauren P (1965) The two histological main types of gastric carcinoma: diffuse and so-called intestinal-type carcinoma. Acta Pathol Microbiol Scand 64:31–49
4. Nakamura K, Sugano H, Takagi K (1968) Carcinoma of the stomach in incipient phase: its histogenesis and histological appearances. Gann 59:251–258
5. Ming SC (1977) Gastric carcinoma. A pathobiological classification. Cancer (Phila) 39: 2475–2485
6. Fenoglio-Preiser C, Carneiro F, Correa P, et al (2000) Gastric carcinoma. In: Hamilton SR, Aaltonen LA (eds) World Health Organization classification of tumours. Pathology & genetics. Tumours of the digestive system. IARC Press, Lyon, pp 39–52
7. Tatematsu M, Katsuyama T, Fukushima S, et al (1980) Mucin histochemistry by paradoxical concanavalin A staining in experimental gastric cancers induced in Wistar rats by *N*-methyl-*N′*-nitro-*N*-nitrosoguanidine or 4-nitroquinoline 1-oxide. J Natl Cancer Inst 64:835–843
8. Katsuyama T, Spicer SS (1978) Histochemical differentiation of complex carbohydrates with variants of the concanavalin A-horseradish peroxidase method. J Histochem Cytochem 26: 233–250
9. Tatematsu M, Katsuyama T, Furihata C, et al (1990) Cellular differentiation and histogenesis of rat glandular stomach cancers. Jpn J Cancer Res 81:760–767
10. Tatematsu M, Furihata C, Katsuyama T, et al (1986) Gastric and intestinal phenotypic expressions of human signet ring cell carcinomas revealed by their biochemistry, mucin histochemistry, and ultrastructure. Cancer Res 46:4866–4872
11. Tatematsu M, Iwata H, Ichinose M, et al (1993) Markers of surface mucous cell type human gastric cancer cells: galactose oxidase-Schiff reactive mucins, monoclonal antibody SH-9 reactive mucins and cathepsin E. Acta Pathol Jpn 43:500–506
12. Hattori T (1985) Morphological range of hyperplastic polyps and carcinomas arising in hyperplastic polyps of the stomach. J Clin Pathol 38:622–630
13. Kushima R, Hattori T (1993) Histogenesis and characteristics of gastric-type adenocarcinomas in the stomach. J Cancer Res Clin Oncol 120:103–111
14. Ishiguro S (1987) Histological significance of foveolar type tubular adenocarcinoma of the stomach (in Japanese with English abstract). Osakadaigaku Igaku Zasshi 39:507–515
15. McIntosh GG, Lodge AJ, Watson P, et al (1999) NCL-CD10-270: a new monoclonal antibody recognizing CD10 in paraffin-embedded tissue. Am J Pathol 154:77–82

16. Nakamura N, Ota H, Katsuyama T, et al (1998) Histochemical reactivity of normal, metaplastic, and neoplastic tissues to alpha-linked *N*-acetylglucosamine residue-specific monoclonal antibody HIK1083. J Histochem Cytochem 46:793–801
17. Reis CA, David L, Nielsen PA, et al (1997) Immunohistochemical study of MUC5AC expression in human gastric carcinomas using a novel monoclonal antibody. Loss of a novel mucin-like epithelial glycoprotein in oral and cervical squamous cell carcinomas. Int J Cancer (Phila) 74:112–121
18. Bara J, Gautier R, Mouradian P, et al (1991) Oncofetal mucin M1 epitope family: characterization and expression during colonic carcinogenesis. Int J Cancer 47:304–310
19. Toribara NW, Roberton AM, Ho SB, et al (1993) Human gastric mucin. Identification of a unique species by expression cloning. J Biol Chem 268:5879–5885
20. Xing PX, Prenzoska J, Layton GT, et al (1992) Second-generation monoclonal antibodies to intestinal MUC2 peptide reactive with colon cancer. J Natl Cancer Inst 84:699–703
21. LeBien TW, McCormack RT (1989) The common acute lymphoblastic leukemia antigen (CD10)—emancipation from a functional enigma. Blood 73:625–635
22. Tajima Y, Shimoda T, Nakanishi Y, et al (2001) Gastric and intestinal phenotypic marker expression in gastric carcinomas and its prognostic significance: immunohistochemical analysis of 136 lesions. Oncology 61:212–220
23. Tsukashita S, Kushima R, Bamba M, et al (2001) MUC gene expression and histogenesis of adenocarcinoma of the stomach. Int J Cancer 94:166–170
24. Takahashi H, Endo T, Yamashita K, et al (2002) Mucin phenotype and microsatellite instability in early multiple gastric cancers. Int J Cancer 100:419–424
25. Pinczower GD, Williams RP, Gianello RD, et al (1996) Characterisation of the tumour-associated carbohydrate epitope recognised by monoclonal antibody 4D3. Int J Cancer 66:636–644
26. Watanabe G, Watanabe H, Ajioka Y, et al (2003) Well-differentiated type adenocarcinomas of gastric mucin phenotype transform into intestinal type carcinomas (in Japanese with English abstract). I To Cho 38:693–700
27. Yao T, Tsutsumi S, Akaiwa Y, et al (2001) Phenotypic expression of colorectal adenocarcinomas with reference to tumor development and biological behavior. Jpn J Cancer Res 92:755–761
28. Ishiguro S, Tsuji N, Terao T, et al (1995) Histological characteristics of differentiated type gastric carcinoma (in Japanese). Byori To Rinsyo 13:10–17
29. Egashira Y, Shimoda T, Ikegami M (1999) Mucin histochemical analysis of minute gastric differentiated adenocarcinoma. Pathol Int 49:55–61
30. Oda I, Gotoda T, Hasuike N, et al (2003) Endoscopic features of differentiated-type early gastric carcinoma with gastric mucin phenotype (in Japanese with English abstract). I To Cho 38:684–690
31. Watanabe H, Kato N, Fuchigami T, et al (1992) Natural history of gastric carcinoma from analysis of microcarcinoma (in Japanese with English abstract). I To Cho 27:59–67
32. Kawachi H, Takizawa T, Eishi Y, et al (2003) Absence of either gastric or intestinal phenotype in microscopic differentiated gastric carcinomas. J Pathol 199:436–446
33. Tatematsu M, Hasegawa R, Ogawa K, et al (1992) Histogenesis of human stomach cancers based on assessment of differentiation. J Clin Gastroenterol 14 (suppl)1:S1–S7
34. Kushima R, Jancic S, Hattori T (1993) Association between expression of sialosyl-Tn antigen and intestinalization of gastric carcinomas. Int J Cancer 55:904–908
35. Hattori T, Kushima R (2001) Das gastral differenzierte Magenadenokarzinom (in German). Pathologe 22:97–104
36. Ito E, Takizawa T (2003) Differentiated adenocarcinoma of the gastric and intestinal phenotype. Histological appearance and biological behavior. I To Cho 38:701–706
37. Tahara E (1993) Molecular mechanism of stomach carcinogenesis. J Cancer Res Clin Oncol 119:265–272
38. Yokozaki H, Yasui W, Tahara E (2001) Genetic and epigenetic changes in stomach cancer. Int Rev Cytol 204:49–95

39. Kihana T, Tsuda H, Hirota T, et al (1991) Point mutation of c-Ki-*ras* oncogene in gastric adenoma and adenocarcinoma with tubular differentiation. Jpn J Cancer Res 82:308–314
40. Kaghad M, Bonnet H, Yang A, et al (1997) Monoallelically expressed gene related to *p53* at 1p36, a region frequently deleted in neuroblastoma and other human cancers. Cell 90: 809–819
41. Jost CA, Marin MC, Kaelin WG Jr (1997) p73 is a human p53-related protein that can induce apoptosis. Nature (Lond) 389:191–194
42. Yokozaki H, Shitara Y, Fujimoto J, et al (1999) Alterations of *p73* preferentially occur in gastric adenocarcinomas with foveolar epithelial phenotype. Int J Cancer 83:192–196
43. Lefebvre O, Chenard MP, Masson R, et al (1996) Gastric mucosa abnormalities and tumorigenesis in mice lacking the pS2 trefoil protein. Science 274:259–262
44. Machado JC, Nogueira AM, Carneiro F, et al (2000) Gastric carcinoma exhibits distinct types of cell differentiation: an immunohistochemical study of trefoil peptides (TFF1 and TFF2) and mucins (MUC1, MUC2, MUC5AC, and MUC6). J Pathol 190:437–443
45. Fishel R, Lescoe MK, Rao MR, et al (1993) The human mutator gene homolog *MSH2* and its association with hereditary nonpolyposis colon cancer. Cell 75:1027–1038
46. Leach FS, Nicolaides NC, Papadopoulos N, et al (1993) Mutations of a *mutS* homolog in hereditary nonpolyposis colorectal cancer. Cell 75:1215–1225
47. Bronner CE, Baker SM, Morrison PT, et al (1994) Mutation in the DNA mismatch repair gene homologue *hMLH1* is associated with hereditary non-polyposis colon cancer. Nature (Lond) 368:258–261
48. Papadopoulos N, Nicolaides NC, Wei YF, et al (1994) Mutation of a *mutL* homolog in hereditary colon cancer. Science 263:1625–1629
49. Aaltonen LA, Peltomaki P, Leach FS, et al (1993) Clues to the pathogenesis of familial colorectal cancer. Science 260:812–816
50. Ionov Y, Peinado MA, Malkhosyan S, et al (1993) Ubiquitous somatic mutations in simple repeated sequences reveal a new mechanism for colonic carcinogenesis. Nature (Lond) 363: 558–561
51. Thibodeau SN, Bren G, Schaid D (1993) Microsatellite instability in cancer of the proximal colon. Science 260:816–819
52. Fleisher AS, Esteller M, Wang S, et al (1999) Hypermethylation of the *hMLH1* gene promoter in human gastric cancers with microsatellite instability. Cancer Res 59:1090–1095
53. Leung SY, Yuen ST, Chung LP, et al (1999) *hMLH1* promoter methylation and lack of hMLH1 expression in sporadic gastric carcinomas with high-frequency microsatellite instability. Cancer Res 59:159–164
54. Toyota M, Ahuja N, Suzuki H, et al (1999) Aberrant methylation in gastric cancer associated with the CpG island methylator phenotype. Cancer Res 59:5438–5442
55. Endoh Y, Sakata K, Tamura G, et al (2000) Cellular phenotypes of differentiated-type adenocarcinomas and precancerous lesions of the stomach are dependent on the genetic pathways. J Pathol 191:257–263
56. Endoh Y, Tamura G, Ajioka Y, et al (2000) Frequent hypermethylation of the *hMLH1* gene promoter in differentiated-type tumors of the stomach with the gastric foveolar phenotype. Am J Pathol 157:717–722
57. Kushima R, Mukaisho K, Tsukashita S, et al (2003) Molecular biological characteristics of early stomach adenocarcinoma of the completely gastric phenotype revealed by laser capture microdissection and comparative genomic hybridization (in Japanese with English abstract). I To Cho 38:707–721

Part 4

Clinical Diagnosis

Endoscopic Diagnosis of Gastric Carcinoma

KATSUHIKO IWAKIRI, YOSHINORI HAYASHI, and CHOITSU SAKAMOTO

Introduction

In Japan, gastric cancer has been the most common cause of death due to cancer. The prognosis of gastric cancer is closely related to the depth of invasion. A new endoscopic classification of early gastric cancer (EGC) was proposed by the Japan Gastroenterological Endoscopy Society in 1962 [1]. EGC was defined by invasion limited to the mucosa and the submucosal layer, irrespective of lymph node involvement [1]. The 5-year survival rate after surgical resection has been very high in patients with EGC; thus, it has become clear that early detection of gastric cancer is an important factor in contributing to any reduction in mortality [2].

Many EGCs are removed by endoscopic mucosal resection (EMR) because endoscopic surgery has improved markedly during the past 10 years. In the Gastric Cancer Treatment Guidelines of the Japanese Gastric Cancer Association [3], the type of gastric cancer amenable to endoscopic treatment is defined as a differentiated, macroscopically diagnosed mucosal cancer 2 cm or less in diameter, and of a protrusion type. In contrast, depressed-type EGC is defined as a differentiated, macroscopically diagnosed mucosal cancer 2 cm or less in diameter without ulcerative findings. To evaluate the indication for EMR and to determine the range of resection, it is important to determine an accurate depth of invasion and the range of the lesion. For this reason, endoscopic diagnosis of EGC has become increasingly significant.

According to the macroscopic classification of gastric cancer (Fig. 1) by the Japanese Gastric Cancer Association [4], Type 0 IIc is the most common type of EGC in Japan [1]. This report relates the characteristic endoscopic findings of EGC to the depth of invasion in 109 patients with Type 0 IIc or Type 0 IIc + III EGC, all of whom were diagnosed by surgical resection in our hospital.

Third Department of Internal Medicine, Nippon Medical School, 1-1-5 Sendagi, Bunkyo-ku, Tokyo 113-8603, Japan
e-mail: k-iwa@nms.ac.jp

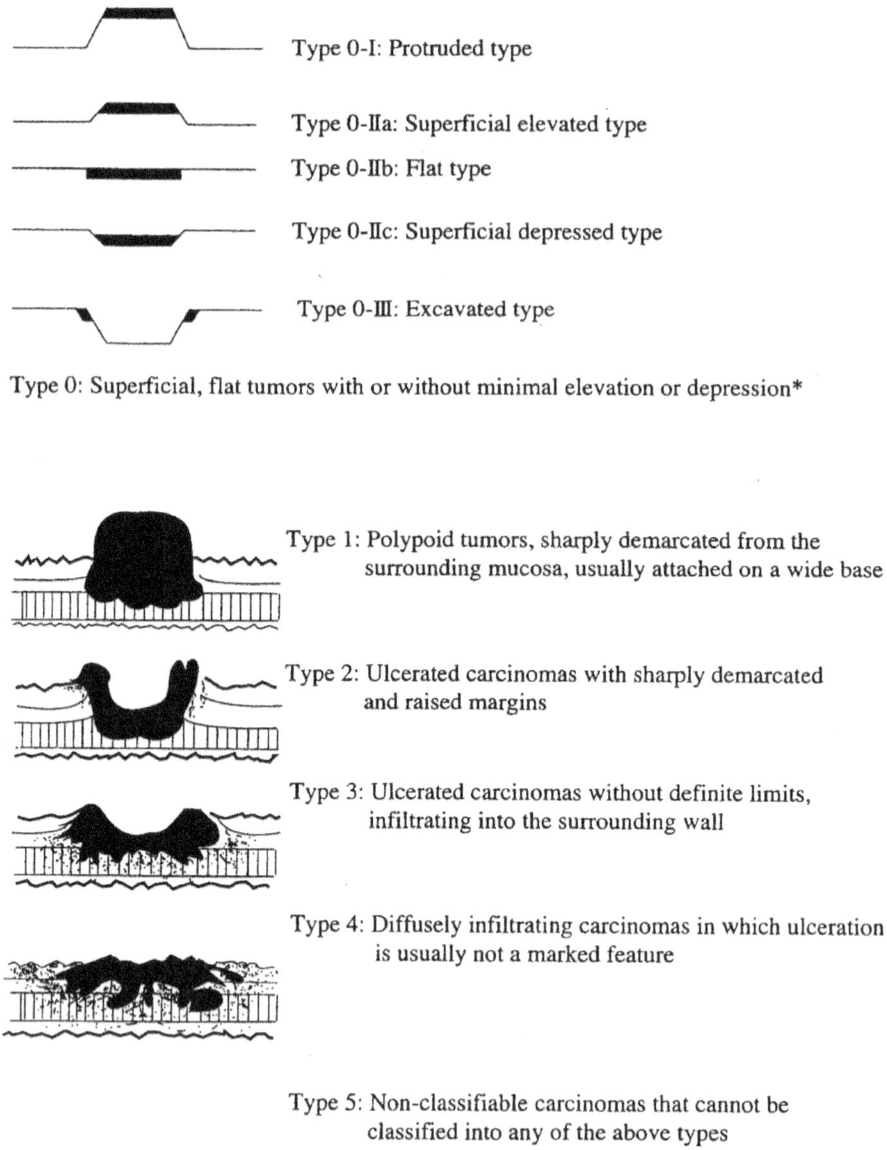

FIG. 1. Macroscopic classification of gastric cancer (Japanese Gastric Cancer Association 2004 [4]). Many early gastric cancers show combined types, e.g., a shallow depression and an ulceration, IIc + III, or a shallow depression and an elevation, IIc + IIa. In the combined types, the type occupying the larger area should be described first, followed by the next type. The definitions of Type 0 I and Type IIa should be as follows. Type 0 I: the lesion has a thickness of more than twice that of the normal mucosa; Type 0 IIa: the lesion has a thickness of twice or less that of the normal mucosa

Characteristic Findings of Superficial Depressed-Type EGC

The subjects of the study were 109 patients with Type 0 IIc or Type 0 IIc + III EGC diagnosed by surgical resection. All patients with superficial depressed-type EGC (Type 0 IIc or Type 0 IIc + III) had a clearly demarcated shallow depression.

Selected Items

The appearance of the overlying mucosa and the demarcation of the depressed area were investigated. Characteristics of the overlying mucosa included (1) surface structure, (2) change in color, (3) thin white coating within the depressed area without ulceration, (4) bleeding, and (5) protrusion in the depressed area. Characteristics of the demarcation area included (1) the area of demarcation between the lesion and the surrounding mucosa, (2) encroachment, (3) marginal elevation, and (4) change in the fold.

The surface structure (Fig. 2) was classified into the following four categories: generally amorphous, partially amorphous, irregular uneven structure, and no change. In addition, colors of the depressed area (Fig. 3) were classified into the following four categories: red, pale, variegated color, and no change. The presence or absence of protrusion (Fig. 4), a thin white coating, and bleeding in the depressed area were investigated. Furthermore, elevation of the whole lesional area also was investigated.

The area of demarcation between the lesion and the surrounding mucosa was classified into three categories: well-demarcated, partially demarcated, and ill-demarcated. Encroachment (Fig. 5) was defined as an irregular sawtooth pattern at the demarcation of the depressed area, including the tip of the fold. The overall marginal elevation of the surrounding mucosa also was investigated. When fold convergence was observed, we evaluated for tapering (Fig. 6), abrupt cessation (Fig. 7), clubbing (Fig. 8), or fusion (Fig. 9) of the folds.

Analysis Methods

Four Board-certified fellows of the Japan Gastroenterological Endoscopy Society (K.I., A.K., Y.H., and M.K.) reviewed the endoscopic photographs obtained on conventional and dye endoscopy and evaluated these for the aforementioned characteristics. An item was judged to be present if findings were obtained on either conventional or dye endoscopy. Data were statistically analyzed using the chi square test.

Results

Findings in Patients with Superficial Depressed-Type (Type 0 IIc) EGC

Findings frequently seen included encroachment, a change in the surface structure, a change in color, abrupt cessation, and tapering of the fold (Table 1). To detect a super-

TABLE 1. Endoscopic findings in 109 patients with Type 0 IIc early gastric cancer

Surface structure in depressed area		
Generally amorphous	13/109	109/109 (100%)
Partially amorphous	47/109	
Irregular, uneven structure	49/109	
No change	0/109	
Change in color in depressed area		
Red	53/109	99/109 (90.8%)
Pale	24/109	
Variegated	22/109	
No change	10/109	
Thin white coating in depressed area		
Positive	24/109 (22.0%)	
Negative	85/109	
Bleeding in depressed area		
Positive	18/109 (16.5%)	
Negative	91/109	
Protrusion in the depressed area		
Positive	25/109 (22.9%)	
Negative	84/109	
Demarcation between the depressed area and surrounding mucosa		
Well-demarcated	55/109	
Partially demarcated	49/109	
Ill-demarcated	5/109	
Encroachment		
Positive	73/109 (67.0%)	
Negative	36/109	
Overall marginal elevation of surrounding mucosa		
Positive	28/109 (25.7%)	
Negative	81/109	
Convergence fold		
Positive	52/109 (47.7%)	
Negative	57/109	
Change in the fold		
Tapering	25/52 (48.1%)	
Abrupt cessation	44/52 (84.6%)	
Clubbing	17/52 (32.7%)	
Fusion	4/52 (7.7%)	

ficial depressed-type EGC, it is important to be aware of the change in color because superficial depressed-type EGC lesions are almost always associated with a change in color to red, pale, or variegated. In case where a change in color is noticed, it is necessary to confirm whether or not there is a depressed lesion in the area of the change in color by inflating and deflating the stomach. A depressed lesion can be located easily by spraying dye on the area that has changed color. By checking the surface of this lesion in conjunction with any encroachment of the margin of the depressed area or tip of the fold convergence, it is possible to distinguish malignant from benign depressed lesions. Even if a depressed lesion is not accompanied by fold convergence, it is possible for the fold to appear quite clearly after the stomach has been inflated and deflated. Fold convergence means that there is a depressed lesion at the end of the fold. If fold convergence is confirmed, it is then necessary to examine for encroachment and any change in the fold (abrupt cessation, clubbing, tapering, fusion). These findings are more easily detectable by spraying dye on the area around the fold. Definitive diagnosis is confirmed by accurate biopsies.

Relationship Between the Depth of Invasion and Findings of Superficial Depressed-Type (Type IIc) EGC

There were significant differences in surface structure, encroachment, converging folds, elevation of the whole lesion, and clubbing of the fold between intramucosal and submucosal invasive cancer (Table 2).

In most patients with intramucosal cancer, the surface structure of the depressed lesion had an irregular, uneven surface. Submucosal invasive cancer had fewer lesions with an irregular, uneven surface; however, lesions with an irregular, uneven, and amorphous surface, or an amorphous surface, were increased significantly. In addition, in patients with submucosal invasive cancer, encroachment or converging folds were observed more frequently. However, in a small number of patients with intramucosal cancer, an amorphous or irregular and amorphous surface structure was seen, and encroachment and converging folds were seen in about 60% and 40% of these patients, respectively. The depth of invasion, therefore, cannot be estimated based solely on the surface structure, encroachment, and converging folds. In contrast, clubbing of the fold rarely was observed in patients with intramucosal cancer, which makes this finding a strong indicator that a lesion is invading the submucosal or a deeper layer. In addition, elevation of the whole lesion indicated submucosal or deeper invasion; there was no elevation in patients with intramucosal cancer. Few patients in the present study exhibited fusion of the folds, and there was no significant difference ($P = 0.053$) for fusion of folds between patients with intramucosal versus submucosal invasive cancer, but this finding also indicated submucosal invasive or deeper-layer cancer because such finding was never detected in intramucosal cancer.

Wall rigidity is also an indicator of depth of invasion. Lesions without ulceration, poor distensibility, and linear contour of the wall after inflating the stomach, are strongly indicative of submucosal invasive or deeper-layer cancer; however, ulcerated lesions may make it difficult to confirm whether wall rigidity exists [5]. Even so, in cases with ulceration, if thickening of the wall is observed at the lesion [5], the cancer was likely to have invaded the submucosa. With respect to lesion size, in lesions greater than 2 cm in diameter, about 50% of these cancers have invaded the submucosa [5]. Furthermore, if the color of the depressed surface is deeply red, the cancer is likely to be submucosal [5]. Photographs taken in typical cases of superficial depressed-type EGC are shown in Figs. 10 through 13.

Differential Diagnosis of Early and Advanced Depressed-Type Gastric Cancer

In cases where fusion of the folds is seen, it is likely that the cancer has invaded the submucosa or deeper layer. With regard to wall rigidity, if, when inflated, there is a

TABLE 2. Relationship between the depth of invasion and endoscopic findings in 109 patients with Type 0 IIc early gastric cancer

		Depth of cancer invasion		P value:
		Intramucosal (M)	Submucosal (SM)	M vs. SM
Surface structure in depressed area				
Generally amorphous		3	10	$P < 0.001$
Partially amorphous		27	22	
Irregular, uneven structure		41	6	
No change		0	0	
Change in color in depressed area				
Red		37	16	$P = 0.066$
Pale		14	8	
Variegated		11	13	
No change		9	1	
Thin white coat in depressed area				
Positive		13	11	$P = 0.2015$
Negative		58	27	
Bleeding in depressed area				
Positive		10	8	$P = 0.2015$
Negative		61	30	
Protrusion in depressed area				
Positive		16	9	$P = 0.892$
Negative		55	29	
Demarcation between the depressed area and surrounding mucosa				
Well-demarcated		36	19	$P = 0.7618$
Partially demarcated		31	18	
Ill-demarcated		4	1	
Encroachment				
Positive		41	32	$P = 0.0051$
Negative		30	6	
Overall marginal elevation of surrounding mucosa				
Positive		19	9	$P = 0.7261$
Negative		52	29	
Elevation of whole lesion				
Positive		0	5	$P = 0.0080$
Negative		71	33	
Convergence fold				
Positive		24	28	$P = 0.0002$
Negative		47	10	
Change in the fold				
Abrupt cessation	Positive	19	25	$P = 0.2814$
	Negative	5	3	
Tapering	Positive	10	15	$P = 0.3917$
	Negative	14	13	
Clubbing	Positive	2	15	$P = 0.0005$
	Negative	22	13	
Fusion	Positive	0	4	$P = 0.053$
	Negative	24	24	

linearized arc of the wall, it is likely that the cancer has invaded the submucosa [5], and if mild elevation of the whole lesion is observed, the cancer is likely to be submucosal [6]. If a very high elevation of the whole lesion is observed, the cancer is likely to have invaded the muscularis propria or deeper (Fig. 14).

Differentiation Between Benign and Cancerous Erosions

Benign erosion is associated with depressions of various shapes with a thin white coating in the active stage and a uniformly red surface in the healing stage. The red surface of benign erosions is flat and smooth. In benign erosion, the demarcation between the depression and the surrounding mucosa is often indistinct, and it is difficult to determine the circumference of the erosion. In contrast, the depression in cancerous erosion is less flat and has an irregular, uneven surface, ranging from finely granular to nodular to amorphous; such features clearly differentiate the surface structure of the cancerous erosion from normal mucosa. The cancerous erosion often is demarcated distinctly from the surrounding mucosa and frequently has encroachment. Benign erosion often occurs as multiple erosions and frequently shows a regular radial or linear arrangement. If erosions differ in shape or size, have an irregular arrangement, or show malignant findings such as distinct demarcation, irregular depressed surface or encroachment, they should be evaluated by biopsy.

Benign erosion is classified into two types, flat or protruding, depending on the marginal elevation. Erosion of the protruding type is observed as a papule, with central erosion; in Japan, this is called verrucous gastritis (raised erosive gastritis in the Sydney system). The surface structure of the verrucous gastritis is smooth, and the tension of the surface remains high. Verrucous gastritis sometimes requires differential diagnosis from Type 0 IIa + IIc EGC. This protruding type of erosion often tends to occur as multiple erosions with similar shape in a regular arrangement; there is little possibility that such erosions are cancerous. When differentiating between benign protruding and malignant erosions, benign erosions are often in the center of the lesion whereas malignant erosions often deviate from the center.

Diagnosis of Protruding-Type EGC

Diagnosis of Type 0 I EGC

Type 0 I EGC is pathologically defined as a protrusion having a thickness of more than twice that of the normal mucosa [3] and is almost always classified histologically as a well-differentiated adenocarcinoma (Figs. 15, 16). Endoscopically, Type 0 I EGC has high protrusions of pedunculated, semipedunculated, or sessile lesions. The surface structure often has an irregular, uneven pattern, and the lesions are well demarcated. The depth of invasion of most Type 0 I pedunculated protruding lesions is the mucosa [7]. The depth of invasion of semipedunculated or sessile protruding lesions can be estimated from their size. A small protruding lesion measuring 20 mm or less in diameter is likely to have invaded the mucosa only, whereas a protruding lesion measuring 30 to 50 mm or more in diameter is likely to represent advanced cancer [5]. Invasion of the submucosa is indicated by a protruding lesion with a depressed or collapsed lesion on the top [5], or one that has deeply reddened overlying mucosa.

Diagnosis of Type 0 IIa EGC

Type 0 IIa EGC is pathologically defined as a protrusion having a thickness of less than twice that of the normal mucosa [3], and it is well demarcated (Figs. 17, 18). The margin of Type 0 IIa is usually irregular. Changes in surface structure associated with a fine-granular to granular pattern are seen in most Type 0 IIa [7]. In many patients, the color of the overlying mucosa is whitish or pale, but in some patients redness is seen. No color change in the overlying mucosa occurs in less than 10% of patients with Type 0 IIa [7]. The depth of invasion of most Type 0 IIa measuring 2 cm or less in diameter is intramucosal [5,7]. Characteristics indicative of invasion into the submucosa include slight depression and erosion or redness at the center of the lesion [5].

Differential Diagnosis of Protruding-Type EGC

Lesions to be differentiated from protruding-type EGC include gastric fundic gland polyp, gastric hyperplastic polyp, and gastric adenoma. Where gastric mucosa without atrophy exists, most protruding lesions are gastric fundic gland polyps, which are seen in the gastric corpus and fundus and often occur as multiple polyps. The surface of the lesion is smooth, and the surface structure of the lesions is no different from the surrounding mucosa.

Gastric hyperplastic polyps are located in the area extending from the gastric antrum to the corpus and are often small and multiple. The surface structure of such polyps is associated with spotted, uneven redness and often is accompanied by erosion and/or bleeding. Smaller hyperplastic polyps are sessile, whereas larger polyps are semipedunculated to pedunculated in accordance with an increase in size. In some larger hyperplastic polyps, it is possible for them to become lobular in shape. The hyperplastic polyp is not thought to be a precursor of gastric cancer; however, malignant transformation has been discovered during endoscopic follow-up in some instances [8,9]. The incidence of the development of gastric cancer appears to be less than 5% [10], and the majority of hyperplastic polyps harboring malignancy have a diameter of greater than or equal to 2 cm [8].

Gastric adenoma is a flat lesion that is broad and raised, of pale color (grayish-white), and usually solitary, although sometimes it occurs in a cluster of two or three. It is necessary that gastric adenoma is differentiated from Type 0 IIa EGC; gastric adenoma is not associated with an irregular granular or nodular surface as seen in gastric cancer [11], and the benign mucosa has an almost smooth or slightly uneven surface with a regular pattern. In cases where a flat lesion is red, the lesion is likely to be Type 0 IIa EGC [11].

Diagnosis of Flat-Type (Type IIb) EGC

Lesions of Type 0 IIb EGC are flat and are detected based on the change in color of the overlying mucosa to a red, pale, or whitish color; these are very rare [12]. Type 0 IIb EGC can be classified into two types, red-type and pale-type. Red-type lesions are dark red or dull red (Figs. 19, 20) but not deeply red, and the lesions are ill demarcated. Lesions of Type 0 IIb EGC have a slightly uneven overlying mucosa. Pale-type lesions are white, or yellowish-white, and grayish, and the lesions are flat and often clearly demarcated (Fig. 21). In both the red and pale types, the visible vascular pattern observed in atrophic gastric mucosa is not seen; it is indistinct or absent in cancerous lesions.

The Latest Advances in Endoscopy

Magnifying Endoscope

With the improved performance of magnifying endoscopes, endoscopic differentiation of minute lesions has become much easier. The shape of the fine surface mucosal pattern, which consists of gastric pits, is classified as A (dotted), B (short-linear), C (striped), D (circular), or mixed patterns AB, BC, and CD [13]. A magnifying endoscope is very useful for identifying differentiated-type gastric cancer because it has a glandular pattern [14]. Sakaki [14] reported that differentiated-type gastric cancer with structural atypia shows a characteristic fine C pattern, and the area of invasion can be diagnosed accurately by using magnifying endoscopy. Undifferentiated-type gastric cancer can be diagnosed from its irregular D pattern, but accurate diagnosis of the spread of cancer is impossible. Therefore, well-differentiated tubular adenocarcinoma treated by EMR is the best indication for magnifying endoscopy.

Magnifying Endoscope with Narrow Band Imaging System

The narrow band imaging (NBI) system is composed of a sequential combination of an electronic endoscope and a light source equipped with different narrow band filters corresponding to red, green, and blue. When the NBI system is used in combination with a magnifying endoscope, capillary network patterns in the superficial layer of the mucosa can be seen clearly [15]. Tajiri et al. [15,16] carried out endoscopy using the NBI system on patients with EGC; they found a fine network capillary pattern in more than half the patients with differentiated cancer, whereas patients with poorly differentiated cancer showed an irregular corkscrew capillary pattern. They concluded that capillary network patterns of intramucosal cancer are specific to the respective histological types of EGC and can be evaluated objectively using magnifying endoscopy with the NBI system.

Conclusion

The Japanese have pioneered research in the field of EGC and have established a universally acceptable macroscopic classification of EGC, which has contributed to the early diagnosis of gastric cancer. This chapter has discussed the endoscopic diagnosis of EGC and the typical cancerous findings of each type of EGC.

References

1. Tasaka T (1962) National questionnaire of gastric cancer in Japan (in Japanese). Gastroenterol Endosc 4:4–14
2. Yoshida S, Yamaguchi H, Saito D, et al (1993) Endoscopic diagnosis: latest trends. In: Nishi M, Ichikawa H, Nakajima T, Tahara E (eds) Gastric cancer. Springer, Tokyo, pp 246–262
3. Japanese Gastric Cancer Association (2001) Gastric cancer treatment guidelines. 1st edn. (in Japanese) Kanehara, Tokyo
4. Japanese Gastric Cancer Association (2004) Gastric cancer treatment guidelines. 2nd edn. (in Japanese) Kanehara, Tokyo
5. Ono H, Yoshida S (2001) Endoscopic diagnosis of the depth of cancer invasion for gastric cancer (in Japanese with English abstract). Stomach Intest (Tokyo) 36:334–340
6. Saigenji K, Ohida M, Koizumi W, et al (2000) Endoscopic diagnosis of early gastric cancer: Diagnosis of IIc type early gastric cancer by conventional and dye endoscopy (in Japanese with English abstract). Stomach Intest (Tokyo) 35:25–36
7. Hosihara Y, Yamamoto T, Hashimoto M, et al (2000) Endoscopic findings and the pitfalls involved when diagnosing elevated-type early gastric carcinomas (in Japanese with English abstract). Stomach Intest (Tokyo) 35:57–64
8. Kamiya T, Morishita T, Asakura H, et al (1981) Histoclinical long-standing follow-up study of hyperplastic polyps of the stomach. Am J Gastroenterol 75:275–281
9. Mizuno H, Kobayashi S, Kasugai T (1975) Endoscopic follow-up of gastric polyps. Gastrointest Endosc 21:112–115
10. Shirasaki S, Hosokawa O, Watanabe K, et al (1989) Malignant transformation of gastric hyperplastic polyp (in Japanese with English abstract). Gastroenterol Endosc 31:848–855
11. Matsumoto H, Hoshihara Y (2003) Type I early gastric cancer (in Japanese). Endosc Dig 15:593–595
12. Suzuki S (1997) Type 0-IIb early gastric cancer. In: Niwa F (ed) Gastric cancer: diagnosis and treatment (in Japanese). Nippon Medical Center, Tokyo, pp 195–206
13. Sakaki N, Iida Y, Saito M, et al (1980) New magnifying endoscopic classification of the fine gastric mucosal pattern (in Japanese with English abstract). Gastroenterol Endosc 22: 377–383
14. Sakaki N (2003) Important points in the diagnosis of gastric cancer using magnifying endoscopy (in Japanese with English abstract). Endosc Dig 15:567–572
15. Tajiri H, Fujisaki J, Nakayoshi T, et al (2003) Recent advances in the endoscopic diagnosis of early gastric cancer (in Japanese with English abstract). Stomach Intest (Tokyo) 38:21–29
16. Tajiri H, Matsuda K, Fujisaki J (2002) What can we see with the endoscope? Present status and future perspectives. Dig Endosc 14:131–137

Color Plates

a,b

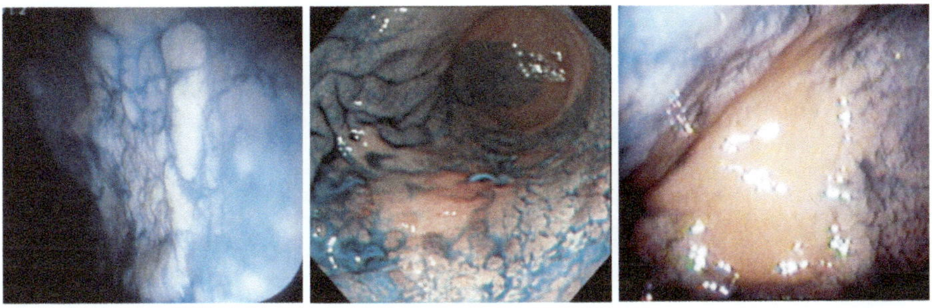

c

FIG. 2a–c. Surface structure in the depressed area. **a** irregular, uneven; **b** partially amorphous; **c** generally amorphous

a,b

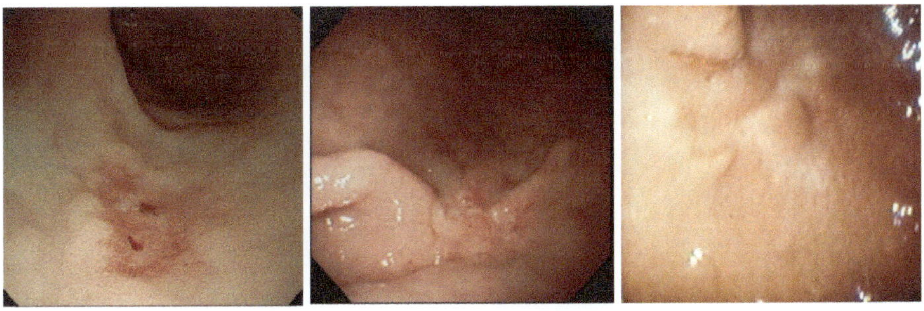

c

FIG. 3a–c. Colors of the depressed area. **a** Red; **b** variegated; **c** pale

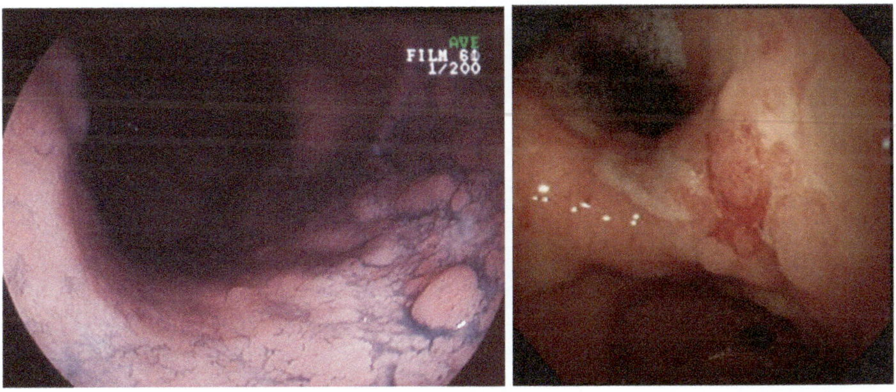

FIG. 4. Protrusion in the depressed area

a 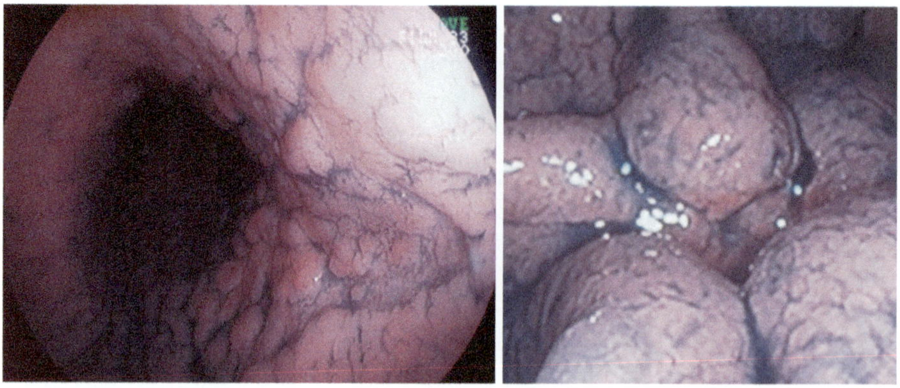 b

Fig. 5. Encroachment observed at the demarcation of the depressed area (**a**) and the tip of the fold (**b**)

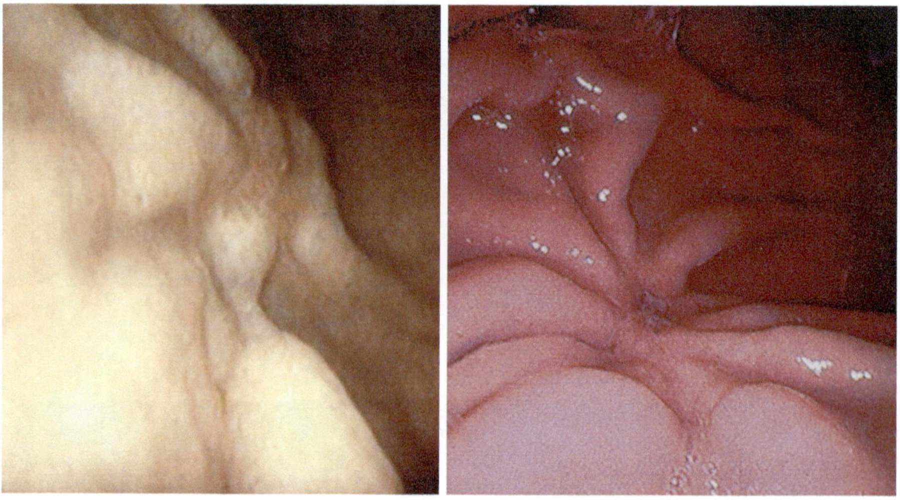

Fig. 6. Tapering of the fold

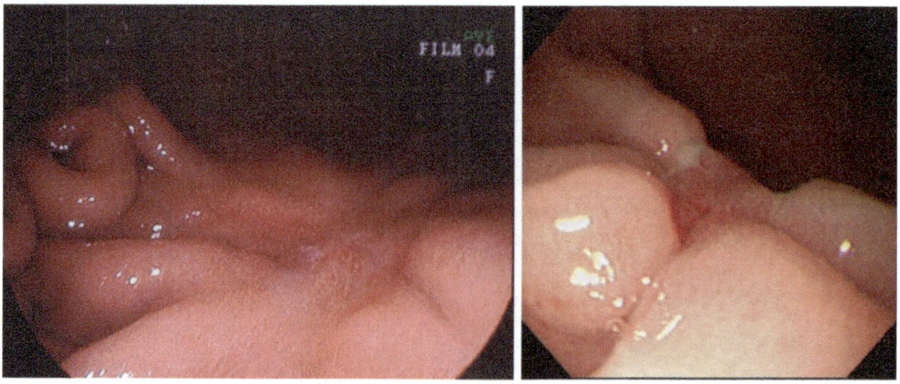

Fig. 7. Abrupt cessation of the fold

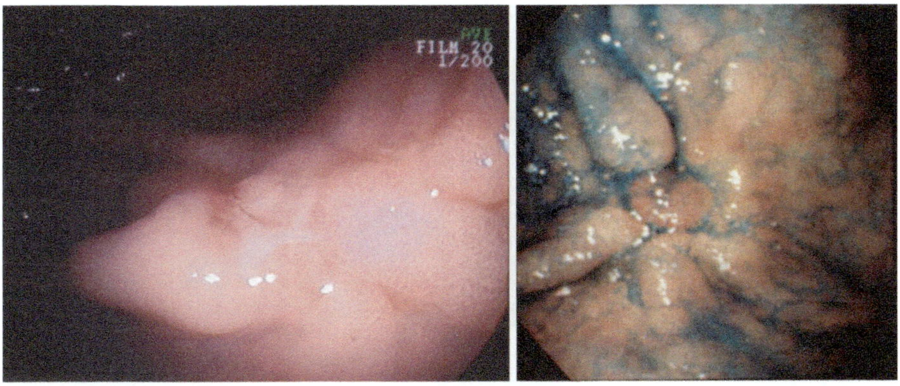

FIG. 8. Clubbing of the fold

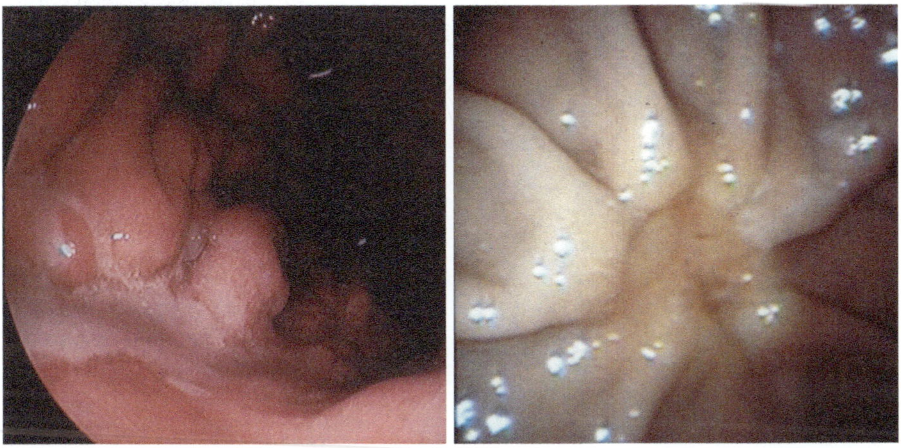

a b

FIG. 9a,b. Fusion of the fold. **a** The depth of the invasion was the submucosa. **b** The depth of the invasion was the muscularis propria

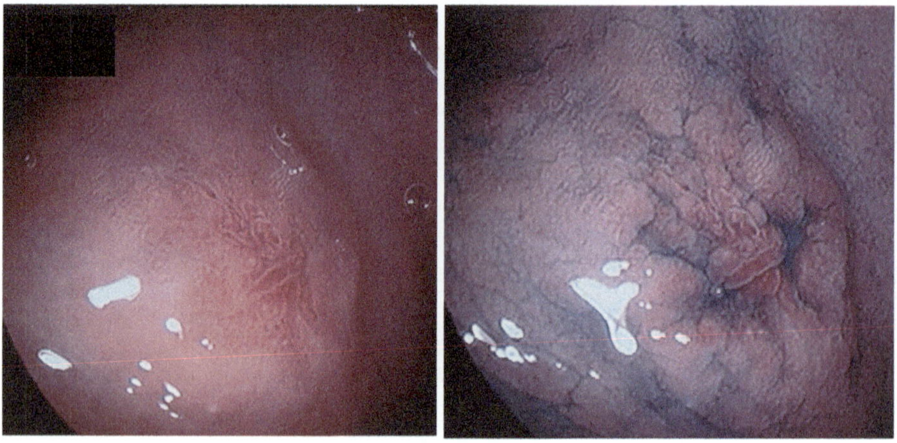

a b

Fig. 10a,b. Type 0 IIc early gastric cancer without converging folds. Histological examination showed a well-differentiated adenocarcinoma, and the depth of the invasion was the intramucosa. **a** Conventional endoscopic finding. **b** Dye endoscopic finding by the indigo-carmine contrast method. In the depressed area, encroachment at the demarcation and an irregular, uneven surface were clearly observed

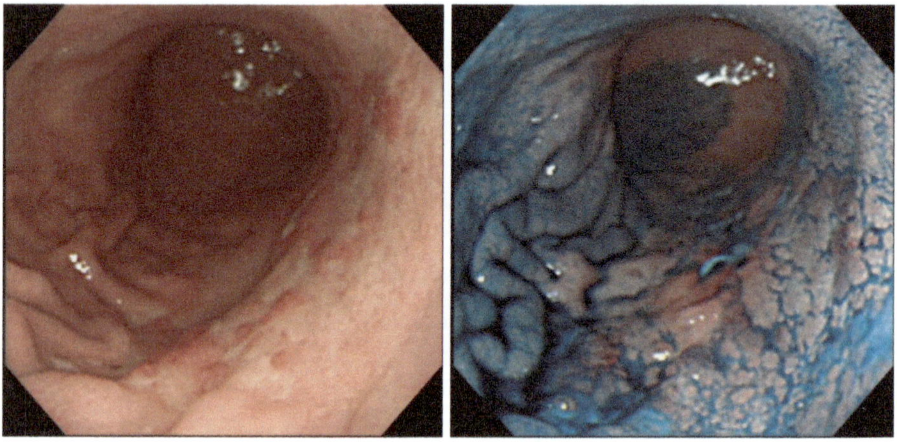

a b

Fig. 11a,b. Type 0 IIc early gastric cancer without converging folds. Histological examination showed an undifferentiated adenocarcinoma, and the depth of the invasion was the submucosa. **a** Conventional endoscopic finding. **b** Dye endoscopic finding by the indigo-carmine contrast method. Partial amorphous structure in the depressed area was clearly observed

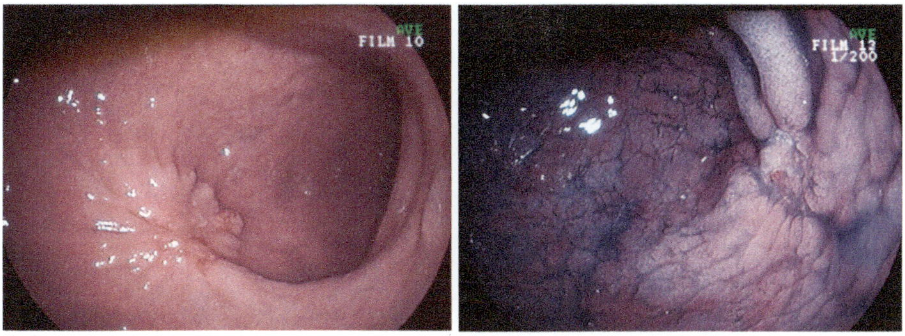

a b

FIG. 12a,b. Type 0 IIc + III early gastric cancer with converging folds. Histological examination showed well-differentiated adenocarcinoma, and the depth of the invasion was the intramucosa. Abrupt cessation and tapering of the fold and encroachment at the demarcation of the depressed area and the tip of the fold were observed. **a** Conventional endoscopic finding. **b** Dye endoscopic finding by indigo-carmine contrast method

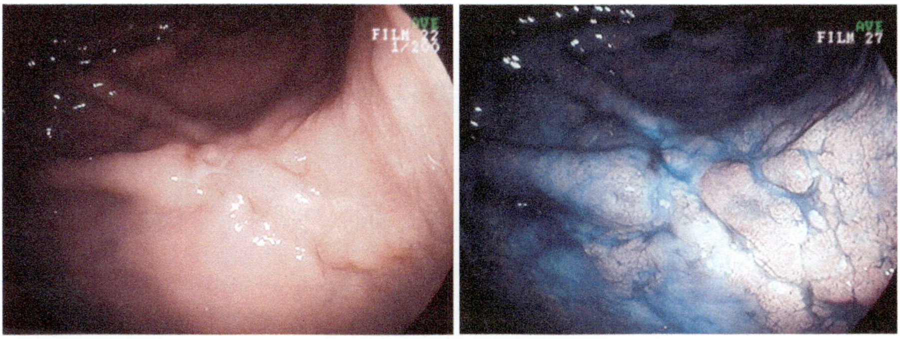

a b

FIG. 13a,b. Type 0 IIc early gastric cancer with converging folds. Histological examination showed an undifferentiated adenocarcinoma, and the depth of the invasion was the submucosa. **a** Conventional endoscopic finding. Clubbing of the fold was observed. **b** Dye endoscopic finding by the indigo-carmine contrast method. Clubbing of the fold and partial amorphous structure in the depressed area were clearly observed

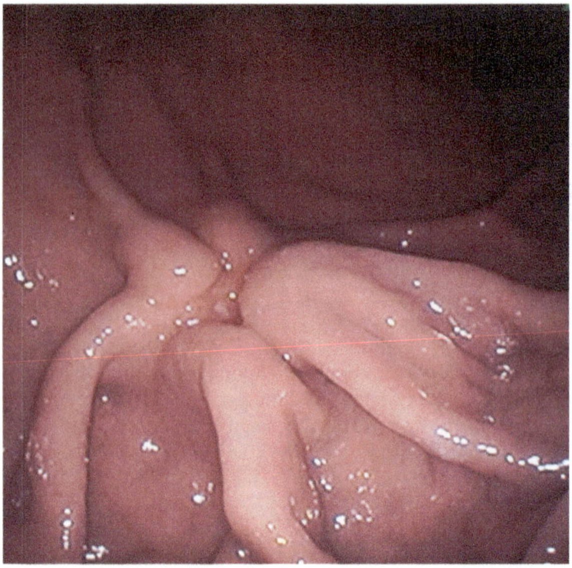

FIG. 14. High elevation of the whole lesion. The depth of the invasion was the subserosa. In addition, clubbing and fusion of the fold were observed

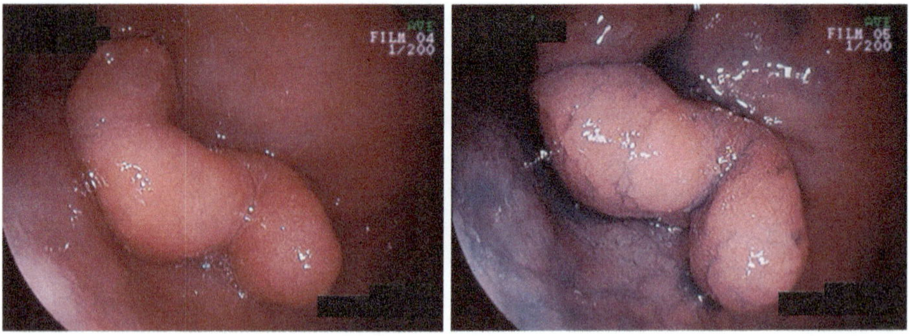

a b

FIG. 15a,b. Type 0 I early gastric cancer. Histological examination showed a well-differentiated adenocarcinoma, and the depth of the invasion was the intramucosa. **a** Conventional endoscopic finding. **b** Dye endoscopic finding by the indigo-carmine contrast method

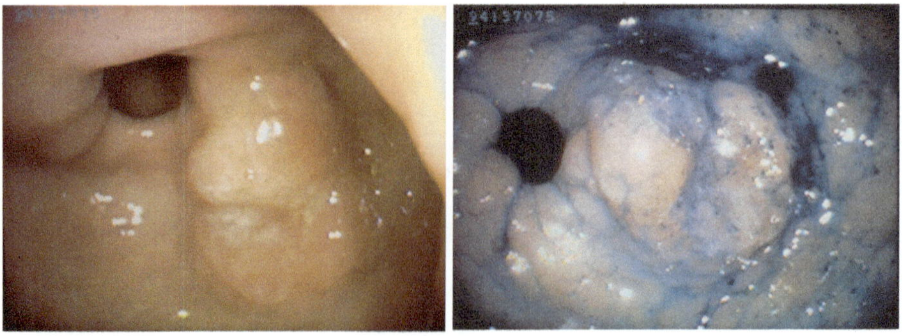

a b

FIG. 16a,b. Type 0 I early gastric cancer. Histological examination showed a well-differentiated adenocarcinoma, and the depth of the invasion was the submucosa. A collapsed lesion on top of the protruding lesion was observed. **a** Conventional endoscopic finding. **b** Dye endoscopic finding by the indigo-carmine contrast method

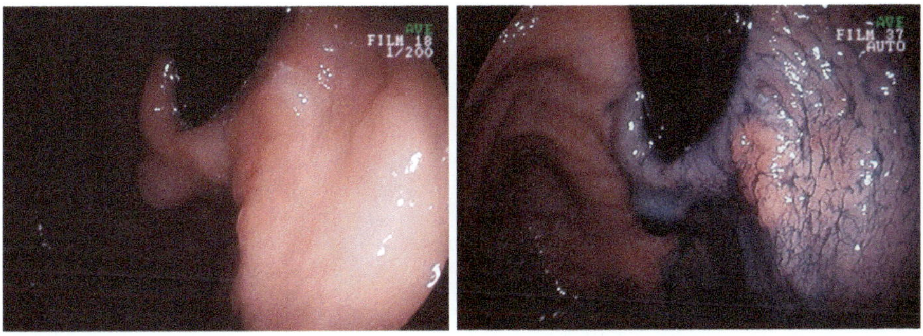

a b

Fig. 17a,b. Type 0 IIa early gastric cancer. Histological examination showed a well-differentiated adenocarcinoma, and the depth of the invasion was the intramucosa. **a** Conventional endoscopic finding. A flat, slightly reddened protruding lesion was observed. **b** Dye endoscopic finding by the indigo-carmine contrast method. Surface structure with granular pattern and a protruding lesion with an irregular margin were clearly observed

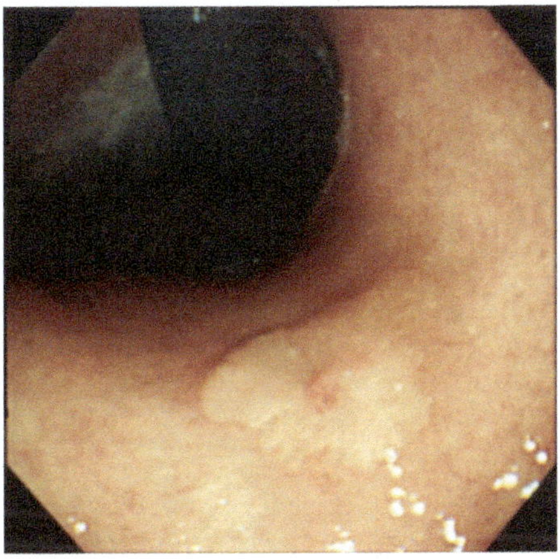

Fig. 18. Type 0 IIa early gastric cancer. Histological examination showed a well-differentiated adenocarcinoma, and the depth of the invasion was the intramucosa. A flat, slightly whitish protruding lesion with an irregular margin was observed

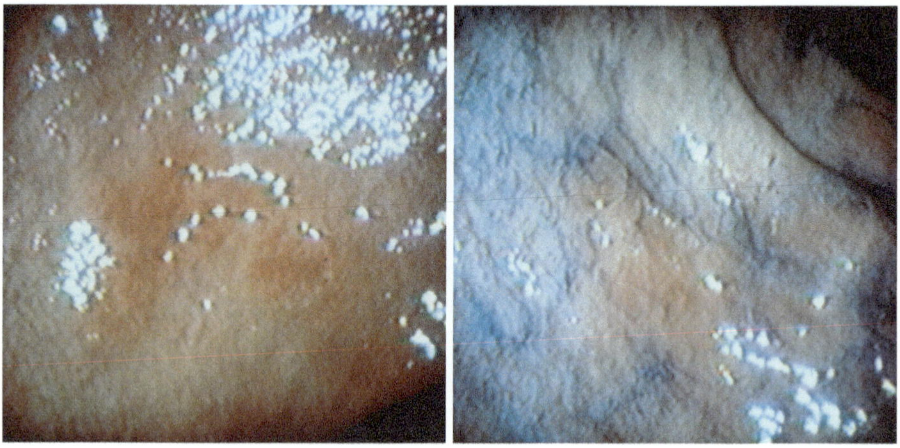

a b

Fig. 19a,b. Type 0 IIb early gastric cancer. Histological examination showed a well-differentiated adenocarcinoma, and the depth of the invasion was the intramucosa. **a** Conventional endoscopic finding. A flat, dull reddish lesion was observed. **b** Dye endoscopic finding by the indigo-carmine contrast method. The surface pattern was clearly different from that of the surrounding mucosa

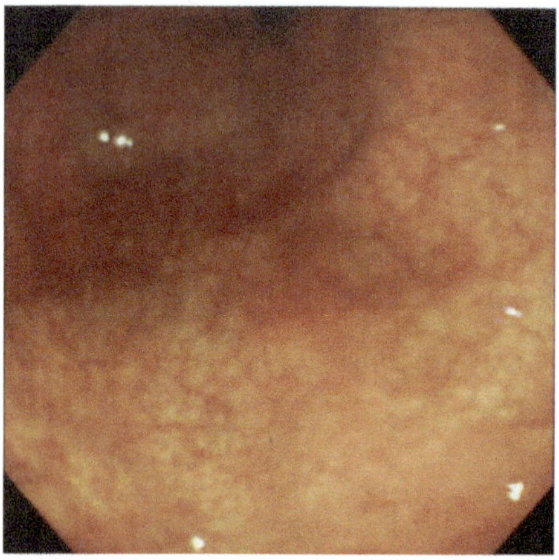

Fig. 20. Type 0 IIb early gastric cancer. Histological examination showed a well-differentiated adenocarcinoma, and the depth of the invasion was the intramucosa. A flat, dull reddish lesion was observed, and the visible vascular pattern, which is observed in atrophic gastritis mucosa, disappeared

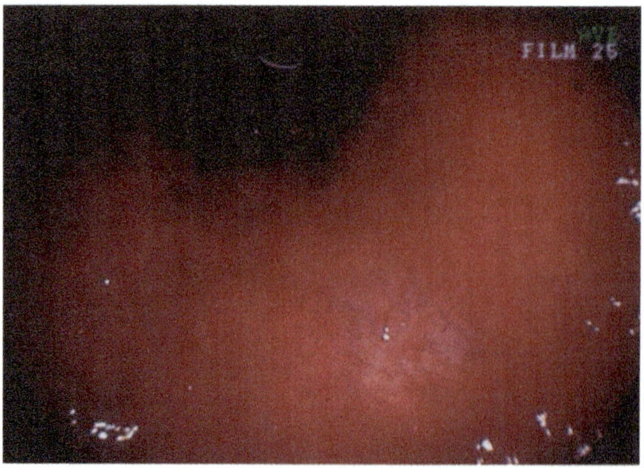

Fig. 21. Type 0 IIb early gastric cancer. Histological examination showed an undifferentiated adenocarcinoma, and the depth of the invasion was the intramucosa. A flat, pale lesion with redness in the center was observed

Ultrasonic Diagnosis of Gastric Cancer

Hidemitsu Yasuda[1], Masanori Hashimoto[1], Shouji Shimoyama[2], and Michio Kaminishi[2]

Introduction

Ultrasonic diagnosis of the digestive tract was first reported in 1976 by Lutz and Petzoldt [1]. and then in 1980 by Morgan et al. [2]. Initial ultrasound devices were limited in their capacity; they were only capable of visualizing hypertrophy and some major changes of the whole intestinal wall. In 1980, Strohm et al. [3] reported their attempt at using a rotating mirror-type ultrasonic endoscope. In the same year, DiMagno et al. [4] conducted an animal experiment with an electronic linear array ultrasonic endoscope. They described its clinical application in 1982 [5]. Following refinements and modifications in the devices used for gastrointestinal ultrasonography, the lamellar structure of the digestive tract began to be discussed.

In Japan, in 1981, Aibe reported his experience with endoscopic ultrasonography. In 1984, he made a detailed report on the relationship between two-dimensional ultrasound images of the digestive tract wall and the histologically observed layers of the digestive tract [6]. In 1982, Yamanaka et al. reported their experience with a 5-MHz electronic linear array ultrasonic endoscope. In 1983, they reported endoscopic ultrasonography of early gastric cancer [7]. From 1983, we began the ultrasonic diagnosis of gastric cancer. We scanned from the surface of the body of the patient. We compared the ultrasonic images scanned before surgery with that of the specimen scanned in a water tank after the surgery.

We also compared the ultrasonic images with pathological findings [8]. In 1986, criteria for evaluation of the invasive depths of gastric tumors were promulgated [9].

Since approximately 1980, various theories have been proposed to interpret ultrasound images of the gastric wall. The view that the gastric wall is usually composed of five layers has been widely accepted [10,11]. According to this view, the gastric wall is composed of three hyperechoic layers and two hypoechoic layers sandwiched between them. Almost universal consensus has been reached about the histological

[1] Department of Surgery, International Medical Center of Japan, 1-21-1 Toyama, Shinjuku-ku, Tokyo 162-8655, Japan
[2] Department of Gastrointestinal Surgery, The University of Tokyo Graduate School of Medicine, Tokyo, Japan
e-mail: hyasuda@imcj.hosp.go.jp

significance of each of these five layers. A hyperechoic layer is sometimes visible near the base of the second layer [12–16]. This structure is viewed either as a boundary echo appearing on the surface of the lamina muscularis mucosae or an echo appearing in the border between the base of the fundic gland and the tissue facing the serosa. If edema is present in the third layer, this layer is sometimes depicted as several stripes.

Among other findings, it is noteworthy that boundary echo, which occurs on the interface of two layers with different sound velocities, is displayed right under the border as a thick beltlike layer. The third layer appears to be bulging out of the submucosal into the muscular layer. As a result, the fourth layer (lamina muscularis propria) is depicted thinner than actually it is. A boundary echo between the internal annular muscle layer and the external longitudinal muscle layer is sometimes depicted within the hypoechoic area of the fourth layer.

Methods

We have examined 581 cases of gastric cancer patients by endoscopic ultrasonography (EUS) before surgery. The ultrasonic apparati that we use are Toshiba SAL-30A (3.5 MHz), SAL-50A (5.0 MHz), SAL-77A, SAL-90A, SAL-250A, and SAL-270A. The ultrasonic endoscopes that we use are Toshiba-Machida EPE-703FL and PEF-703FA.

Ultrasonic Anatomy of the Gastric Wall

The normal digestive tract is usually composed of the following five layers when observed by ultrasonography (Figs. 1, 2): first layer (foveolar, epithelium, scanned as a hyperechoic layer, including the boundary echo between the intraluminal medium and the foveolar epithelium); second layer (lamina propria mucosae, scanned as a

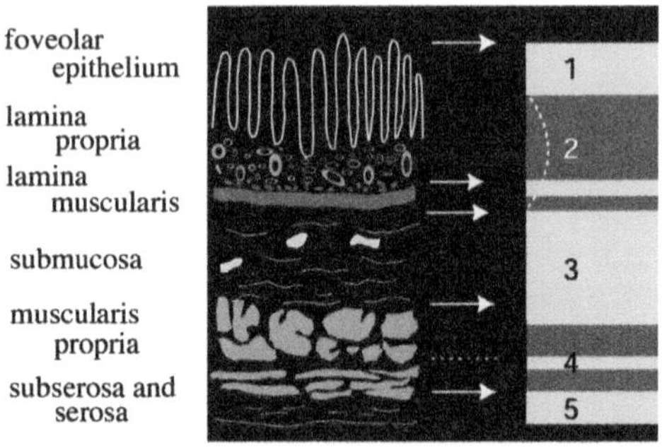

Fig. 1. Ultrasonographic anatomy of the gastric wall. Consistently observed: first layer (hyperechoic); foveolar epithelium (M)/boundary echo; second layer (hypoechoic); lamina propria mucosae (M); third layer (hyperechoic); submucosa (SM); fourth layer (hypoechoic); lamina muscularis propria (MP); fifth layer (hyperechoic); subserosa and serosa (SS + S)/boundary echo. Occasionally observed: hyperechoic area within the second layer; surface of lamina muscularis mucosae (MM); a hyperechoic layer within the fourth layer; border between the internal annular muscle layer and the external longitudinal muscle layer

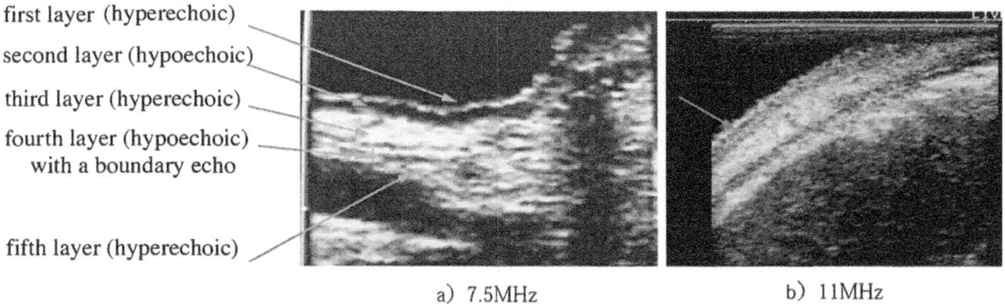

FIG. 2. Ultrasonic images of the normal gastric wall (electronic linear array ultrasonic endoscope); endoscopic ultrasonography (EUS) image of the gastric wall at 7.5 MHz (*left*) and 11 MHz (*right*). The *arrow* in **b** indicates a hyperechoic layer within the second layer. This echo appears to arise from the surface of the lamina muscularis mucosae

hypoechoic layer, including the lamina muscularis mucosae as well); third layer (submucosa, a relatively wide hyperechoic layer in the middle of the wall); fourth layer (lamina muscularis propria, a hypoechoic layer, including the boundary echo between the internal annular muscle layer and the external longitudinal muscle layer); and fifth layer (subserosa and serosa, a hyperechoic layer, including the boundary echo between the gastric wall and surrounding tissue).

Evaluation of the Depth of Gastric Tumor Invasion

The depth of tumor invasion is evaluated on the basis of ultrasonic features of the gastric wall. Figure 3 shows the basic criteria for tumor depth evaluation. Depth "M" means the absence of changes in the third layer; depth "SM" indicates the finding of a defect (hypoechoic) in the third layer; depth "MP" refers to marked interruption of the third layer with no change in the fifth layer; depth "SS" means smooth displacement of the fifth layer; and depth "SE" indicates interruption of the fifth layer by a hypoechoic area and the presence of an irregular outer margin. In type 4 cases, hypertrophy of all layers (particularly marked in the third layer) is seen and the echo level of the third layer is lower, with less clear borders between the third and other layers.

Results

Accuracy Rate of the Depth of Gastric Cancer Invasion by EUS

When our 518 cases were examined, the predictive value of EUS was 76.8% for M cases and 57.0% for SM cases (Table 1). The predictive value was 94.6% for early gastric cancer and 82% for advanced gastric cancer. For the 32 patients with early gastric cancer for whom preoperative endoscopy and intraoperative assessment of induration of gastric tumor were performed, the accurate diagnosis rate for M cases was 72% with intraoperative diagnosis, 75% with EUS, and 70% with endoscopy [13–16].

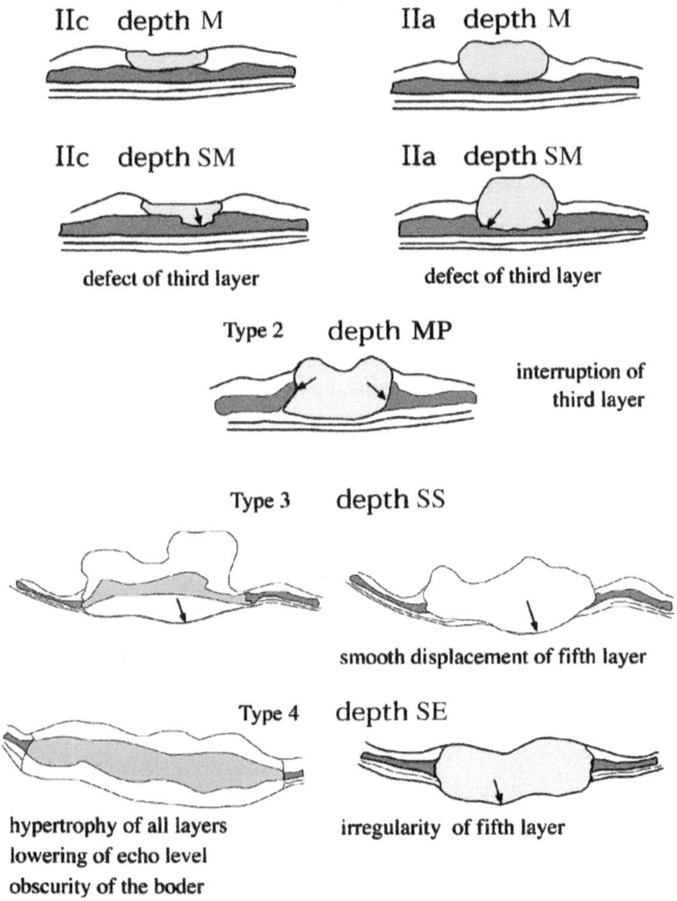

FIG. 3. Evaluation of the depth of gastric tumor invasion by ultrasonic method

Echo Levels of Gastric Cancer and Ulcer Scars

The echo levels within the gastric cancer-affected area and the ulcer scar-affected area were analyzed. Figure 4 shows a frequency distribution graph (bar graph) with an overlapping normal distribution curve calculated from the mean and variance for the 60 gastric cancer cases and 27 cases with ulcer scars. On this graph, the distribution of the echo level of gastric cancer was shifted toward lower levels as compared to the echo level for the second layer (the 15th grade), whereas the distribution of ulcer scars was shifted to higher levels. The echo level inside the gastric cancer was slightly lower than that for the lamina propria mucosae (the second layer). The echo level inside the ulcer scars was significantly higher than the echo level of the lamina propria mucosae.

TABLE 1. Accuracy rate of the ultrasonic depth diagnosis of gastric cancer invasion by endoscopic ultrasonography (EUS)

Pathological diagnosis on EUS	M	SM	MP	SS	SE	Accuracy (%) *1 SS/SE	Accuracy (%) *2 SS + SE	Accuracy (%) *3 early/advanced
M	136	36	3	2		76.8 (136/177)		94.6 (295/312)
SM	46	77	10	1	1	57.0 (77/135)		
MP	3	17	21	2	1	47.7 (21/44)		82.0 (169/206)
SS	1	8	9	14	9	34.1 (14/41)	77.2 (125/162)	
SE	3	5	11	53	49	40.5 (49/121)		
Accuracy (%): retrospective	72.0	53.8	38.9	19.4	81.7	57.3 (189/518)	69.3 (359/518)	89.6 (464/518)

When our 518 cases were examined, the predictive value of EUS was 76.8% for M cases and 57.0% for SM cases; the predictive value was 94.6% for early cancer and 82% for advanced cancer

M, absence of changes in third layer; SM, hypoechoic defect in third layer; MP, interrupted third layer; SS, smooth displacement of fifth layer; SE, fifth layer interrupted by hypoechoic area plus irregular outer margin; accuracy *1, distinguish depth SS from depth SE; accuracy *2, diagnose depth SS and depth SE as depth s; accuracy *3, diagnose depth M and SM as early; diagnose depth MP, SS, and SE as advanced

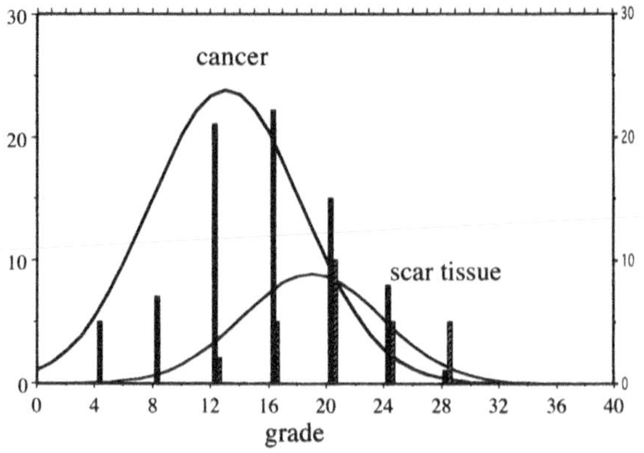

FIG. 4. Echo levels of gastric cancer and ulcer scars. *Black bars* indicate frequency distributuion of mean echo levels of gastric *cancer*; *blue shaded bars* indicate frequency distributuion of mean echo levels of *scar tissue*. Two normal distribution curves are overlapped to the bar graph

Evaluation of Blood Flow Through Gastric Cancer and Ulcer Scars

Endoscopic ultrasonography using the two-dimensional color Doppler method is also useful in evaluating upper digestive tract diseases. The size and number of blood vessels greater than 100 μm in size in gastric cancers were examined using an image analyzer and then compared with histological findings. The blood flow detection rate by the Doppler method rose when the maximum diameter of blood vessels within a lesion was greater than 400–500 μm or the total area of vascular cross section per 1 cm^2 was more than 1 mm^2. The vascular diameter and area per unit area differed significantly among the M, SM, and advanced cancer groups. This result suggests that SM cancer can be distinguished from advanced cancer by the current Doppler method.

The group rated as positive by the Doppler study had a significantly elevated incidence of tumor metastasis to lymph nodes (33.4%). Postoperative remote metastasis was noted in 4 (6.6%) of the 61 cases rated as positive by the Doppler test. In contrast, no remote metastasis was found in 56 of the 61 cases rated as negative. These results suggest that evaluation of blood flow in the tumor by the Doppler method can predict the risk for remote metastasis to some extent.

Lymph Node Metastasis

Body Surface Scanning

Group 1. Lymph nodes are easier to identify if the patient drinks water before scanning. Arteries and veins of the greater omentum can be checked by the color Doppler method, although swelling of lymph nodes does not readily allow a diagnosis of lymph node metastasis. Thick lymph nodes, assuming a quasispherical form, are suspected of representing tumor metastasis (Fig. 5).

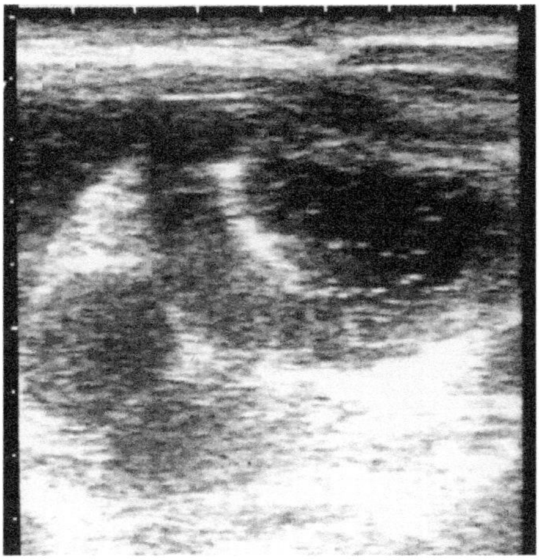

Fig. 5. Two swollen lymph nodes detected along the lesser curvature of the middle gastric body by scanning from body surface after water intake

Group 2. Lymph nodes around the celiac artery, the common hepatic artery, the splenic artery, etc., can be clearly scanned from the body surface. To identify these lymph nodes, it is better to scan without having the patient ingest water, because the air swallowed with water can hamper their detection. Care is taken to avoid mistaking the accessory spleen for swollen lymph nodes.

Group 3. Swollen lymph nodes around the aorta and on the dorsal side of the pancreatic head can also be clearly visualized by ultrasonic scanning from the body surface.

Endoscopic Ultrasound Scanning

The lymph nodes around the stomach and the esophagus are scanned. Because swelling of lymph nodes can represent inflammation, we cannot make a definite diagnosis as to the presence or absence of lymph node metastasis on the basis of morphological features alone. However, normal lymph nodes tend to be flat and show a homogeneous internal echo, whereas lymph nodes with a spherical form, irregular edges, and nonhomogeneous internal echo may reflect tumor metastasis (Fig. 6).

Clinical Cases

O-IIa Type (Depth, M)

Preoperative EUS image (Fig. 7a): The hypoechoic area within the second layer (M layer) is thickened (the area between white arrows). The third layer shows no change (black arrow). The hyperechoic area within the third layer (SM layer) is slightly depressed at the point of the black arrow, but the displacement is smooth, ruling out cancer invasion. The depth is thus rated as M.

Pathological findings (Fig. 7b): Well-differentiated adenocarcinoma, consistent with the ultrasound image. Depth is rated as M.

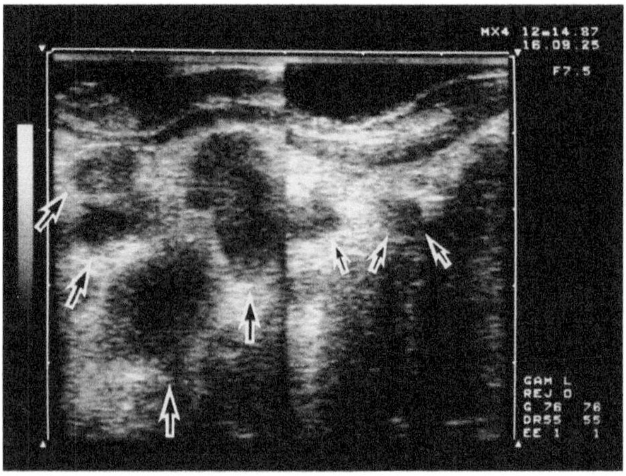

Fig. 6. Swollen lymph node along the greater curvature of the cardia depicted by EUS scanning

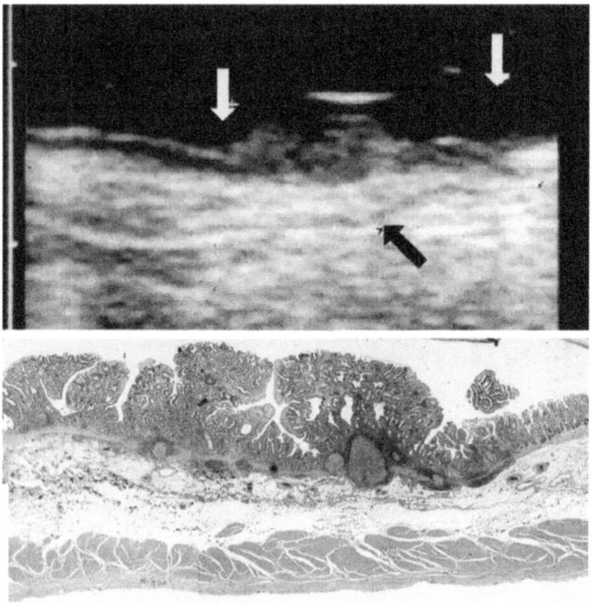

Fig. 7. O-IIa type (depth, M). **a** Preoperative EUS image. *White arrows* indicate the range of IIa lesion. *Black arrow* shows shallow depression of the third layer representing the lymphoid follicle. **b** Pathological findings. (H&E, original magnification: ×20)

O-IIc + (III) Type (depth, M)

Preoperative EUS image (Fig. 8a): A lesion is visible between the descending arrows. The first layer (corresponding to the foveolar epithelium) is not clear. The third layer shows mild wavy hypertrophy. No echo level reduction is visible (the area between the ascending black arrows). Because the IIc plane was wide, the lesion was attributed to insufficient dilatation of the gastric wall. Depth was rated as M preoperatively.

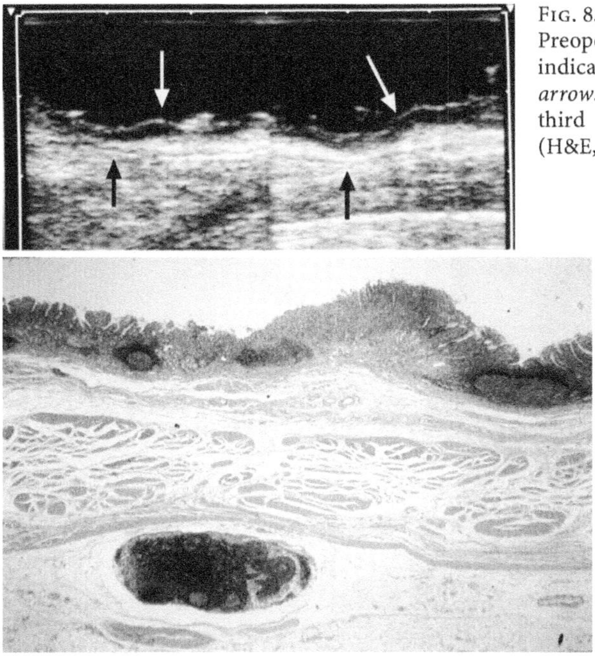

a

b

FIG. 8. O-IIc + (III) type (depth, M). **a** Preoperative EUS image. *White arrows* indicate the range of IIc lesion. *Black arrows* show slightly narrowing of the third layer. **b** Histological findings. (H&E, original magnification: ×20)

Histological findings (Fig. 8b): Signet-ring cell carcinoma. Mild fibrosis is visible in the submucosa. Depth was rated as M.

O-IIc + (III) Type: (Depth, M) (Smooth Tapering)

Preoperative EUS image (Fig. 9a): The center of the third layer in the affected region shows a gradual decrease in thickness (smooth tapering). The echo level has decreased to a level intermediate between the levels of the third and second layers; this is a typical EUS image of an O-IIc + (III) tumor. The mild decrease in echo level suggests ulcer scars.

Histological findings (Fig. 9b): Ulcer scars, extending to the muscular layer, are visible, but the cancer remains within the mucosa.

O-IIc Type (Depth, SM)

Preoperative EUS image (Fig. 10a): A defect of the third layer is visible (between the white arrows). The depth of invasion is rated as SM on the EUS image.

Pathological findings (Fig. 10b): A focus of cancer is visible in the submucosa (between the arrows). It is histologically rated as signet-ring cell carcinoma. The pathological features are consistent with those seen on the EUS image. The submucosal invasion is 2 mm in width and about 1 mm in depth. This is the minimal tumor invasion detectable by the current EUS technique.

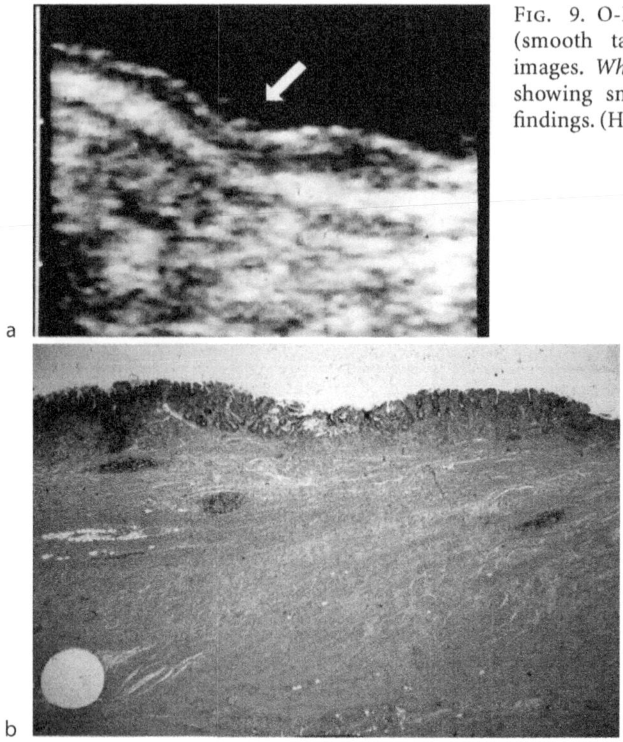

FIG. 9. O-IIc + (III) type: (depth, M) (smooth tapering). **a** Preoperative EUS images. *White arrow* indicates the region showing smooth tapering. **b** Histological findings. (H&E, original magnification: ×40)

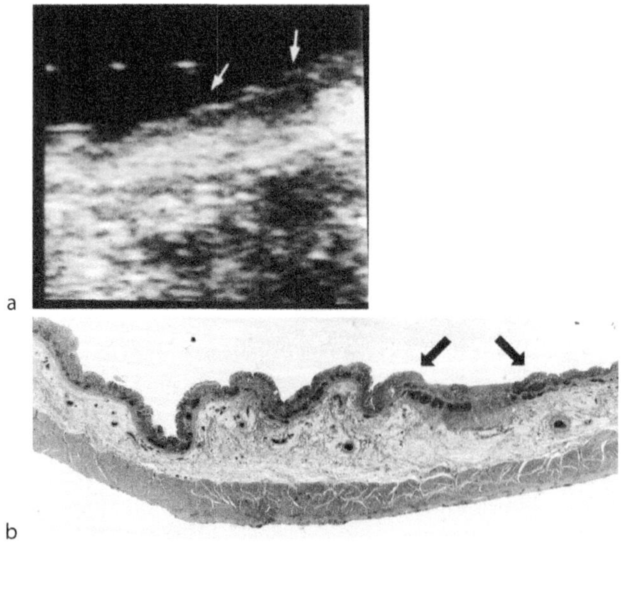

FIG. 10. O-IIc type (depth, SM). **a** Preoperative EUS image. *White arrows* indicate the defect of the third layer. **b** Pathological findings. *Black arrows* indicate a focus of a cancer in the submucosa. (H&E, original magnification: ×20)

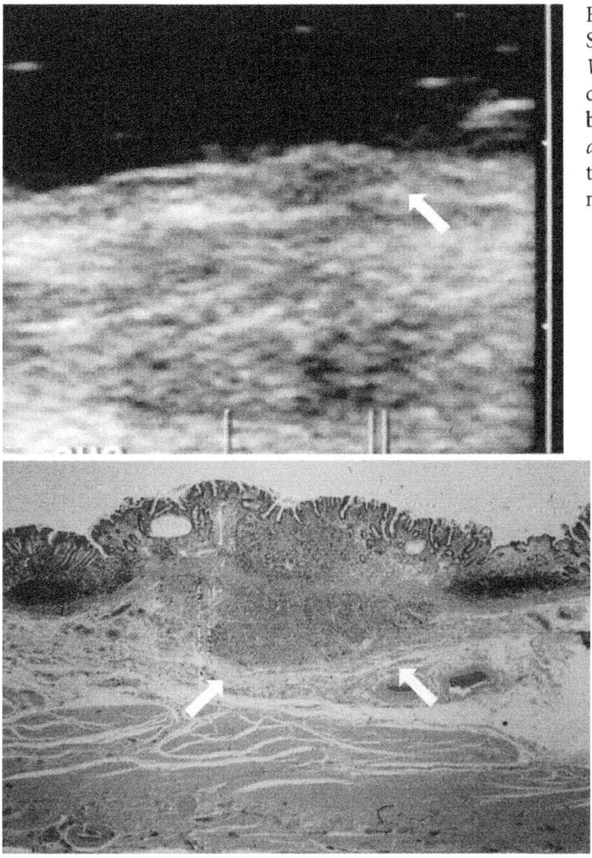
a
b

FIG. 11. O-IIc + (III) type (depth, SM). **a** Preoperative EUS image. *White arrow* indicates a hypoechoic area in the third layer. **b** Pathological findings. *White arrows* indicate a cancer lesion in the submucosa. (H&E, original magnification: ×40)

O-IIc + (III) Type (Depth, SM)

Preoperative EUS image (Fig. 11a): Although the depth of invasion is rated as M by preoperative EUS, retrospective observation yields a slightly invasive hypoechoic area in the third layer (arrow), suggesting tumor invasion with a depth of SM.

Pathological findings (Fig. 11b): The tumor is rated as tub2, with an invasive depth of SM. Histopathological features are quite consistent with the EUS findings.

O-IIa + IIc Type Lesion (Depth, SM)

Preoperative EUS image (Fig. 12a): A hypoechoic area, evidently occupying the third layer, is noted. As the deepest part of the third layer remains intact, the depth of invasion is rated as SM.

Pathological findings (Fig. 12b): The tumor is rated as signet-ring cell carcinoma, with an invasive depth of SM. The small space (200 µm) between the submucosal focus and the muscular layer is less than the ultrasound device's resolution of distance, but a hyperechoic layer is visible, slightly protruding from the third layer to the fourth

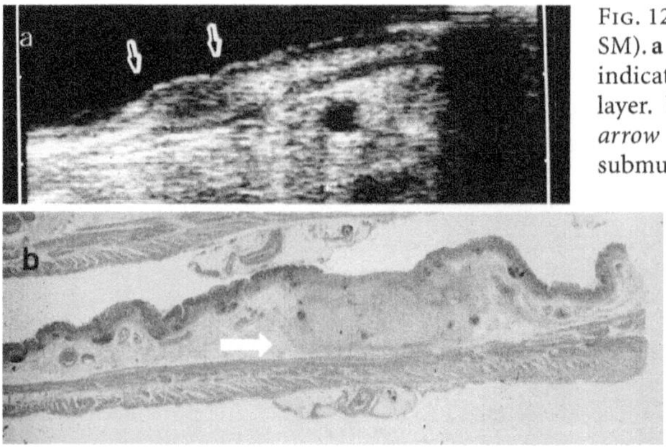

Fig. 12. O-IIa + IIc type lesion (depth, SM). **a** Preoperative EUS image. *Arrows* indicate a hypoechoic area in the third layer. **b** Pathological findings. *White arrow* indicates a cancer lesion in the submucosa

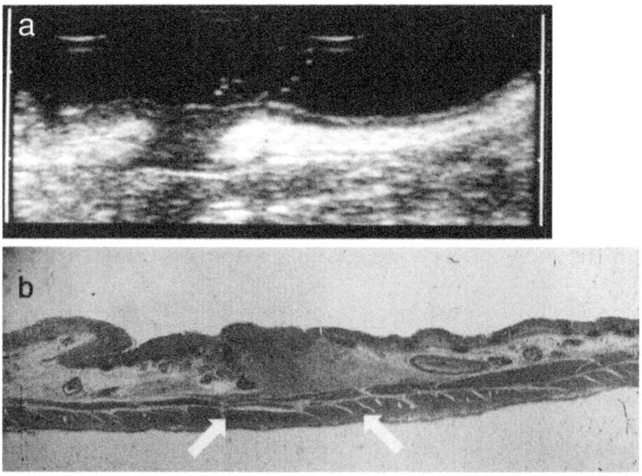

Fig. 13. O-IIa + IIc type lesion (depth, SM). **a** Preoperative EUS image; **b** Pathological findings. *White arrows* indicate a cancer lesion in the submucosa

layer. This is a typical case in which the border is visible, although the width of the border layer is less than ultrasonic resolution.

O-IIa + IIc Type Lesion (Depth, SM)

Preoperative EUS image (Fig. 13a): A hypoechoic area, occupying the third layer, is visible. Because this area contacts the fourth layer, a diagnosis of slight invasion of the MP is made.

Pathological findings (Fig. 13b): The tumor is rated as tub2, with the depth of invasion being SM. The cancer focus remains in the submucosa, but the focus in the submucosa is in direct contact with the muscularis propria. Because the acoustic impedance differs little between the cancer focus and the muscularis propria, the cancer appears to be continued with the muscularis propria on the ultrasound image.

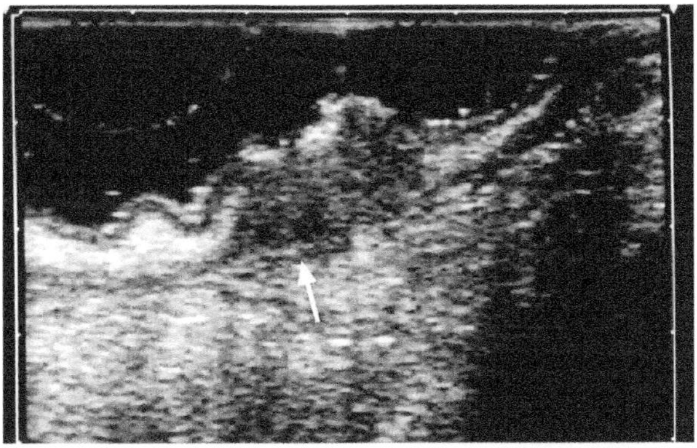

FIG. 14. EUS image of type 2 advanced gastric cancer (depth, MP). *White arrow* indicates a boundary echo within the lamina muscularis propria

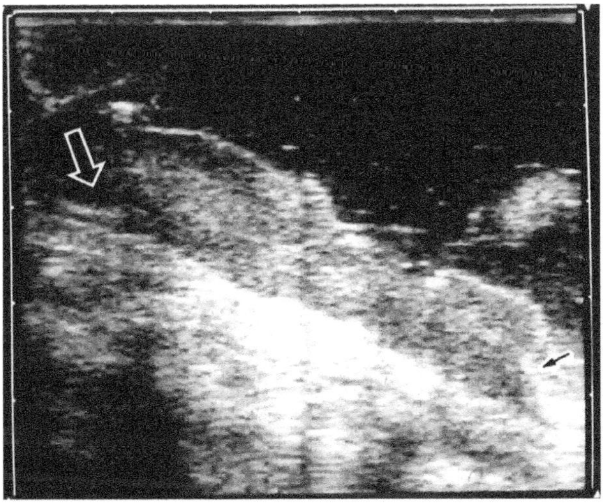

FIG. 15. EUS image of type 3 advanced cancer (depth, SS). *Two arrows* indicate the interrupted points of normal third layer

Type 2 Advanced Cancer (Depth, MP)

EUS image (Fig. 14): A typical Preoperative EUS image of MP cancer. The third layer (SM) is interrupted at both ends of the tumor. A boundary echo within the fourth layer musculature (arrow) is retained in the center of the lesion. The cancer has invaded the superficial muscular layer.

Type 3 Advanced Cancer (Depth, SS)

EUS image (Fig. 15): Irregular hypoechoic areas are visible across all layers of the gastric wall. The fifth layer shows smooth displacement. The normal third layer is interrupted at the point indicated by the arrow. Diffuse hypertrophy, primarily in the third layer at the tumor center, is characteristic of scirrhous-type gastric cancer. Diffuse hypertrophy of the gastric wall is visible around the lesion. This is a type 3 advanced cancer.

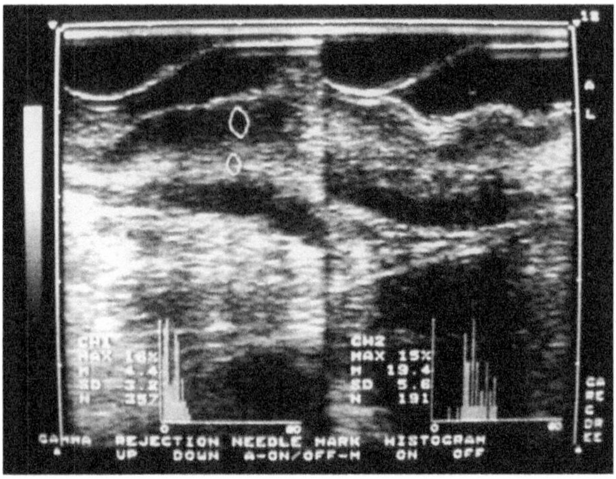

Fig. 16. EUS image of type 4 advanced cancer (depth, SS)

Type 4 Advanced Cancer (Depth, SS)

EUS image (Fig. 16): Severe hypertrophy is visible in the second, third, and fourth layers. Tumor invasion is suggested in the hypertrophic areas. Tumor invasion reduces the echo level. Because the bright third layer is thickened, there is an impression that the overall echo level has risen. In fact, however, the echo level of the third layer of the lesion has decreased to a level intermediate between the normal second and third layers.

Discussion

Devices

There are two types of ultrasonic endoscope. One is composed of an ultrasound probe attached to the tip of an endoscope, and the other is a small-diameter probe (miniature probe) that can be inserted through the forceps channel of an ordinary endoscope. The special device can be divided into a mechanical radial scanner and an electronic linear or convex probe. The mechanical radial scanner can yield real-time images (movie) with the probe rotating for a 360° range. This type of device provides a wide visual field, but the interval between two beams becomes wider as the object is further away, resulting in lower resolution. The electronic linear or convex probe switches the scanning lines electrically and yields real-time images along a given cross section. The linear type is composed of linearly arrayed probes. The convex type is composed of probes arranged in an archlike form. Spatial resolution is high with the electronic linear or convex probe, but the scanned area is narrower. The special device first mentioned can be used for two-dimensional color Doppler evaluation of blood flow through the digestive tract wall and inside the tumor. Some types of this device allow puncture cytology and histological examination under ultrasound guidance (Olympus GF UC240P-AL5, GF UTC240-AL5, GF UMP230; Pentax EG-3630U, FG-34UX, etc.; Toshiba PEF-708FA, etc.).

The miniature probe is easy to use and can be applied to many purposes. However, it is susceptible to the influence of fiber torsion. Furthermore, fine adjustment of the tip angle of this type of probe to the curve of the gastric wall is sometimes difficult. In the high-frequency range (above 12 MHz), this type of probe can yield detailed cross-sectional images (Olympus UM-S30-25R), but when used for thick lesions the power of the ultrasound will attenuate, reducing the accuracy of information on the deeper side of the tissue. The Fujinon miniature probe is characterized by the ability to perform radial scanning and to yield linear images by mechanical pullout manipulation. When using this probe manually, care must be taken regarding the speed of pullout manipulation and to avoid distortion of the scanned cross section. New probes are marketed that can evaluate three-dimensional structures (UM-3D2R and UM-3D3R). These probes are used in combination with EU-IP2 to obtain three-dimensional images.

Depth Diagnosis

Yoshino et al. [17] reported that the rate of accurate determination of the depth of tumor invasion in 204 gastric cancer cases was 85.3%. For the 109 early gastric cancer cases, the accuracy was 85.3% for those rated as M and 67.3% for those rated as SM. Chonan et al. [18] reported accuracy for 100 cases of type IIc early gastric cancer (pM-SM1), 96.2% with EUS and 94.2% with endoscopy. For 5 pSM2 cases, the accuracy was 62.5% with EUS and 75% with endoscopy. The accuracy will rise to 80%, approximately, when EUS images are analyzed in comparison to the pathology, including review of cases with overdiagnosis resulting from micro-invasion and ulceration [19–21]. The ability to detect cancer tissue in the submucosal layer and ulcer scar (information essential for endoscopic mucosal resection) will exceed 90%, excluding microinvasion. EUS often provides valuable information on lesions of the upper part of the gastric body in cases presenting ectopic glands in the submucosal layer, and also in cases showing small amounts of tumor invasion into the submucosal layer. On the other hand, endoscopy allows a higher accurate diagnosis rate in cases in which extension of the gastric wall is insufficient (e.g., IIa + IIc lesions at the pylorus). The accurate diagnosis rate for SM cases was markedly higher, if the two diagnoses yielded the same results.

Factors Hampering Accurate Diagnosis

Attenuation of Ultrasound

When a miniature probe is used, ultrasound attenuation raises a significant problem, particularly in cases in which the lesion is thick (greater than 10 mm). In such cases, it is advisable to use a conventional type of EUS. If the lesion has a pedicle, it is worthwhile to attempt to place the probe at the base of the pedicle or compress the lesion with a balloon.

Fibrosis

Fibrosis and inflammatory cell infiltration can also lead to overdiagnosis. Depending on the severity of inflammation and the timing of ulceration, the echo pattern of fibrous tissue sometimes differs from the echo pattern of cancerous tissue. Ulcer scar tissues show a rise in echo level as they heal.[2,3] Signs of inflammatory changes include (1) a higher echo level as compared to cancerous tissue, (2) a symmetrical pattern that tends to concentrate at a single point, and (3) slight destruction of the gastric wall. When an ultrasound device is capable of detecting blood flow in the digestive tract wall or tumor by the two-dimensional color Doppler method, blood flow tends to be more abundant in cancerous than in fibrous tissue. However, at present, it is not easy to distinguish cancerous tissue from fibrous tissue on ultrasound images.

Microinvasion

The resolution of endoscopic ultrasonography is determined by the axial resolution, lateral resolution, and slice thickness of ultrasonic beam. It can also vary depending on the frequency of the ultrasound used and the type of scanning (mechanical radial scanning or electronic scanning). It is in the order of several hundreds of micrometers. With the ultrasound devices currently available, it is difficult to detect tumor invasion in some glands.

Essential Points in EUS Procedure

1. Accurate localization of lesions. It is essential to confirm that the lesion is accurately scanned.
2. Minimization of contamination of deaerated water by residue and air. Bubbles and food residues attenuate ultrasound beams, making it difficult to evaluate the continuity of layers.
3. The angle must be adjusted so that ultrasound beams can be applied perpendicularly to the layers of the lesion. When a cross section is scanned obliquely, the resultant image sometimes shows thickening or partial breakage of the normal layers. If the dose level of the antispasmodic is insufficient, accurate cross-sectional images are difficult to obtain due to movement of the wall.
4. A reduction in echo level of the submucosa due to fibrosis or edema needs to be distinguished from a reduced echo level caused by cancer invasion. Locally thickened muscularis propria or submucosa, caused by contraction of the digestive tract wall, must be distinguished from cancer invasion.

Conclusion

In conclusion, endoscopic ultrasonography yielded valuable information on the deeper mucosal layers and blood flow in gastric cancer and wall. Endoscopic ultrasonography also allowed puncture under ultrasonic guidance. This technique may thus become indispensable for the diagnosis and treatment of gastric cancer.

References

1. Lutz HT, Petzoldt R (1976) Ultrasonic patterns of space-occupying lesions of the stomach and the intestine. Ultrasound Med Biol 2:129–132

2. Morgan CL, Trought WS, Oddson TA, et al (1980) Ultrasound patterns of disorder affecting the gastrointestinal tract. Radiology 135:129
3. Strohm WD, Phillip J, Hagenmuller F, et al (1980) Ultrasonic tomography by means of an ultrasonic fiber-endoscopy. Endoscopy 12:241
4. DiMagno EP, Buxton JL, Regan PT (1980) Ultrasonic endoscopy. Lancet 1:629
5. DiMagno EP, Regan PT, Clain JL, et al (1982) Human endoscopic ultrasonography. Gastroenterology 83:824
6. Aibe T (1984) A study on the structure of layers of the gastrointestinal wall visualized by means of the ultrasonic endoscope. (1) The structure of layers of the gastric wall. Gastroenterol Endosc 26:1447–1464
7. Yamanaka T, Yoshida Y, Seki H, et al (1983) Ultrasonic diagnosis of invasion of early gastric cancer by means of ultrasonic endoscope. Nippon Shokakibyo Gakkai Zasshi 80:122
8. Jyojima Y, Yasuda H, Shimazu R, et al (1985) The diagnosis of the depth of invasion of gastric cancer. Jpn J Med Ultrasonics 12, (suppl I): 859–860
9. Yasuda H (1986) The diagnosis of the depth of gastric cancer invasion by ultrasonic method. J Jpn Surg Soc 87:608–625
10. Bolondi L, Casanova P, Santi V, et al (1986) Sonographic appearance of the normal gastric wall: an in vitro study. Ultrasound Med Biol 12:991–998
11. Tio TI, Tygat GN (1986) Endoscopic ultrasonography of normal and pathological upper gastrointestinal wall structure: comparision of studies in vivo and vitro with histology. Scand J Gastroenterol Suppl 21:27–33
12. Yasuda H, Hashimoto M, Tsuji E, et al (1999) Evaluation of the ultrasonic tomography of the gastric wall using a high resolution annular array probe; particularly lamina muscularis mucosa. Gastroenterol Endosc 41:2212–2223.
13. Shimoyama S, Seto Y, Yasuda H, et al (2000) Wider indications for the local resection of gastric cancer by adjacent lymphadenectomy. J Surg Oncol 75:157–164
14. Shimoyama S, Yasuda H, Mafune K, et al (2002) Indications of a minimized scope of lymphadenectomy for submucosal gastric cancer. Ann Surg Oncol 9:625–631
15. Shimoyama S, Joujima Y, Yasuda H, et al (2002) Prospectively performed modified D1 lymphadenectomy for clinically diagnosed mucosal, node negative gastric cancer: findings over the past decade. Int Surg 85:202–208
16. Shimoyama S, Yasuda H, Hashimoto M, et al (2004) Accuracy of linear-array EUS for preoperative staging of gastric cardia cancer. Gastrointest Endosc 60:50–55
17. Yoshino J, Inui K, Wakabayashi T, et al (2003) Standard technique in endoscopic ultrasonography for assessment of the depth of invasion of gastric cancer. Endosc Dig 15:553–558
18. Chonan A, Mishima T, Mochizuki F, et al (2001) Endoscopic ultrasonographic diagnosis of the depth of invasion of early gastric cancer for determining the indication for endoscpic mucosal resection. Stomach Intest 36:1625–1632
19. Yanai H, Noguchi T, Mizumachi S, et al (1999) A blind comparison of the effectiveness of endoscopic ultrasonography and endoscopy in staging early gastric cancer. Gut 44:361–365
20. Nomura N, Goto H, Niwa Y, et al (1999) Usefulness of contrast-enhanced EUS in the diagnosis of upper GI tract disease. Gastrointest Endosc 50:555–560
21. Habermann CR, Weiss F, Riecken R, et al (2004) Preoperative staging of gastric adenocarcinoma: comparison of helical CT and endoscopic US. Radiology 230:465–471

Recent Advances in Radiology for the Diagnosis of Gastric Carcinoma

Gen Iinuma[1], Hideto Tomimatsu[1], Yukio Muramatsu[1], Noriyuki Moriyama[1], Toshiaki Kobayashi[2], Hiroshi Saito[2], Tetsuo Maeda[3], Kunihisa Miyakawa[3], Fumihiko Wakao[3], Mitsuo Satake[3], and Yasuaki Arai[3]

Introduction

Radiographic diagnosis of gastric carcinoma [1] was first introduced in the 1960s in Japan, which led the world in the early diagnosis of gastric carcinoma by double-contrast method using film-screen systems (FSS) [2,3]. Qualitative diagnostics, including diagnosis of the depth of tumor invasion, were explored thoroughly in the 1970s, and it could be claimed that the radiographic diagnosis of gastric carcinoma was completely established by the beginning of the 1980s [4]. Gastric radiography has now become a standard examination modality in the screening and preoperative staging of gastric carcinoma and is widely used across the globe. The mortality rate from gastric carcinoma is especially high in Japan, and gastric radiography has made a substantial contribution to the detection of gastric carcinoma in mass screening. With recent advances in endoscopic techniques, the primary role in the diagnosis of gastric carcinoma, including its early diagnosis, has been inherited by endoscopy, but it is also a fact that radiography is still widely used in clinical diagnosis in screening and preoperative staging [5]. The demand for computerization of medical information grew in the 1980s, and against a background of advances in image engineering, the digitalization of medical images has proceeded apace [6,7]. In gastric radiography, too, digitalization via digital radiography (DR) using high-resolution charge-coupled device (CCD) cameras (CCD-DR) has been established and disseminated rapidly, and we also have reported its usefulness in the diagnosis of gastric carcinoma [8]. Meanwhile, a recent major development in the field of radiology has been the emergence of multidetector row computed tomography (CT) (MDCT) [9]. With the advent of MDCT in the second half of the 1990s, CT has achieved increased efficiencies and improved image quality in a revolutionary scanning modality [10]. In the preoperative staging of gastric carcinoma, it is now possible to accurately evaluate local inva-

[1] Cancer Screening Division, Research Center for Cancer Prevention and Screening, [2] Cancer Screening Technology Division, Research Center for Cancer Prevention and Screening, [3] Diagnostic Radiology Division, National Cancer Center Hospital, National Cancer Center, 5-1-1 Tsukiji, Chuo-ku, Tokyo 104-0045, Japan
e-mail: giinuma@gan2.ncc.go.jp

sion and small metastases, and three-dimensional (3D) MDCT imaging (MDCT gastrography) has arrived on the scene as a new diagnostic tool for primary lesions.

In this chapter, we describe the present status of radiologic diagnosis of gastric carcinoma using CCD-DR at our center, report our experience of MDCT gastrography in the preoperative staging of gastric carcinoma, and discuss the future prospects for radiographic diagnosis of gastric carcinoma using these new diagnostic techniques.

Advanced Digital Radiographic Systems for Gastric Diagnosis

In our hospital, images yielded by radiography of the gastrointestinal tract became completely digitalized with the adoption of CCD-DR (DR-2000H; Hitachi Medical, Tokyo, Japan) in 1999. At present, hard copies of diagnostic images are prepared for interpretation, but monitor-based diagnosis is yet to become a reality. Our radiographic investigations of the gastrointestinal tract use three CCD-DR systems: one C-arm type, one over-tube type, and one under-tube type. Each CCD-DR is connected by a DR network to two laser printers and an image server, and in parallel with the scanning procedure, reference images are forwarded to the hospital information system via a gateway after DICOM (digital imaging and communication in medicine) conversion at the same time as the diagnostic images are processed. After DICOM

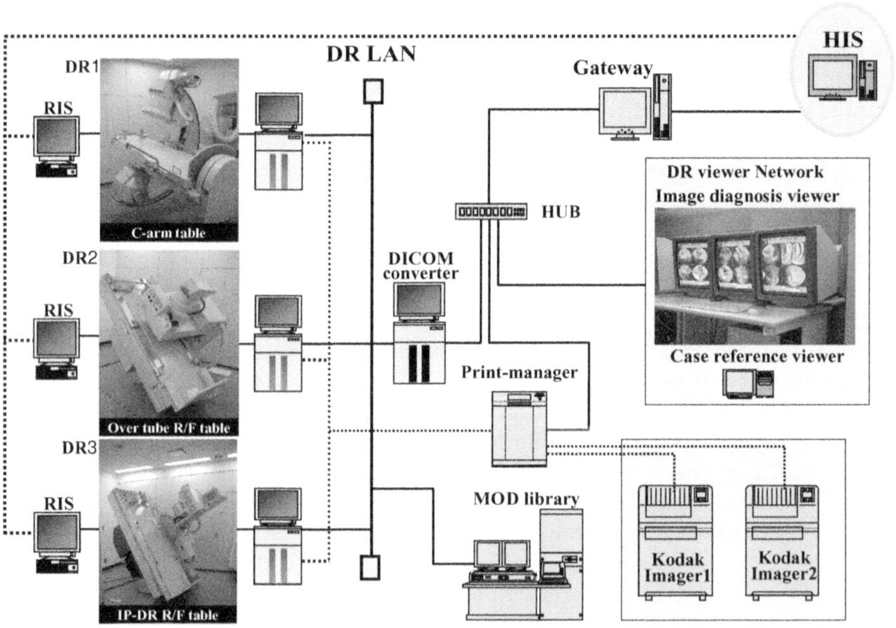

Fig. 1. Advanced digital radiography system for gastric diagnosis. Three charge-coupled device-digital radiography (CCD-DR) units are routinely used for gastric examinations in our hospital. Each unit connects with a DR network, and the images can be diagnosed on an image workstation

conversion, the images are accessible for monitor diagnosis at an image workstation with three viewers (Fig. 1).

The Status of CCD-DR-Based Radiographic Examination of Gastric Carcinoma

At our center, we use 250–300 ml barium at a 130–140 w/v% concentration in gastric radiographic studies. The scanning methods employed are the filling method, double-contrast radiography, and the compression method, but the core diagnostic technique in radiographic diagnosis of gastric carcinoma is double-contrast imaging obtained with barium (positive contrast medium) and gas (negative contrast medium). After barium is swallowed, the patient is given 5 g of a foaming agent, and by distending the stomach via the CO_2 gas so produced, we are able to easily obtain double-contrast images. The barium contained in the gas-distended stomach moves with changes in posture, and double-contrast images of excellent quality are obtained by ensuring that the barium adheres uniformly to the mucosal surfaces. Unlike the filling and compression methods, double-contrast imaging is indispensable for the visualization of early gastric carcinoma, which is characterized by few irregularities of the mucosal surfaces (Fig. 2). With gastric radiography based on the double-contrast method, we can easily identify the macroscopic types of gastric carcinomas, their exact extensions and locations in the stomach (Figs. 3–6). However, viewing double-contrast images obtained with contrast provided by gas and barium requires a broad dynamic range. The dynamic range for CCD-DR images adequately covers the image quality required for gastric radiography, and the image quality matches that in conventional FSS. Additionally, CCD-DR digital images also enable the optimization of image quality via image processing after scanning and, compared with FSS, are relatively well matched image by image and allow standardized diagnostic images to be obtained.

Comparative Evaluation of FSS and CCD-DR in the Diagnosis of Gastric Carcinoma

We conducted a prospective study to evaluate the difference in diagnostic accuracy between FSS and CCD-DR, and reported in a publication of *Radiology* [8]. From January to February 1997, we randomly assigned patients scheduled for gastric radiography to either FSS or CCD-DR; 112 patients were examined by FSS and 113 by CCD-DR. Six radiologists who were blinded to the clinical details assessed the films for each patient with a six-level confidence rating for the presence or absence of gastric carcinoma. The CCD-DR images in this study were prepared as hard copies for diagnosis. The diagnoses for each patient were rated against those produced by three other radiologists who conducted the actual radiographic examinations and were aware of all clinical data, such as endoscopic findings and the pathology of biopsy specimens. The sensitivity and specificity of FSS and CCD-DR for gastric carcinoma were determined from the assessments obtained, the difference between the two modalities was statistically analyzed, and a comparison was performed by receiver-operating characteristic (ROC) analysis. The study yielded a diagnosis of gastric carcinoma by FSS in 24 patients and by CCD-DR in 27 patients; the sensitivity for diagnosing the presence of gastric carcinoma was 64.6% and 75.3%, respectively

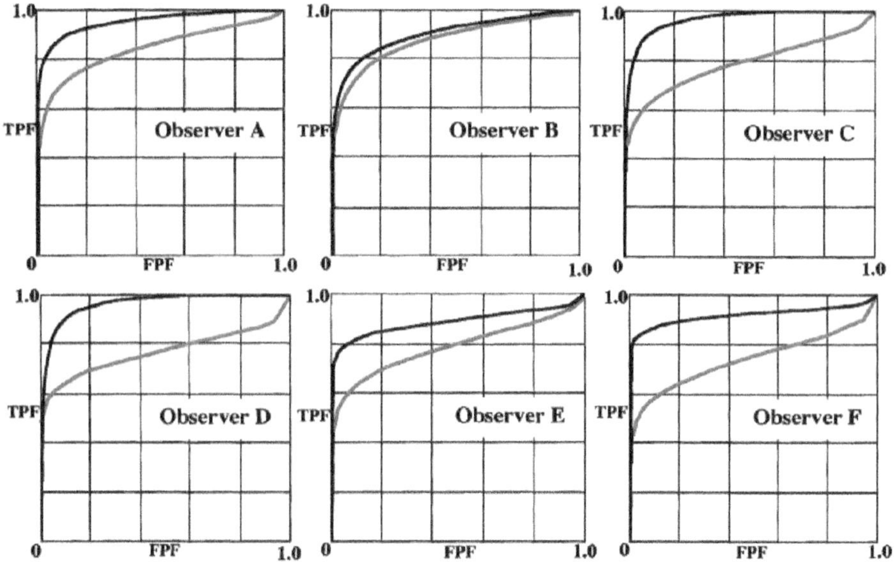

FIG. 7. Receiver operating characteristic (ROC) curves obtained from six observers. All observers achieved more accurate results with CCD-DR than with conventional radiography. Diagnostic accuracy of CCD-DR is clearly superior to that of conventional radiography. (Used with permission from Radiological Society of North America)

($P = 0.278$), and the specificity was 84.5% and 90.5%, respectively ($P = 0.011$). The ROC analysis [11] also showed that the diagnostic performance of CCD-DR was clearly superior (Fig. 7).

Usefulness of Radiography of Gastric Carcinoma by CCD-DR

The diagnostic performance of CCD-DR for gastric carcinoma is adequately comparable to that of FSS, indicating that the digitalization of images in gastric radiography is entirely feasible. The future adoption of diagnosis by monitor display will make possible the real-time display and optimization of diagnostic images and enable greater ease of image storage and retrieval. Capitalizing on these advantages of digitalization promises to yield an efficient and effective diagnostic environment for screening and preoperative staging, as compared with the conventional FSS modality.

Preoperative Evaluation of Gastric Carcinoma Using MDCT

To date, the role of radiographic CT studies in the preoperative staging of gastric carcinoma has primarily involved evaluating invasion of surrounding organs or metastasis to lymph nodes or other organs, and it was rare for it to be used for evaluation of the primary tumor itself [12,13]. However, the advent of MDCT has made possible the arrival of full-scale volume scans, facilitating high-speed, detailed image acquisition over an extensive area. The degree of resolution of CT images has improved dramatically with MDCT, enabling the detailed evaluation of local lesions and the detection of small metastases, even in ordinary axial images [14]. Moreover, workstations that are capable of processing the massive quantities of image data produced by MDCT have been developed, and the three-dimensional CT visualization of gastric lesions, which is called MDCT gastrography, has become straightforward. This trend is fairly flourishing in the diagnosis of colorectal cancer as MDCT colonography, which is considered to have a great potential of being a modality for colorectal cancer screening [15–17].

Three-Dimensional Visualization of the Stomach by MDCT Gastrography

To visualize gastric lesions in three dimensions using MDCT, it is necessary to distend the gastric lumen with a foaming agent (CO_2 gas). As a consequence of the contrast between the gas and the inner gastric surface, owing to the substantial difference in density, it is possible to effortlessly prepare 3D images of the inner gastric surface. MDCT gastrography employs two methods for visualization, virtual endoscopic views and 3D gas insufflation views, obtained by 3D processing of the CT image data (Fig. 8).

Evaluation of the Detectability of Gastric Carcinoma by MDCT Gastrography

In the 3-month period between March and June 2003, we evaluated 4-row MDCT (Aquilion; Toshiba Medical Systems, Tokyo, Japan) in 84 gastric carcinoma patients who underwent MDCT for preoperative staging. Each scan was performed with the standard abdominal scan parameter settings for preoperative staging using automatic exposure control [18]. We prepared virtual endoscopic and 3D gas insufflation views from the image data obtained for each patient by MDCT volume scans, and two radiologists prepared responses on the basis of all clinical data for each patient, including gastroscopic findings, and the detectability of gastric carcinoma was evaluated by consensus for each display method. Eighty-six gastric carcinoma lesions (44 early and 42 advanced lesions) were diagnosed in the 84 patients. The detectability by virtual endoscopic and 3D gas insufflation views by MDCT gastrography was 47.7% and 40.9%, respectively, for early lesions (Table 1), and 59.5% and 76.2% for advanced lesions (Table 2). Hence, the detectability was less than 50% for early lesions, but about 60%–70% for advanced lesions of gastric carcinoma [19]. Especially in early lesions, all protruded-type lesions could be recognized, while less than half of depressed-type lesions, which is a common type of early gastric carcinoma, were missed (Figs. 9, 10).

TABLE 1. Detectability for 44 early gastric carcinomas by multidetector row computed tomography (MDCT) gastrography

	Protruded type	Flat elevated type	Depressed type	Total
Virtual endoscopic views	100% (2/2)	50.0% (1/2)	45.0% (18/40)	47.7% (21/44)
Three-dimensional gas insufflation views	100% (2/2)	50.0% (1/2)	37.5% (15/40)	40.9% (18/44)

Table 2. Detectability for 42 advanced gastric cancers by MDCT gastrography

	Borrman I type	Borrman II type	Borrman III type	Borrman IV type	Total
Virtual endoscopic view	0% (0/1)	84.6% (11/13)	68.8% (11/16)	25.0% (3/12)	59.5% (25/42)
Three-dimensional gas insufflation view	0% (0/1)	76.9% (10/13)	68.8% (11/16)	91.7% (11/12)	76.2% (32/42)

MDCT gastrography is presently inadequate for the detection of gastric carcinoma and its potential for clinical application is low.

Potential for MDCT Gastrography in Preoperative Staging for Gastric Carcinoma

MDCT gastrography is simpler and less invasive than endoscopy and radiography, and permits evaluation of the stomach overall in an examination of short duration. Detection of early lesions is challenging, and although it therefore has low potential as a screening method, it is capable of detecting lesions that are advanced to a certain extent, and also of simultaneously detecting lesions in other organs of the abdomen. In preoperative staging, as for radiography, it is capable of objectively ascertaining the position and overall picture of the primary lesion, and of diagnosing the relations between the degree of extramural invasion and surrounding organs. With the axial images of MDCT, representing a quantum leap in resolution compared with normal CT, it was possible to also diagnose correctly lymph node metastasis. Because MDCT itself is an examination method required for the preoperative diagnosis of local spread or remote metastasis of gastric carcinoma, it is highly likely at present that it can partially replace the role of radiography or ultrasound endoscopy. As well, because the image data of MDCT is digitalized density information, it is possible to selectively visualize 3D information in a manner that is effective for diagnosis, and has a great potential of being a modality for computer-aided diagnosis [20]. By digitally combining the 3D view of the primary lesion and the 3D image data of diagnosed lymph node metastasis, it will be possible to provide surgeons with effective preoperative 3D views of gastric carcinoma (Fig. 11).

Conclusions

As a result of future advancements in image engineering and computer technology, digital radiographic systems and MDCT systems will continue to evolve, and it can be predicted that new diagnostic methods that utilize the advantages of digitalization in the radiological diagnosis of gastric carcinoma will also be developed. MDCT gastrography has little potential at present as a diagnostic method for the primary lesions of gastric carcinoma. However, with further advances in MDCT, higher-speed examinations, improved image quality, and optimization of exposure dose, it appears certain that MDCT gastrography will gradually replace radiography, endoscopy, and ultrasound endoscopy.

Acknowledgments. This work was supported by Grants for Scientific Research Expenses for Health and Welfare Programs and the Foundation for the Promotion of Cancer Research, and by the 3rd-term Comprehensive 10-year Strategy for Cancer Control from the Ministry of Health, Labor and Welfare.

References

1. Templeton FE (1964) X-ray examination of the stomach, rev edn. University of Chicago Press, Chicago
2. Kuru M (1966) X-ray diagnosis. In: Atlas of early gastric carcinoma of the stomach. Nakayama-Shoten, Tokyo, pp 219–223
3. Shirakabe H, Ichikwa H, Kumakura K, et al (1966) Atlas of X-ray diagnosis of early gastric cancer. Igaku Shoin, Tokyo
4. Ichikawa H (1993) X-ray diagnosis of early gastric cancer. Gastric cancer. Springer-Verlag, Tokyo, pp 232–245
5. Okumura T, Maruyama M (1993) A prospective study on advanced gastric cancer detection by mass screening. Gastric Cancer. Springer-Verlag, Tokyo, pp 263–277
6. Sonoda M, Takano M, Miyahara J, et al (1983) Computed radiography utilizing scanning laser stimulated luminescence. Radiology 148:833–838
7. Hillman BJ, Ovitt TW, Nudelman S, et al (1981) Digital video subtraction angiography of renal vascular abnormalities. Radiology 139:277–280
8. Iinuma G, Ushio K, Ishikawa T, et al (2001) Diagnosis of gastric cancers: comparison of conventional radiography with a 4 million-pixels charge-coupled device. Radiology 214: 497–502
9. Berland LL, Smith JK (1998) Multidetector-array CT: once again, technology creates new opportunities. Radiology 209:327–329
10. Hu H, He HD, Foley WD, Fox SH (2000) Four multidetector-row helical CT: image quality and volume coverage speed. Radiology 215:55–62
11. Metz CE, Goodenough DJ, Rossmann K (1973) Evaluation of receiver operating characteristic curve data in terms of information theory, with applications in radiography. Radiology 109:297–303
12. Botet JF, Lightdale CJ, Zauber AG, et al (1991) Preoperative staging of gastric cancer: comparison of endoscopic US and dynamic CT. Radiology 181:426–432
13. Habermann RC, Weiss F, Riecken R, et al (2004) Preoperative staging of gastric adenocarcinoma: comparison of helical CT and endoscopic US. Radiology 230:465–471
14. Ba-Ssalamah A, Prokop M, Uffmann M, et al (2003) Dedicated multidetector CT of the stomach: spectrum of diseases. *Radiographics* 181:426–432
15. Dachman A (2003) Atlas of virtual colonoscopy. Springer-Verlag, New York
16. Iannaccone R, Laghi A, Catalano C, et al (2003) Detection of colorectal lesions: lower-dose multi-detector row helical CT colonography compared with conventional colonoscopy. Radiology 229:775–781
17. Macari M, Bini EJ, Jacobs SL, et al (2004) Colorectal polyps and cancers in asymptomatic average-risk patients: evaluation with CT colonography. Radiology 230:629–636
18. Itoh S, Ikeda M, Mori Y, et al (2002) Lung: feasibility of a method for changing tube current during low-dose helical CT. Radiology 224:905–912
19. Iinuma G, Moriyama N (2004) Clinical potential of CT gastrography for visualization of gastric cancers. In: Recent advances in gastric cancers: the 17th International Symposium of Foundation for Promotion of Cancer Research, pp 37–38
20. Summers RM (2003) Road maps for advancement of radiologic computer-aided detection in the 21st century. *Radiology* 229:11–13

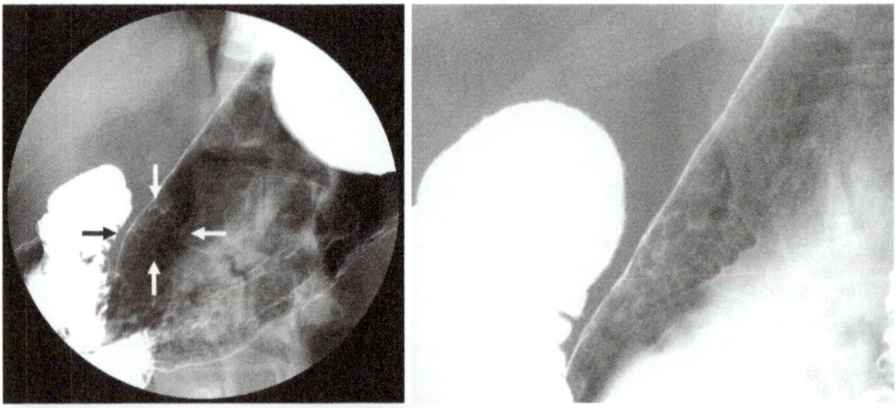

a b

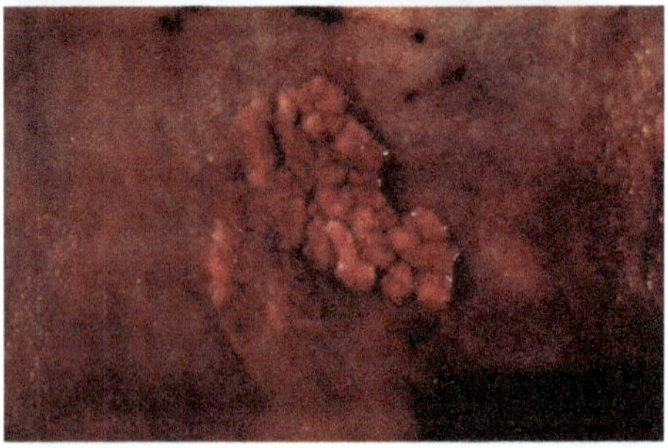

c

FIG. 2. A 55-year-old man. A flat lesion is visualized at the lesser curvature side of the lower gastric body (**a**, *arrows*). CCD-DR clearly delineates the irregular surface of the lesion (**b**). Gross specimen shows a flat type of early gastric cancer, 2.5 × 1.5 cm in size (**c**)

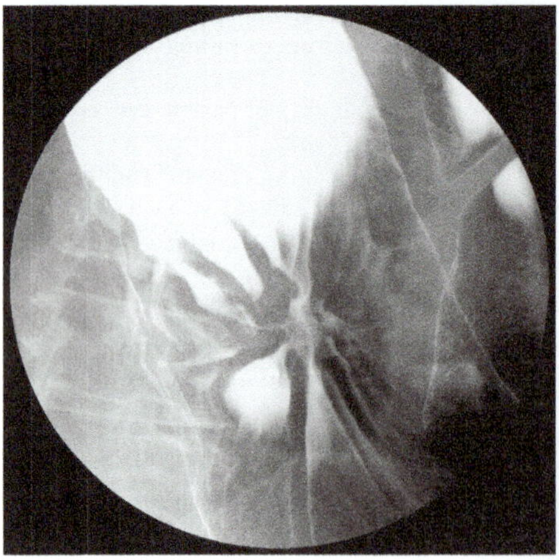

a

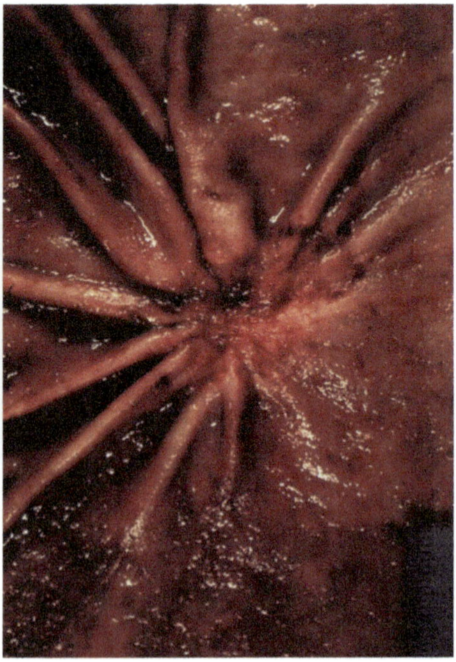

b

FIG. 3. A 65-year-old woman. A depressed type of advanced cancer with converging folds is clearly demonstrated by CCD-DR at the anterior wall of the middle gastric body (**a**). Gross specimen shows a relatively deep carcinomatous erosion of 5.5 × 4.5 cm. The converging folds partially make some protuberance at the margin of the lesion (**b**)

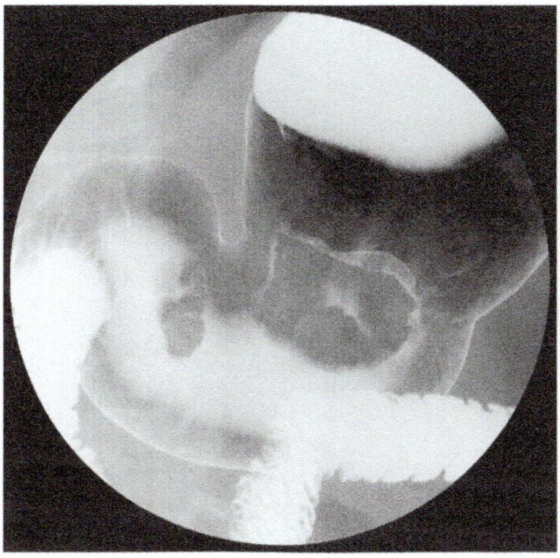
a

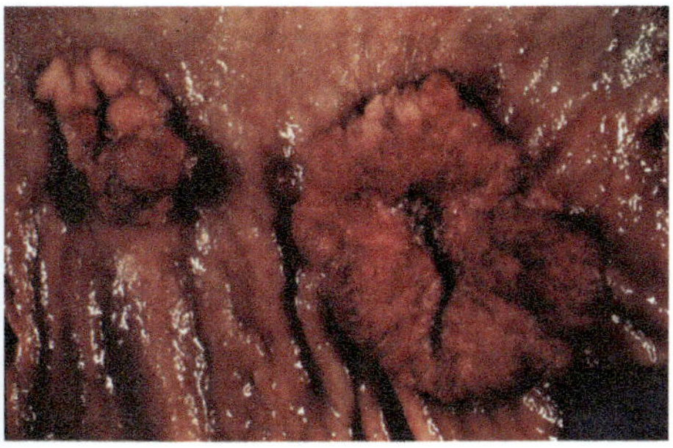
b

FIG. 4. A 70-year-old man. CCD-DR visualizes two gastric cancers at the posterior of the lower gastric body to the antrum (**a**). Gross specimen demonstrates a protruded advanced cancer with central ulceration measuring 4.0 cm and a protruded type of early cancer measuring 2.0 cm (**b**)

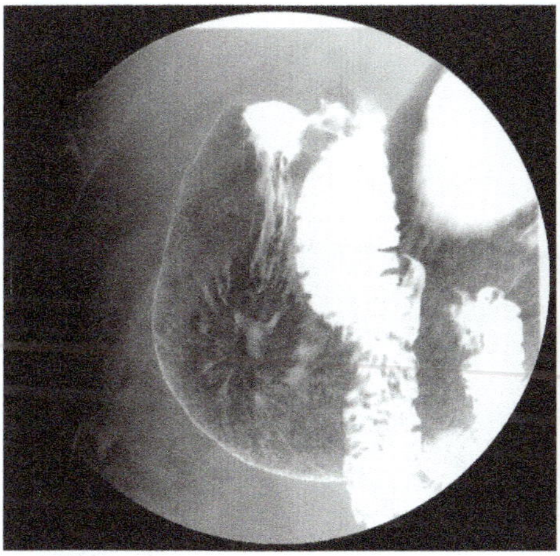
a

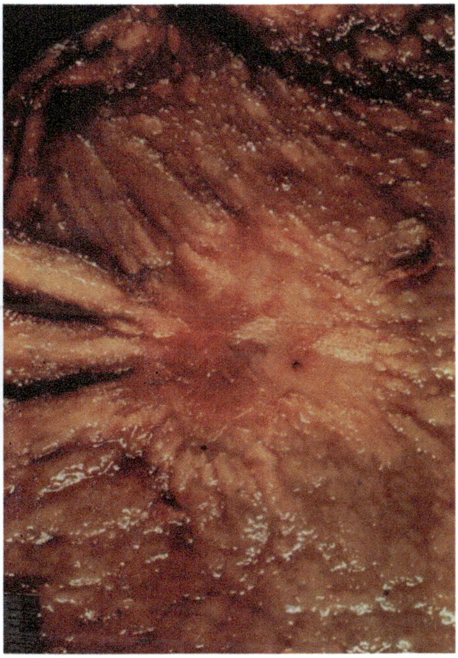
b

FIG. 5. A 55-year-old man. CCD-DR demonstrates a depressed type of gastric cancer at the posterior wall of the antrum (**a**). Gross specimen shows a depressed type of advanced cancer 5.0 × 4.5 cm in size (**b**)

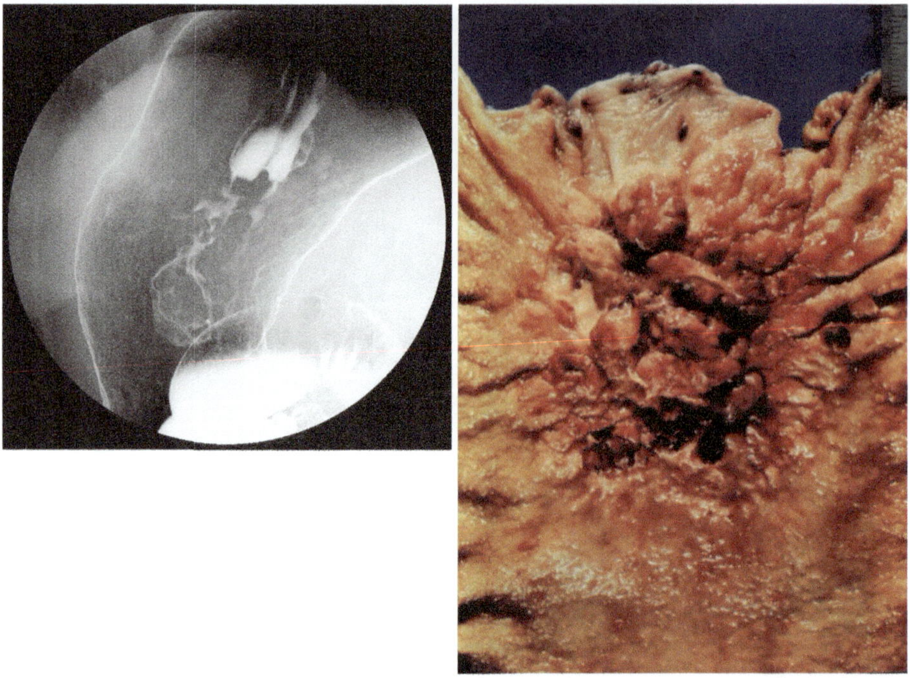

a b

Fig. 6. A 71-year-old man. An advanced cancer is demonstrated by CCD-DR just below the cardia (**a**). Gross specimen shows an ulcerative type of advanced gastric cancer 6.0 cm in diameter (**b**)

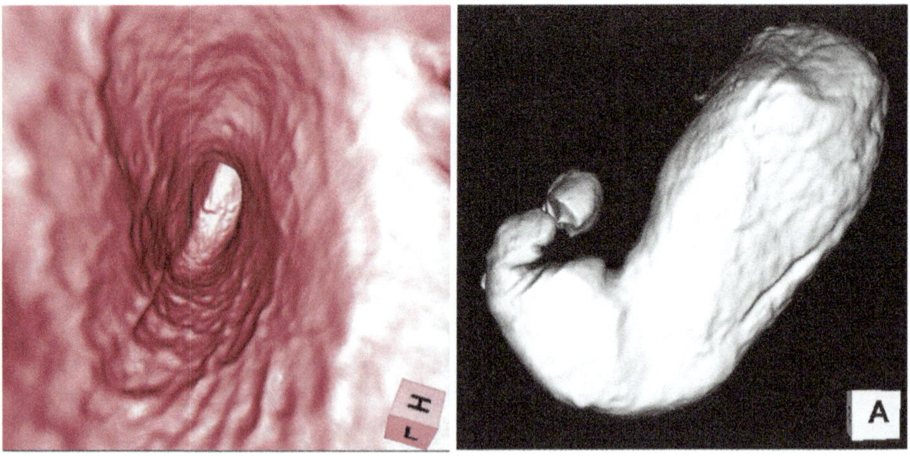

a b

Fig. 8. Two imaging modes of multidetector row computed tomography (MDCT) gastrography. **a** A representative virtual endoscopic view, resembling gastroscopic images. **b** A representative 3D gas insufflation view, resembling radiographic images

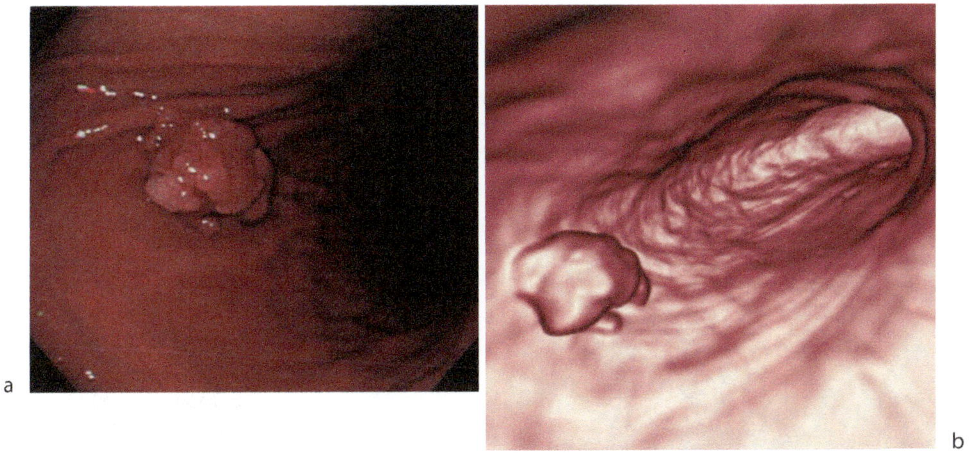

Fig. 9. A 63-year-old man. Conventional endoscopy demonstrates a protruded type of early gastric cancer 2 cm in size at the greater curvature side of the upper gastric body (**a**). The lesion is clearly visualized by virtual endoscopic view (**b**)

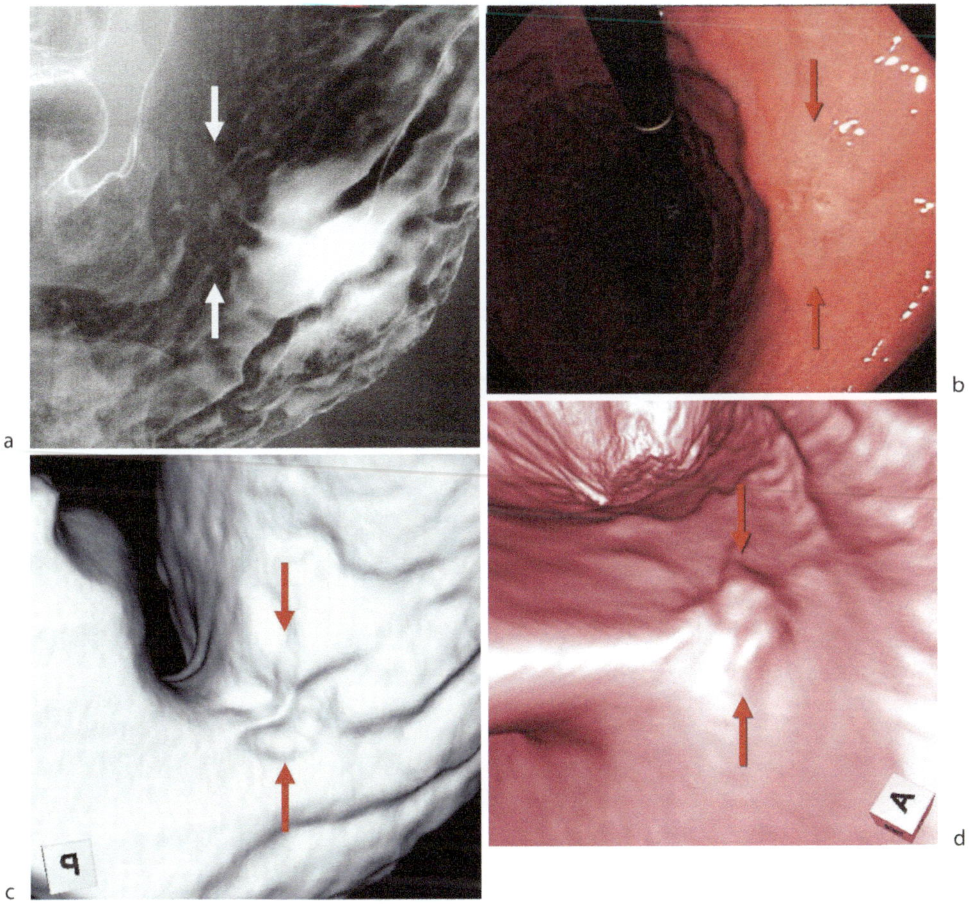

Fig. 10. A 33-year-old man. A small depressed type of early gastric cancer measuring 1.5 cm is identified at the posterior side of the gastric angle by gastric radiography and gastroscopy (*arrows* in **a, b**). The lesion can barely be recognized by virtual endoscopic and 3D views of MDCT gastrography (*arrows* in **c, d**)

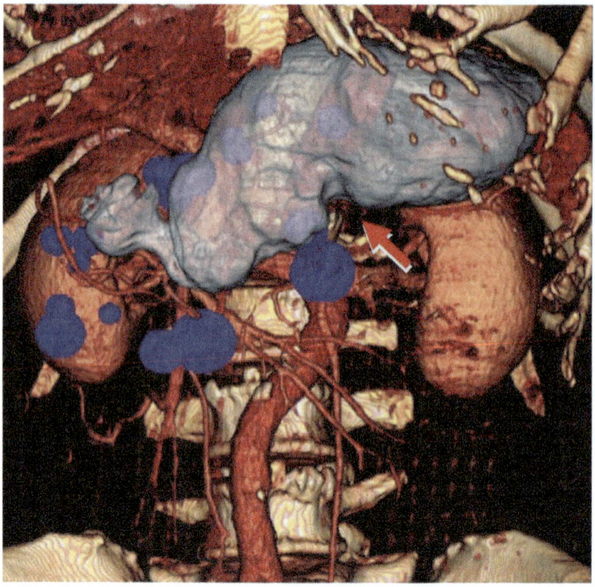

Fig. 11. Three-dimensional imaging of a gastric cancer and lymph node metastases. The 3D view of the primary lesion (*arrow*) and the 3D image data of diagnosed lymph node metastases can be combined digitally to produce effective 3D views of gastric carcinoma in the preoperative staging

Part 5

Therapy for Gastric Carcinoma

The Gastric Cancer Treatment Guideline

Mitsuru Sasako

Introduction

The Japan Gastric Cancer Association issued the first edition of the *Gastric Cancer Treatment Guideline* in March 2001 [1]. Based on new evidence, the second edition was issued in April 2004 [2]. In this chapter, the content of this guideline is introduced.

Background of the Japanese Guideline

Gastric cancer remains the most common cancer in Japan, although it surrendered first place of the high annual mortality rate to lung cancer. The mortality rate of gastric cancer is seven times higher in Japan than in the United States and three times higher than in the UK [3]. Consequently, gastric cancer patients are treated not only in cancer specialist hospitals but also in most university hospitals and general hospitals, even in rural areas. In more than 100 Japanese hospitals, more than 100 patients undergo gastrectomy for gastric cancer every year. Even in other hospitals, the hospital volume is much higher than in most European hospitals.

The second unique situation in Japan is that more than half the patients have T1 tumors, that is, early gastric cancer. This result is partly due to the mass screening system, which covers actually as little as 10% of the entire population over 40 years old [4]. On the whole, the knowledge of the high risk of gastric cancer among general practitioners and even among the common citizen seems more important for early detection of this disease. Most Japanese tend to undergo endoscopy when they have even minimum symptoms of the upper gastrointestinal tract. We have accumulated an enormous database using the common rule, The General Rules for the Gastric Cancer Study issued by the Japanese Research Society for Gastric Cancer in 1962. According to the large database, the incidence of lymph node metastasis increases by

Gastric Surgery Division, National Cancer Center Hospital, 5-1-1 Tsukiji, Chuo-ku, Tokyo 104-0045, Japan
Japan Gastric Cancer Association, c/o Digestive Surgery Department, Kyoto Prefectural University of Medicine, Kawaramachi Hirokoji, Kamigyo-ku, Kyoto, Japan
e-mail: msasako@gan2.ncc.go.jp

tumor depth, and the deeper the tumor invasion, the more distant regional lymph nodes become metastatic. The incidence of nodal metastasis was just 2%–3% in T1 mucosal cancer and 15%–20% in T1 submucosal cancer [5]. Using this database, it was possible to select patients with T1 tumors who have negligible risk of lymph node metastasis. Together with the development of the instruments and technique of endoscopic mucosal resection (EMR), many of these mucosal cancers with minimal risk of nodal metastasis are now treated endoscopically [6]. In the year 2003, approximately 350 patients with T1 tumor underwent an EMR as definitive treatment, whereas about 300 underwent open surgery at National Cancer Center Hospital, Tokyo.

One of the reasons for this high incidence of early gastric cancer (EGC) is that the diagnostic criteria of gastric carcinoma are slightly different in Japan from those in the West [7]. Many Western pathologists diagnose the lesions without definite invasion as dysplasia, whereas they are diagnosed as well-differentiated adenocarcinoma in Japan if they have cellular and structural atypia compatible with adenocarcinoma. As biopsy specimens are usually taken from the surface of the lesions, they cannot prove deeper invasion of the lesions. Therefore, many of these "dyplasia" actually invade into the submucosal layer or even deeper when they are resected and histologically examined [8].

The most common type of surgery for curable gastric cancer in Japan is a gastrectomy with D2 lymph node dissection. In many Western countries, surgeons refrain from this procedure due to higher mortality than limited surgery (D0/1) and uncertain efficacy [9]. This contrast is partly explained by the high incidence of the disease and subsequent high hospital and surgeon volume in Japan, but also by the relatively low body mass index of the average Japanese. Difficulty and efficacy of abdominal surgery are somewhat affected by the volume of intraabdominal adipose tissue. In obese patients, generally speaking, a complicated surgery is much more difficult than in slim patients. Less than 1% of patients have body mass index over 30 in Japan, whereas more than 20% are obese in the United States. This fact makes surgeons more conservative in use of an aggressive type of surgery in the West.

Principles: Basic Structure of the Guideline

This guideline shows the standard treatments and reasonable options for each stage. They are clearly separated into two groups, the standard treatments or the treatments under investigation (Tables 1, 2). As treatment strategy varies widely in EGCs, the standard treatment is indicated with detailed conditions in stage Ia and Ib tumors. Unlike many other guidelines, the algorithm system is not used.

Treatment of Early Gastric Cancer

A wide resection with lymphadenectomy remains the gold standard treatment for gastric cancer, even for T1 gastric cancers, 10% of which have lymph node metastasis. In the guideline, standard radical gastrectomy is defined as a gastrectomy of more than two-thirds of the stomach with D2 lymph node dissection. However, patients with negligible risk of having nodal metastasis can be treated by a mere wide resection, avoiding a gastrectomy, which makes a serious change of eating habits obligatory.

Table 1. Stage-specific standards of care by the Japanese Guideline

	N0	N1	N2	N3
T1(M)	EMR, ModA	ModB	STD	Ext Palliative surgery CTX
T1(SM)	ModA ModB	STD		
T2	STD	STD	STD	Radiation therapy
T3	STD	STD	STD	Palliative care
T4	Ext (C.R)	Ext (C.R)		
M1				

MER, endoscopic mucosal resection; ModA, modified gastrectomy A; ModB, modified gastrectomy B; STD, standard gastrectomy; Ext (C.R), extended gastrectomy with combined resection of involved organs; EXT, extended gastrectomy including extended lymphadenectomy, combined organ resection for lymphadenectomy; CTX, chemotherapy

Table 2. Treatments in clinical research by the Japanese Guideline

	N0	N1	N2	N3
T1(M)	EMR*	LADG		Ext Reduction surgery CTX HTCTX
T1(SM)	LADG LR, SG			
T2	LADG	ACTX	ACTX	
T3	ACTX	D3 ACTX	D3 ACTX	
T4	CTX, ACTX Rad	Ext CTX ACTX		
M1				

EMR*, extended indication for EMR; LADG, laparoscopy-assisted distal gastrectomy; LR, local resection wedge resection; SG, segmental gastrectomy; ACTX, adjuvant chemotherapy; D3, D3 lymphadenectomy; HTCTX, hyperthermochemotherapy

The endoscopic mucosal resection (EMR) is the most beneficial method for patients because they do not have to undergo laparotomy or general anesthesia [6]. Theoretically, several groups of patients have very limited probability of nodal metastasis [10]. If the lesion is a mucosal cancer of differentiated histology without either lymphatic or vascular involvement, and without ulcerative change, the probability of lymph nodal metastasis is less than 0.3%. If the lesions fulfill the criteria, except that there is ulcerative change inside the lesion, only those that are 3 cm or less in size can be regarded as node negative (less than 0.8%). For lesions showing minimal submucosal invasion, less than 500 μm in depth, without lymphatic or vascular involvement, with size 3 cm or less, the upper limit of 95% confidence interval of the probability of nodal metastasis is 2.5%.

However, EMR for a large lesion is technically demanding and it is not easy to remove lesions larger than 2 cm in one piece by the strip biopsy method. In this regard, EMR using a specially invented knife or hook to dissect the entire submucosal layer from the surface of the proper muscle layer is becoming more and more popular because it enables one-piece resection with full mucosal and submucosal layers of large size, up to even 10 cm. The term endoscopic submucosal dissection (ESD) is recently being used for this technique with the intention of discriminating it from EMR by strip biopsy technique using a snare [6]. At the moment, ESD is not for every gastroenterologist or surgeon. Therefore, the indication for EMR is described as follows in the Japanese Guideline: mucosal cancer, differentiated-type histology, smaller than 2 cm, without ulcer or ulcer scar in the lesion. These criteria should be confirmed by histological evaluation of the endoscopically resected specimen. To be accurate in evaluating the whole specimen, it is strongly advised to carry out a one-piece resection. For this meaning, EMR for T1 tumors other than those described in the guideline are regarded as treatment under investigation.

T1 tumors that do not meet the criteria for EMR or ESD should be treated by surgery. Two types of modification of D2 gastrectomy are recommended in the Japanese Guideline, because of low incidence of lymph node metastasis to the second tier nodal stations [11]. The area of resection is the same as the standard gastrectomy, but with D1 (including all perigastric lymph nodes of the relevant part of the stomach) plus the left gastric artery nodes is one option for clinically T1 (mucosal) and pN0 cancer of differentiated type larger than 2 cm or of undifferentiated histology of any size. For clinically T1 (submucosal) and pN0 cancer or clinically T1 (mucosal) and pN1 cancer, two-thirds or wider gastrectomy with D1 plus the left gastric, the common hepatic, and the celiac artery nodes is the recommended option. The indication of the modified procedures is based on the clinical and surgical diagnosis and therefore contains some risk of underestimation. The guideline gives caution of this risk. Other T1 tumors should be treated by the standard D2 gastrectomy. Laparoscopic gastrectomy with D1 or D2 lymph node dissection is nominated as a treatment under investigation.

Treatment of Curable Advanced Gastric Cancer

For sT2 and sN0–2 tumors and sT3 and sN0–2 tumors, the standard D2 gastrectomy is the gold standard in the Japanese Guideline. For sT4 and sN0–2 tumors, the standard D2 gastrectomy with additional resection of the involved organ is regarded as the standard [13]. If published results of clinical studies evaluating the efficacy of D2 dissection are reviewed, the majority of them showed negative results [12–14]. However, all these negative studies were heavily criticized regarding the quality of surgery given in the D2 arm [15,16]. These results were understandable if the concepts of hospital volume and learning curve are incorporated.

The clinical trial (phase III) carried out by the Japan Clinical Oncology Group (JCOG) to evaluate the efficacy of paraaortic lymph node dissection has been closed and the survival results are awaited [17].

Another JCOG clinical trial on gastric cancer invading the lower esophagus proved that the abdominal-only approach should be used for these tumors whose esophageal invasion is 3 cm or less. Therefore, the majority of patients with type II or III tumors of the Siewert classification should be treated through laparotomy and the trans-diaphragmatic approach [18]. Thorough mediastinal node dissection by thoracotomy is not needed to treat these tumors.

Just as in Europe, any kind of adjuvant treatment is regarded as a treatment under investigation. Although many meta-analyses of adjuvant chemotherapy show a small but significant benefit of adjuvant chemotherapy over surgery alone, treatment regimens of these analyses are widely heterogeneous. Similar to the conclusions of all these meta-analyses, adjuvant chemotherapy after curative surgery is regarded as under investigation and should be evaluated exclusively in clinical trials with surgery alone as the control [19–21]. Also, the guideline advocates RCT on adjuvant chemotherapy for curable gastric cancer, both pre- and postoperatively.

In the United States, an adjuvant chemoradiotherapy (CRT) after curative surgery is now regarded as the standard treatment [22]. However, in the clinical trial that proved the benefit of CRT over surgery alone, the type of lymph node dissection was just D0 (almost without nodal dissection) for 54% of patients, D1 for 36%, and D2 dissection for 10% of the patients. This finding means that 90% of the patients underwent surgery with insufficient local control in terms of lymph node dissection. Together with the fact that adjuvant chemotherapy alone could not prove a benefit over surgery alone, this trial proved the efficacy and importance of local control for the treatment of gastric cancer. Because the standard surgery for curable tumors in Japan includes much wider lymph node dissection and the stage-specific survival results of this trial were still worse than those of Japanese data, these results supporting the efficacy of CRT cannot be applied to Japanese patients. The effect of CRT after D2 dissection remains uncertain. In the Japanese guideline, the standard treatment for curable advanced gastric cancer is still D2 gastrectomy alone. Any kind of adjuvant treatment is regarded as investigational.

Treatment of Incurable Gastric Cancer

Only those who can undergo R0 resection have a possibility of cure depending on the tumor stage, that is, T factor and N factor. Patients with nonresectable disease or with distant metastasis are incurable and are primarily treated by chemotherapy if they do not have serious symptoms such as massive bleeding or stenosis hindering oral intake. In the guideline, resection of primary gastric tumor in patients with distant metastasis is defined as reduction surgery and is regarded as investigational treatment. This reduction surgery has often been carried out in Japan without any evidence of advantage for the patients.

Similarly, the majority of recurrences are nonresectable and are treated by chemotherapy. However, at the moment, there is no standard chemotherapy regimen for nonresectable or recurrent gastric cancer. In the United States, the combination chemotherapy using fluorouracil and cisplatin plus docetaxel (5-FU + CDDP + docetaxel) is now regarded as the standard [23]. In Europe, on the other hand, epirubicin

+ CDDP + 5FU is recommended as the standard regimen [24]. These two newly developed regimens are highly toxic, and their efficacy and safety are not yet confirmed in Japanese patients. Actually, combination chemotherapy including TS-1, CPT-11, paclitaxel, 5-Fu, or CDDP is under investigation with the expectation of a longer survival period than with 5-FU alone.

References

1. Japanese Gastric Cancer Association (2001) Gastric cancer treatment guideline, 1st edn. Kanehara, Tokyo
2. Japanese Gastric Cancer Association (2004) Gastric cancer treatment guideline, 2nd edn. Kanehara, Tokyo
3. Japanese Cancer Association (2004) Tajima K, Kuroishi T, Oshima A eds. Cancer mortality and morbidity statistics, Japan and the world—2004. Japan Scientific Society Press, Tokyo, pp 176–177
4. Tsubono Y, Hisamichi S (2000) Screening for gastric cancer in Japan. Gastric Cancer 3:9–18
5. Sasako M (2000) What is reasonable treatment for gastric adenocarcinoma? J Gastroenterol 35(suppl XII):116–120
6. Gotoda T (2004) Endoscopic diagnosis and treatment for early gastric cancer. Cancer Rev 2:17–37
7. Schlemper RJ, Itabashi M, Kato Y, et al (1997) Differences in diagnostic criteria for gastric carcinoma between Japanese and Western pathologists. Lancet 349:1725–1729
8. Lansdown M, Quirke P, Dixon MF, et al (1989) High grade dysplasia of the gastric mucosa: a marker for gastric carcinoma. Gut 31:977–983
9. Hundahl SA, Macdonald JS, Benedetti J, et al (2002) Surgical treatment variation in a prospective, randomized trial of chemoradiotherapy in gastric cancer: the effect of undertreatment. Ann Surg Oncol 9:278–286
10. Gotoda T, Yanagisawa A, Sasako M, et al (2000) Incidence of lymph node metastasis from early gastric cancer: estimation with a large number of cases at two large centers. Gastric Cancer 3:219–225
11. Sasako M (2003) Principles of surgical treatment for curable gastric cancer. J Clin Oncol 21: 274s–275s
12. Bonenkamp JJ, Hermans J, Sasako M, et al (1999) Extended lymph-node dissection for gastric cancer. New Engl J Med 340:908–914
13. Cuschieri A, Weeden S, Fielding J, et al (1999) Patient survival after D1 and D2 resection for gastric cancer: long-term results of the MRC randomized surgical trial. Br J Cancer 79: 1522–1530
14. Dent DM, Madden MV, Price SK (1988) Randomized comparison of R1 and R2 gastrectomy for gastric carcinoma. Br J Surg 75:110–112
15. Sue-Ling H, Johnston D (1995) D1 versus D2 dissection for gastric cancer. Letter to editor. Lancet 345:1515–1516
16. MuCulloch P (1995) D1 versus D2 dissection for gastric cancer. Letter to editor. Lancet 345: 1516–1517
17. Sano T, Sasako M, Yamamoto S (2004) Gastric cancer surgery: morbidity and mortality results from a prospective randomized controlled trial comparing D2 and extended para-aortic lymphadenectomy—Japan Clinical Oncology Group Study 9501. J Clin Oncol 22: 2767–2773
18. Sasako M, Sano T, Sairenji M, et al (2004) Left thoracoabdominal approach compared with abdominal and transhiatal approach for cardia or subcardia cancer. Results of a surgical randomized controlled trial (JCOG-9502). Proc ASCO 2004:314
19. Hermans J, Bonenkamp JJ, Boon MC, et al (1993) Adjuvant therapy after curative resection for gastric cancer: meta-analysis of randomized trials. J Clin Oncol 11:1441–1447

20. Panzini I, Gianni L, Fattori PP, et al (2002) Adjuvant chemotherapy in gastric cancer: a meta-analysis of randomized trials and a comparison with previous meta-analyses. Tumori 88: 21–27
21. Mari E, Floriani I, Tinazzi A, et al (2000) Efficacy of adjuvant chemotherapy after curative resection for gastric cancer: a meta-analysis of published randomised trials. A study of the GISCAD. Ann Oncol 11:837–843
22. Macdonald JS, Smalley SR, Benedetti J, et al (2001) Chemoradiotherapy after surgery compared with surgery alone for adenocarcinoma of the stomach or gastroesophageal junction. N Engl J Med 345:725–730
23. Ajani JA, Van Custem E, Moiseyenko V, et al (2003) Docetaxel, cisplatin, 5-fluorouracil compare to cisplatin and 5-fluorouracil for chemotherapy naïve patients with metastatic or locally recurrent, unresectable gastric carcinoma: interim results of a randomized phase III trial (V325). Proc ASCO 2003:249
24. Findlay M, Cunningham D, Norman A, et al (1994) A phase II study in advanced gastro-esophageal cancer using epirubicin and cisplatin in combination with continuous infusion 5-fluorouracil (ECF). Ann Oncol 5:609–616

Endoscopic Resection for Early Gastric Cancer

Mitsuhiro Fujishiro

Introduction

Endoscopic resection of early gastric cancers (EGC) originated from the development of a polypectomy technique using high-frequency current to gastric polyps in 1968 [1,2], and it became popular as endoscopic mucosal resection (EMR) after the birth of a strip biopsy method in 1984 [3]. Endoscopic resection mainly has been developed not in Western countries but in Japan, probably because the incidence of gastric cancer and the tumor description are different between them [4]. Although decreasing in number, the incidence of gastric cancer was approximately 80 patients per 100 000 population in Japan and nearly half the patients had EGC [5]. The increasing ratio of EGC accelerates the development of various novel endoscopic resection techniques and, now, EGC with ulcer findings or with a large size, in any location, can be resected endoscopically using advanced techniques. In this section, indication, techniques, outcomes, and future perspectives of endoscopic resection are summarized.

Indication for Endoscopic Resection

Although various EMR methods had been developed and a large number of EGC had been resected endoscopically, however, surprisingly, there had been no official guidelines available for the treatment of EGC before the late 1990s and institutional differences in the selection of EMR candidates existed for a long time [6–10]. Empirical indication for EMR was intestinal-type mucosal cancers without ulcerative findings, ≤2 cm in size if elevated or ≤1 cm in size if depressed or flat. The Japanese Gastric Cancer Association issued the first version of their gastric cancer treatment guidelines in 2001, which showed that endoscopic resection was indicated for intestinal-type mucosal cancers without ulcerative findings, ≤2 cm in size, regardless of tumor morphology [11]. These criteria were determined by considering two aspects: being free of lymph node metastasis and the probability of successful en bloc resection. Con-

Department of Gastroenterology, The University of Tokyo Graduate School of Medicine, 7-3-1 Hongo, Bunkyo-ku, Tokyo, Japan
e-mail: mtfujish kkr@umin.ac.jp

Table 1. Frequency of lymph node metastases in early gastric cancer

Criteria	Frequency (no. with metastasis/total number)	95% confidence interval
Intramucosal cancer Differentiated adenocarcinoma, no lymphatic vascular invasion, irrespective of ulcer findings, tumor ≤3 cm	0/1230	0%–0.3%
Intramucosal cancer Differentiated adenocarcinoma, no lymphatic vascular invasion, without ulcer findings, irrespective of tumor size	0/929	0%–0.4%
Intramucosal cancer Undifferentiated adenocarcinoma, no lymphatic vascular invasion, without ulcer findings, tumor ≤2 cm	0/141	0%–2.6%
Cancer with minute submucosal penetration (≤500 μm) Differentiated adenocarcinoma, no lymphatic vascular invasion, irrespective of ulcer findings, tumor ≤3 cm	0/145	0%–2.5%

Source: From Ref. [12]

sidering patient quality of life, technical factors should be excluded from determining the indication criteria of EMR as much as possible. If the technical problems are overcome, indication could be expanded to all those tumors that have been described as node-negative tumors (Table 1) [12]. Newly developed EMR methods using cutting devices, which is categorized as endoscopic submucosal dissection (ESD) to date, has great impact on the indication of endoscopic resection for EGC, and some institutions with ESD techniques expand their indication criteria to the condition of node-negative tumors as clinical trials.

Techniques of Endoscopic Resection

Various endoscopic resection techniques are described in Table 2. Major techniques are as follows: (1) the just cut, or lift and cut technique; (2) the inject, lift, and cut technique, such as strip biopsy [3] (Fig. 1); (3) the inject, suck, and cut technique, such as endoscopic mucosal resection with cap (EMRC) [13] (Fig. 2); and (4) inject, incise the mucosa, and dissect the submucosa, that is, ESD [14–20] (Fig. 3).

Polypectomy is usually applied to the resection of protruded tumors with a narrow base or a stalk. The inject, lift, and cut technique requires a double-channel endoscope, and both the snare and the grasping forceps are advanced through the working channels. This technique is applied to the resection of small tumors without ulcer findings regardless of morphology. The disadvantages of this technique are requirement of two assistants and existence of locations impossible for resection due to short working range of the endoscope, angulation of the gastric wall, etc.

The inject, suck, and cut technique can be performed by a single-channel endoscope but requires a specialized transparent plastic cap that is fitted to the tip of an endoscope. Looping of the snare into the groove of the rim of the cap is necessary

TABLE 2. Techniques of endoscopic resection

- Just cut, or lift and cut
  - Polypectomy [1,2]
  - Endoscopic double-snare polypectomy (EDSP) [7]
- Inject, lift, and cut
  - Strip biopsy [3]
  - Four-point fixation endoscopic mucosal resection [33]
- Inject, suck, and cut [cap-assisted endoscopic mucosal resection (EMR)]
  - EMR with cap (EMRC) [13]
  - Endoscopic aspiration mucosectomy (EAM) [34]
  - EMR with ligation (EMRL) [35]
- Inject, incise the mucosa, dissect the submucosa [endoscopic submucosal dissection (ESD)]
  - Endoscopic resection with hypertonic saline-epinephrine solution (ERHSE) [14, 37]
  - EMR with an insulation-tipped (IT) electrosurgical knife (IT-EMR) [15,16,36]
  - EMR with sodium hyaluronate solution (EMRSH) [20, 21, 27]
  - Endoscopic resection with a hook knife [17]
  - Endoscopic resection with the tip of an electrosurgical snare (thin type)/a flex knife [18]
  - Endoscopic resection with a triangle-tipped knife [19]

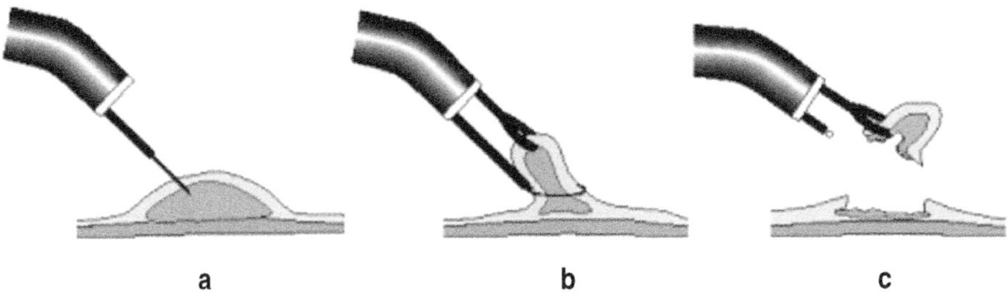

FIG. 1. Strip biopsy. **a** Submucosal fluid injection. **b** The lesion is lifted with a pair of grasping forceps and the snare is closed snugly. **c** The lesion is resected and retrieved by the grasping forceps

before starting resection. This technique is also applied to the resection of small tumors without ulcer findings regardless of morphology. The advantages of this technique over the inject, lift, and cut technique are requirement of only one assistant, applicability even in a narrow and angular space, convenience for beginners, etc.

ESD requires special cutting knives, such as a needle knife [14], an insulation-tipped (IT) electrosurgical knife [15,16], a hook knife [17], a flex knife [18], and a triangle-tipped knife [19], or special devices such as a small-caliber tip transparent (ST) hood [20] (Fig. 4). The major advantages of this technique in comparison with the others are (1) the resected size and shape can be controlled; (2) en bloc resection is possible even in a large tumor; and (3) tumors with ulcerative findings are also resectable. Thus, this technique can be applied to the resection of complex tumors such as large tumors, ulcerative nonlifting tumors, and recurrent tumors (Figs. 5–7). The disadvantages of this technique are the requirement of two or more assistants; also, it is time consuming, and much more bleeding and a little higher perforation rate are seen

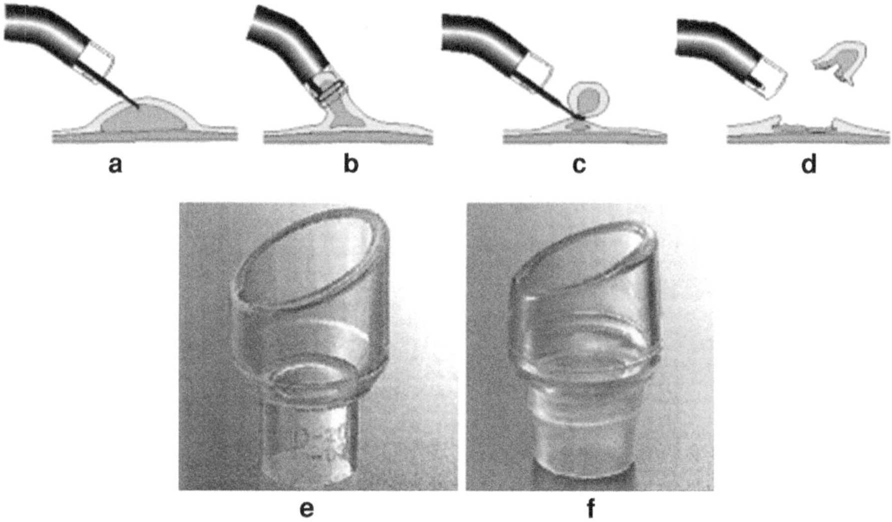

Fig. 2. Endoscopic mucosal resection with cap (EMRC). **a** Submucosal fluid injection. **b** The lesion is drawn into the cap by suction and the snare is closed snugly. **c** The snared lesion is released from the cap. **d** The lesion is resected. **e** Newly designed prelooped soft cap 18 mm in outer diameter (D-206; Olympus, Tokyo, Japan). **f** Conventional hard prelooped cap 16.5 mm in outer diameter (MAJ-296; Olympus)

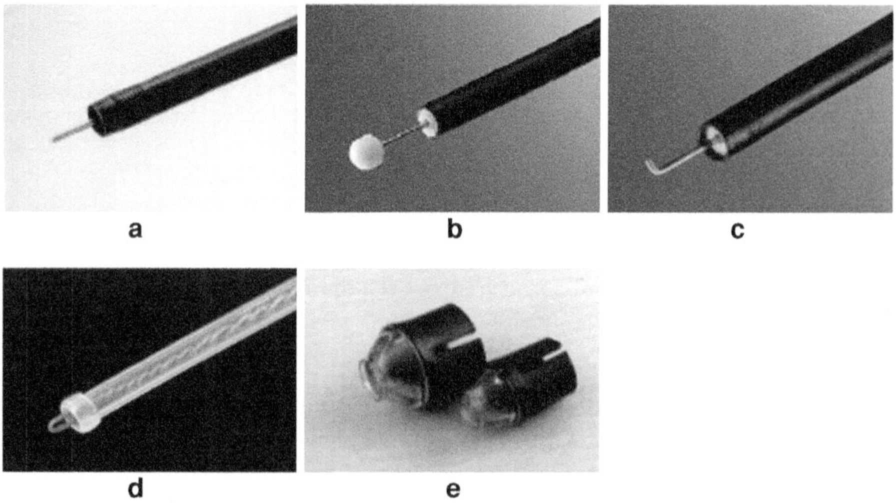

Fig. 4. Commercializ devices for endoscopic submucosal dissection (ESD). **a** Needle knife (KD-1L-1; Olympus, Tokyo, Japan). **b** Insulation-tipped (IT) electrosurgical knife (KD-610L; Olympus). **c** Hook knife (KD-620LR; Olympus). **d** Flex knife (KD-630L; Olympus). **e** Small-caliber-tip transparent (ST) hood (DH-15GR, 15CR; Fujinon Toshiba ES Systems, Tokyo, Japan)

than in the other methods. In case of bleeding, hemostatic forceps or hot biopsy forceps are used instead of hemoclips, because they disturb the subsequent procedures. It is preferable to use a special endoscope that can splash water from the tip by a foot-switch for identification of bleeding vessels. To prevent perforation, investigations of submucosal injection solutions have been actively done. It is described that a hyaluronic acid solution makes a better long-lasting submucosal cushion than other available solutions [21–23]. As a further improvement of hyaluronic acid solution, the usefulness of a mixture of a high molecular weight hayaluronic acid and a glycerin plus sugar solution is reported [24].

Outcomes of Endoscopic Resection

The outcomes of endoscopic resection reported until 1999 are described in Table 3 [25]. The inject, lift, and cut technique resulted in a little higher en bloc resection rate than the inject, suck, and cut technique for tumors ≥11 mm and ≤20 mm in size. However, if the tumors exceeded 20 mm in size, en bloc resection rates became extremely low in both techniques. Local recurrent rates were around 10% in the former, but local recurrent rates of the latter were less than 5%. In immature stages of ESD, en bloc resection rates were not as good in comparison with those of the other techniques. After maturity of the techniques of ESD, en bloc resection rates became greater than 90%, regardless of size, and local recurrence rates became almost zero (Table 4).

Complications of endoscopic resection include pain, bleeding, perforation, and stricture formation. Bleeding is the most common complication and is typically minor and treatable with endoscopy. The risks vary according to the definition of bleeding.

TABLE 3. Outcomes of endoscopic resection before 2000

	En bloc resection rate			Local recurrence rate	Complication rate	
Techniques	≤10 mm	11–20 mm	≥21 mm		Bleeding	Perforation
Strip biopsy	70% (421/599)		—	11% (63/599)	1.3% (8/599)	0.2% (1/599)
Strip biopsy	87% (123/141)	61% (27/44)	25% (2/8)	12% (23/193)	—	—
Four-point fixation EMR	71% (30/42)	72% (21/29)	14% (2/14)	—	20% (14/70)	0% (0/70)
EMRC	80% (44/55)	42% (24/57)	0% (0/9)	1.7% (2/118)	15% (18/121)	0% (0/121)
EAM	84% (52/62)		—	4.8% (3/62)	7.4% (9/121)	0.8% (1/121)
ERHSE	63% (123/196)	44% (60/136)	19% (7/37)	2.3% (8/349)	6.7% (25/373)	2.9% (11/373)
IT-EMR	87% (45/52)	74% (28/38)	42% (13/31)	—	—	5.6% (77/1386)

Source: From Ref. [25]

TABLE 4. Recent outcomes of endoscopic resection

Techniques	En bloc resection rate ≤20 mm	En bloc resection rate >21 mm	Local recurrent rate	Complication rate: Bleeding	Complication rate: Perforation
IT-EMR [36]	97% (231/238)	94% (141/150)	—	—	—
ESD with the tip of an electrosurgical snare (thin type)/a flex knife [18]	95% (56/59)		—	1.7% (1/59)	3.4% (2/59)
ESD with sodium hyaluronate and small-caliber-tip transparent hood [27]	100% (37/37)	97% (32/33)	—	1% (1/70)	0% (0/70)
ESD with a hook knife [17]	95% (194/204)		0.5% (1/204)	—	1.5% (3/204)
S-ERHSE [37]	—	79% (27/34)	0% (0/34)	0% (0/34)	12% (4/34)

S-ERHSE, submucosal-endoscopic resection with hypertonic saline-epinephrine solution

Most bleeding occurs during the procedure or within 24h. One recent study demonstrated that the administration of proton pump inhibitors might be minimally effective for ulcer healing of endoscopic resection or only effective for bleeding complications after the procedure [26]. Perforation is uncommon with endoscopic resection except for ESD, and the perforation rates of ESD also have lessened to acceptable levels from recent reports [16–18,27]. Furthermore, recent case series suggest that immediately recognized perforation can be successfully sealed with endoclips and conservatively observed without emergency laparotomy by endoscopic clipping, nasogastric suction, decompression of pneumoperitoneum, and antibiotics [28,29].

Future Perspectives Expanding Indication of Endoscopic Resection

Endoscopic resection has been developed as a reasonable and convenient diagnostic and treatment modality because histological information about the whole tumor can be obtained; furthermore, a curative treatment is achieved in case of localized tumors without lymph node metastasis, preserving the whole stomach. Furthermore, preoperative prediction of fulfillment of indication criteria, especially in tumor depth, has been reported as, at most, 90% [30,31]. En bloc resection is absolutely desirable for precise histological evaluation, and ESD has enabled us to succeed with en bloc resection. The progress of therapeutic endoscopy has also brought us the concept of diagnostic endoscopic resection for some tumors clinically diagnosed as submucosal invasive cancers, because histopathological diagnosis of submucosal invasive cancers lacks consistency with clinical diagnosis in 66% of cases [32]. If we can perform thorough and precise histopathological investigations using the resected specimens of endoscopic resection, there is no way to deny the application of endoscopic resection as the first step before gastrectomy, which would consequently avoid unnecessary gastrectomy.

Will much further expansion of the indication criteria of endoscopic resection be possible in the future? The answer must be "Yes." The incidence of lymph node metastasis from submucosal invasive cancers is at most 20%, which means that 80% of them might be cured by local treatment. Even in advanced cancers, not all cases have lymph node metastasis. If we have the skill to accomplish en bloc resection for all gastric tumors endoscopically and to distinguish node-negative tumors from node-positive tumors, it is possible to preserve most of the healthy remnant stomach in all patients with node-negative tumors.

It may be a dream so far, but in the future we will be able to avoid unnecessary gastrectomy, using prediction of lymph node metastasis by other unknown predictive markers, for example, using gene analysis of biopsy samples or resected specimens by endoscopic resection. Furthermore, combination with chemo-/radio-therapy may avoid gastrectomy with lymph node dissection for the tumors that are clinically negative for lymph node metastases but have the possibilities of lymph node metastases as seen by histology. A new generation of endoscopic resection has already come!

References

1. Niwa H (1968) Improvement of fibrogastroscope for biopsy and application of color television and high frequent currents for endoscopic biopsy (in Japanese). Gastroenterol Endosc 10:315
2. Tsuneoka K, Uchida T (1969) Fibergastroscopic polypectomy with snare method and its significance developed in our department: polyp resection and recovery instruments (in Japanese with English abstract). Gastroenterol Endosc 11:174–184
3. Tada M, Shimada M, Murakami F, et al (1984) Development of the strip-off biopsy (in Japanese with English abstract). Gastroenterol Endosc 26:833–839
4. Schlemper RJ, Itabashi M, Kato Y, et al (1997) Differences in diagnosis criteria for gastric carcinoma between Japanese and Western pathologists. Lancet 349:1725–1729
5. Tominaga S (ed) (1999) The research group for population-based cancer registration in Japan: cancer incidence in Japan. Cancer mortality and morbidity statistics, Japan and the world—1999. Japan Scientific Societies Press, Tokyo, pp 83–144
6. Ooshiba S, Ashida K, Tanaka M, et al (1993) Curative endscopic resection of early gastric cancer: the possibility of extending its indications (in Japanese with English abstract). Stomach Intest 28:1421–1426
7. Takekoshi T, Fujii A, Takagi K, et al (1988) The indication for endoscopic double snare polypectomy of gastric lesions (in Japanese with English abstract). Stomach Intest 23: 387–398
8. Tada M, Karita M, Yanai H, et al (1988) Evaluation of endoscopic strip biopsy therapeutically used for early gastric cancer (in Japanese with English abstract). Stomach Intest 23: 373–385
9. Oguro H (1995) Progess in treatments for early gastric cancer; indication for endoscopic resection of early gastric cancer (in Japanese). Clin Gastroenterol 10:85–93
10. Hiki N (1996) Endoscopic mucosal resection (EMR) for early gastric cancer (in Japanese with English abstract). Jpn J Surg 97:273–278

11. The Japanese Gastric Cancer Association (ed) (2001) Guidelines for gastric cancer treatment. Kanahara-shuppan, Tokyo
12. Gotoda T, Yanagisawa A, Sasako M, et al (2000) Incidence of lymph node metastasis from early gastric cancer: estimation with a large number of cases at two large centers. Gastric Cancer 3:219–225
13. Inoue H, Takeshita K, Hori H, et al (1993) Endoscopic mucosal resection with a cap-fitted panendoscope for esophagus, stomach, and colon mucosal lesions. Gastrointest Endosc 39:58–62
14. Hirao M, Masuda K, Asanuma T, et al (1988) Endoscopic resection of early gastric cancer and other tumors with local injection of hypertonic saline-epinephrine. Gastrointest Endosc 34:264–269
15. Ookuwa M, Hosokawa K, Boku N, et al (2001) New endoscopic treatment for intramucosal tumors using an insulated-tip diathermic knife. Endoscopy 33:221–226
16. Miyamoto S, Muto M, Hamamoto Y, et al (2002) A new technique for endoscopic mucosal resection with an insulated-tip electrosurgical knife improves the completeness of resection of intramucosal gastric neoplasms. Gastrointest Endosc 55:576–581
17. Oyama T, Hotta Y, Hirasawa D, et al (2003) Endoscopic submucosal dissection using a hook knife (abstract in Japanese). Gastroenterol Endosc 45:1525
18. Yahagi N, Fujishiro M, Kakushima N, et al (2004) Endoscopic submucosal dissection for early gastric cancer using the tip of an electro-surgical snare (thin type). Dig Endosc 16:34–38
19. Inoue H, Kudo S (2003) A novel procedure of en bloc EMR using triangle-tipped knife (abstract). Gastrointest Endosc 57:494
20. Yamamoto H, Kawata H, Sunada K, et al (2003) Successful en-bloc resection of large superficial tumors in the stomach and colon using sodium hyaluronate and small-caliber-tip transparent hood. Endoscopy 35:690–694
21. Yamamoto H, Yube T, Isoda N, et al (1999) A novel method of endoscopic mucosal resection using sodium hyaluronate. Gastrointest Endosc 50:251–256
22. Fujishiro M, Yahagi N, Kashimura K, et al (2004) Comparison of various submucosal injection solutions for maintaining mucosal elevation during endoscopic mucosal resection. Endoscopy 36:579–583
23. Conio M, Rajan E, Sorbi D, et al (2002) Comparative performance in the porcine esophagus of different solutions used for submucosal injection. Gastrointest Endosc 56:513–516
24. Fujishiro M, Yahagi N, Kashimura K, et al (2004) Different mixtures of sodium hyaluronate and their ability to create submucosal fluid cushions for endoscopic mucosal resection. Endoscopy 36:584–589
25. Ida K, Kato T, Nakajima T, et al (2002) Outcome after using EMR according to standard guidelines for endoscopic treatment of early gastric cancer (in Japanese with English abstract). Stomach Intest 37:1137–1143
26. Lee SY, Kim JJ, Lee JH, et al (2004) Healing rate of EMR-induced ulcer in relation to the duration of treatment with omeprazole. Gastrointest Endosc 60:213–217
27. Yamamoto H (2002) Endoscopic mucosal resection using sodium hyaluronate (EMRSH) for early gastric cancer (in Japanese with English abstract). Dig Endosc 14:1759–1765
28. Tsunada S, Ogata S, Ohyama T, et al (2003) Endoscopic closure of perforations caused by EMR in the stomach by application of metallic clips. Gastrointest Endosc 57:948–951
29. Ono H, Kondo H, Gotoda T, et al (2001) Endoscopic mucosal resection for treatment of early gastric cancer. Gut 48:225–229
30. Sano T, Okuyama Y, Kobori O, et al (1990) Early gastric cancer; endoscopic diagnosis of depth of invasion. Digest Dis Sci 35:1335–1340
31. Ohashi S, Segawa K, Okumura S, et al (1999) The utility of endoscopic ultrasonography and endoscopy in the endoscopic mucosal resection of early gastric cancer. Gut 45:599–604
32. Ono H, Yoshida S (2001) Endoscopic diagnosis of the depth of cancer invasion for gastric cancer (in Japanese with English abstract). Stomach Intest 36:334–340

33. Tanaka M, Inatsuchi S (1997) A four-point fixation method for the resection of early gastric cancer, with particular reference to the analysis of cases of incomplete resection. Surg Endosc 11:295–298.
34. Torii A, Sakai M, Kajiyama T, et al (1995) Endoscopic aspiration mucosectomy as curative endoscopic surgery; analysis of 24 cases of early gastric cancer. Gastrointest Endosc 42:475–479
35. Masuda K, Fujisaki J, Suzuki H, et al (1993) Endoscopic mucosal resection using ligating device (EMRL) (in Japanese). Dig Endosc 5:1215–1219
36. Gotoda T, Ono H, Oda I, et al (2002) The importance of histological evaluation and the necessity of one-piece resection for endoscopic gastric mucosal resection (in Japanese with English abstract). Stomach Intest 37:1145–1154
37. Ishigooka M, Uchisawa M, Kusama K, et al (2002) Endoscopic resection for early gastric cancer by direct incision of the submucosa, with local injection of HSE solution (in Japanese with English abstract). Stomach Intest 37:1163–1168

Color Plates

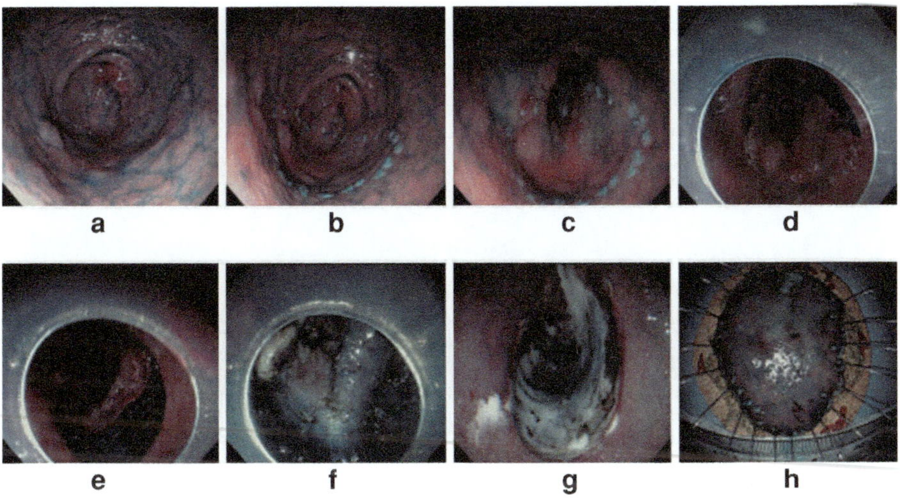

FIG. 3. Endoscopic submucosal dissection (ESD). **a** Chromoendoscopy reveals margins of the lesion clearly. **b** Marking dots are made on the circumference of the lesion. **c** Submucosal fluid injection is done to the distal margins of the lesion. **d** The mucosa around the marking dots of the distal margins is incised. **e** After submucosal injection of the proximal margins of the lesion, circumferential mucosal incision is completed and the lesion is separated from the surrounding nonneoplastic area. **f** Submucosal dissection is started from the proximal edges. **g** The lesion is completely detached from the muscle layer, and sucralfate is sprayed for comfirmation of hemostasis. **h** The resected specimen (including all the marking dots) shows en bloc resection of the lesion

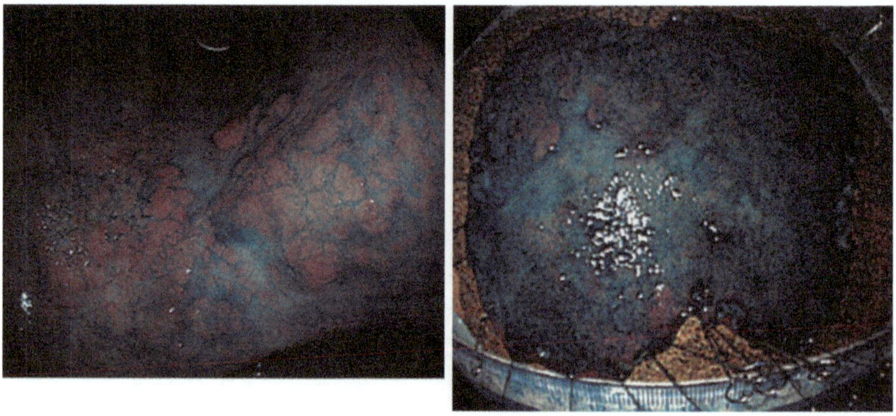

a b

FIG. 5. Large gastric tumor. **a** Endoscopic view. **b** Resected specimen

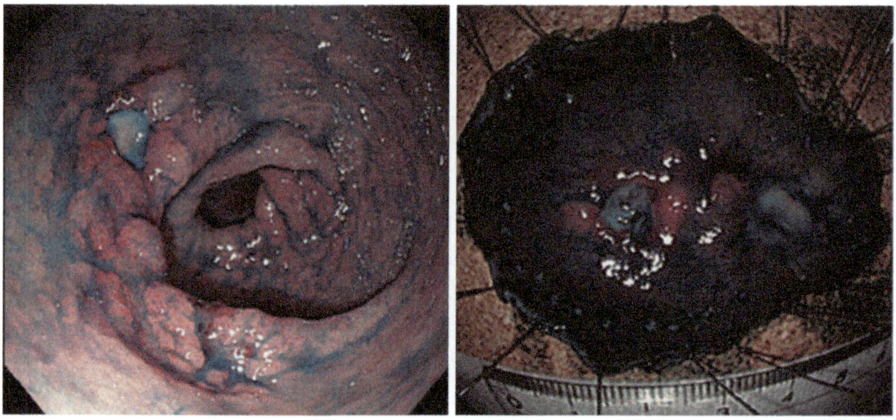

a b

FIG. 6. Ulcerative gastric tumor. **a** Endoscopic view. **b** Resected specimen

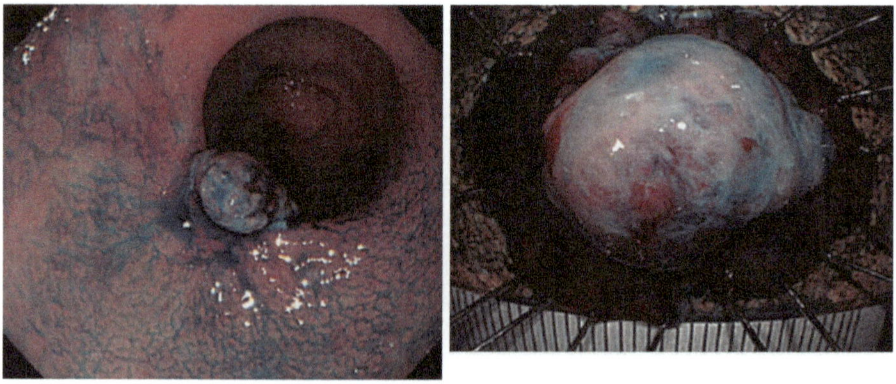

a b

FIG. 7. Recurrent gastric tumor. **a** Endoscopic view. **b** Resected specimen

Current Treatment Strategies for Early Gastric Cancer

Shouji Shimoyama and Michio Kaminishi

Introduction

Most surgeons in Japan have long considered extended lymphadenectomy (D2 dissection) as an essential part of surgical treatment for gastric cancer (GC) to clear completely the possible involved nodes. Accordingly, more than two-thirds gastrectomy is thought to be a necessary procedure, even for early gastric cancer (EGC). This radical surgery for EGC can, as a consequence, achieve excellent 5-year survival rates of greater than 90% [1,2]. The accumulation of EGC patient records undergoing a D2 dissection, both from individual institutional records [3–10] and from a nation-wide archive [11], subsequently revealed that the incidences of positive nodes among mucosal and submucosal GC, respectively, ranged from 1.8%–5% to 10%–25%. However, almost all node-positive mucosal GC patients and approximately 70% of node-positive submucosal GC patients exhibited perigastric node involvement, suggesting that EGC rarely spreads beyond the perigastric area. These site-specific analyses of positive nodes have subsequently changed the concept of surgical strategy for EGC in that a uniform D2 dissection is not always necessary.

On the other hand, it has been established that various degrees of physiological and nutritional disorders develop in a large proportion of patients following gastrectomy. These postgastrectomy sequelae include early and late dumping syndromes, reflux esophagitis and gastritis, alkaline regurgitation, weight loss, malabsorption, vitamin and mineral deficiencies, anemia, and metabolic bone diseases [12]. These sequelae are often symptomatic and cannot be ignored. Gastrectomy in association with a certain amount of lymphadenectomy results in a loss or decreased reservoir size, abnormalities in gastric emptying (either too rapid or delayed), a loss of pyloric function that causes alkaline regurgitation, decreased caloric intake, and a loss of gastric motility. Each status, sometimes in combination or sometimes as a group, is responsible for the postgastrectomy sequelae, which often aggravate the patient's postoperative quality of life. Against the background of the above excellent surgical outcomes and preferential node involvement in most EGC patients, current surgical trends for EGC have shifted

Department of Gastrointestinal Surgery, The University of Tokyo Graduate School of Medicine, 7-3-1 Hongo, Bunkyo-ku, Tokyo 113-8655, Japan
e-mail: shimoyama-tky@umin.ac.jp

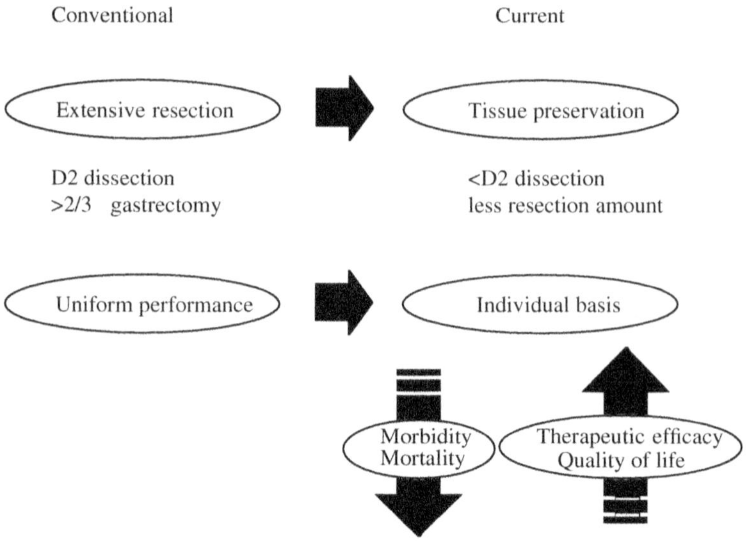

FIG. 1. Current surgical trends and changing attitudes for early gastric cancer treatment

from an extensive resection to the preservation of as much tissue as possible to provide a better postoperative quality of life (Fig. 1). The preservation of tissues in this regard means an optimization of the resection amount, which has two different aspects: one is a "reduced" scope of lymphadenectomy, and the other is a "reduced" resection of the stomach. These concepts are termed a "less invasive" surgery.

The Japanese Gastric Cancer Association (JGCA) published guidelines for the treatment of GC in 2001 [13]. Along with the foregoing shift in trends, the guideline introduces various types of treatment for EGC as "recommended options" as well as "allowed but investigational options." Minimizing surgical trauma (morbidity and mortality) while maximizing patient quality of life and therapeutic effects, which should be at least equal to the currently achieved patient survivals, forms the main goal of the less invasive strategies (Fig. 1); thus, such optimizations should be considered on a stage-specific and individual basis. Therefore, accurate staging performance and careful patient selection procedures are mandatory. However, it is also a fact that the current staging is not absolutely accurate even by the introduction of routine use (7.5 MHz) or higher resolution (15–20 MHz) endoscopic ultrasonography. Individually based treatment strategies therefore face practical but unavoidable problems where underestimation phenomenon do occur in some instances, that is, a certain lesser extent of surgery, which is preoperatively considered to be optimal, proves to be insufficient for those patients who were postoperatively proved to have more advanced diseases. Therefore, survival outcomes encompassing underestimated patients constitute a substantial concern for evaluating the actual rationality of each less invasive strategy. This chapter introduces a spectrum of current less invasive surgical strategies for EGC and their comprehensive evaluations, such as their indications, survival outcomes, surgical invasiveness, and quality of life.

Definitions and Documentation of Clinicopathological Factors

Clinicopathological factors for considerations of less invasive surgery included cancer depth (T), nodal involvement (N), scope of lymphadenectomy (D), gross form, and histological type.

EGC (T1 cancer) was further divided into mucosal (T1-M) and submucosal (T1-SM) cancers. Nodal involvement followed the updated definitions of the Japanese Gastric Cancer Association [14], and was classified into four degrees—N0, N1, N2, and N3—according to the highest tier of positive nodes [14]. The JGCA classification is based on the anatomical considerations of node positivity, not on the numerical considerations of positive nodes as proposed in the revised (5th edition) UICC classification. Clinical (pre- and intraoperative) and pathological (postoperative) T and N classifications were independently documented and were notated by prefixes c and p, respectively (e.g., cTcN and pTpN). Scope of lymphadenectomy (D number: D0, D1, D2, and D3) corresponds to the dissected node tier.

Definitions of "Less Invasive" and a "Standard" Surgery

As stated earlier, less invasive surgical strategies for EGC consist of a "reduced" scope of lymphadenectomy and a "reduced" resection of the stomach. In this context, a "standard" extent of surgery should be first defined.

With regard to the standard scope of lymphadenectomy, currently available prospective randomized trials, which were conducted in South Africa [15], Hong Kong [16], the United Kingdom [17], and the Netherlands [18], have not reported any therapeutic benefit from a D2 over a D1 dissection. At present, therefore, a D2 dissection fails to gain global acceptance as a recommended procedure. Nevertheless, a number of Western experts seem to consider that the negative impact of a D2 dissection is not yet conclusive, and controversies still exist as to the optimal extent of a lymphadenectomy, because several observational studies from Japan [19,20] as well as from the specialized Western institutes [21–24] demonstrated that a substantial segment of patients (T2–3 and/or stage II–III) benefitted from a D2 dissection. Surprisingly, these results are also supported by updated data from the Dutch trial [25]. These findings clearly indicate that a D2 dissection is necessary in a substantial proportion of GC patients. The failure to gain any survival benefit from a D2 dissection in two recently randomized trials is attributable to technical variabilities among participating surgeons less familiar with a D2 dissection, to a routine performance of a distal pancreaticosplenectomy [26,27], or to the Western habitus and large amount of fat connective tissues that preclude extensive resections, which leads to an increase in short-term morbidity and in-hospital mortality that might nullify its anticipated therapeutic efficacy. These considerations are supported by the fact that lesser surgical volumes or splenectomy is one of the causes of increasing morbidity and mortality [28–30]. In this regard, it should be noted that several Western specialists have demonstrated, even during the earlier period, the safe performance of a D2 dissection with 22%–54% morbidity and 0%–8% mortality, which were equivalent to those of a D1

Table 1. Surgical invasiveness of a D1 or a D2 dissection

Author [reference]	Year	D1 No.	D1 Morbidity	D1 Mortality	D2 No.	D2 Morbidity	D2 Mortality
D1/D2 experiences							
Pacelli et al. [31]	1993	163	28%	7.4%	157	22%	3.8%
Sierra et al. [32]	2003	85	48%	2.3%	71	54%	0%
Siewert et al. [33]	1993	558	29%	5.2%	1096	31%	5%
Lewis et al. [34]	2002	50	36%	12%	72	28%	8%
Smith et al. [35]	1991	62	34%	0%	123	43%	2%
D2 experiences							
Roukos et al. [22]	2000	NA	NA	NA	35	20%	2.8%
Degiuli et al. [39]	1998	NA	NA	NA	191	21%	3.1%
Roviello et al. [40]	2002	NA	NA	NA	451	17%	2%
Jentschura et al. [41]	1997	NA	NA	NA	532	NA	4.5%

NA, not available

dissection (28%–48% morbidity and 0%–12% mortality) [31–35] (Table 1). Furthermore, postoperative quality of life was not influenced by a D2 dissection [36–38]. Recently, much lower morbidity (17%–21%) and mortality (2%–5%) after a D2 dissection have been reported according to accumulating surgical experiences [22,39–41] (Table 1), which can be kept at levels comparable to those in the control arms of the British and Dutch trials (25%–28% morbidity and 4%–7% mortality). A D2 dissection is, therefore, justified after adequate experience and its adaptation as a standard procedure [42].

This professional stance, that the safe performance of a D2 dissection is without increasing adverse events, allows the augmentation of its therapeutic efficacy by a clearance of the positive nodes in the advanced stage GC. In Japan, a systematic lymphadenectomy is recognized as a safe procedure with 1.0% mortality [2]. Therefore, a "standard" extent of surgery in this chapter means a conventional D2 dissection in association with more than two-thirds gastrectomy, and less invasive surgery is positioned as a lesser extent of resection than a "standard" extent of surgery. Because a reduced amount of resection of the stomach inevitably limits the scope of a lymphadenectomy, the establishment of indications of a less-invasive surgery for EGC should be considered by answering the following questions: the amount by which the scope of a lymphadenectomy can be reduced, the patients for whom this would be most suitable, the amount of reduction for the resected stomach when the scope of a lymphadenectomy can be reduced, and whether the "less invasive" surgery maintains survival outcomes.

We should remember that even node-negative EGC patients by routine histology do have micrometastases at considerable incidences (12%–25%). These findings further suggest that cT1cN0 patients have potential risks of micrometastasis in the first-tier nodes (potentially pN1). The conceptual basis of node dissection is a clearance of one or more stations beyond the most distant node(s) occupied by cancer; thus, a D-number should in principle be larger than a cN-number to avoid leaving microinvolved nodes. The "reduced" scope of lymphadenectomy (<D2) should therefore be justified at this moment only for cN0 patients to encompass the possibly microinvolved first-tier nodes.

Reduced Scope of Lymphadenectomy

Modified D1 Dissection

Oohara previously found distinct evidence that node-negative mucosal GC patients who underwent a D1 dissection showed equal survival outcomes to those undergoing a D2 or wider dissection [43]. Furthermore, node-positive stations of mucosal GC were confined to the perigastric area (pN1) or, if at all present, to the root of the left gastric artery (station no. 7) with the observed risk at 0.7% [43]. These facts prompted them to establish a concept of a minimized scope of lymphadenectomy, that is, a lymphadenectomy of the perigastric nodes as well as around the left gastric artery (modified D1 lymphadenectomy), and this has been actually performed in a prospective manner since 1987 for clinically mucosal, node-negative, nonpalpable GC [44]. Notwithstanding the fact that an intraoperative palpation is a subjective finding, these investigators believe that it provides us an important information concerning unexpected submucosal or deeper cancer invasion, or a deep peptic ulcer inside the cancer, or both, all of which are potential risk factors of lymph node metastasis. A peptic ulcer inside the cancer is a predominant characteristic of node-positive mucosal GC because the destruction of the muscularis mucosa facilitates cancer cell entry into the lymphatic network [45]. Furthermore, the frequency of nodal involvement increases in proportion to the degree of submucosal invasion. As already stated, an underestimation could inevitably occur so that palpation could be one of the compensatory procedures for the imperfect staging performance. This procedure could, therefore, exclude such underestimated patients from candidates for a modified D1 dissection.

The surgical qualities of a modified D1 dissection according to each institutional criterion have been reported by several investigators [44,46] (Table 2). In one report, underestimation was actually observed even by the introduction of endoscopic ultrasound (EUS); however, the incidences of such underestimation gradually decreased according to the progression of the investigational period, suggesting that a learning curve for TN staging performance was observed. The excellent 5-year disease-specific survival rates (100%) including the underestimated patients suggests the rationality of both the staging performance and indications of the procedure.

The contribution toward improving patient quality of life by a modified D1 dissection has been rarely reported, presumably because even a D2 dissection can be performed safely in Japan. The authors have observed 16% morbidity and 0% mortality after a modified D1 dissection (unpublished data), which are lower than those figures of a radical D2 dissection reported by other specialists (28%–54% morbidity and

TABLE 2. Treatment results of a modified D1 dissection[a] in publications

Authors [reference]	Period	No. of patrents	Underestimation: SM invasion[a]	Underestimation: Node positivity	5y-SR
Shimoyama et al. [44]	1987–1996	138	20%	3%	100%
Kubota et al. [46]	1977–1982	185	NA	NA	100%

SM, submucosal; 5y-SR, 5-year disease-specific survival rate; NA, not available
[a] The indications are mucosal, node-negative, nonpalpable gastric carcinonia (GC)

0%–8% mortality). This result suggests the lower surgical invasiveness of a modified D1 dissection [31–35].

The modified D1 dissection has now been placed as a "recommended" option in the JGCA guidelines, and nation-wide performance of a modified D1 dissection is anticipated. The treatment results from a large archive are not currently available; however, the pioneering investigators [44,46] have proved its rationale by demonstrating their prospective audits of more than 5 years of experience.

Modified D2 Dissection

Under the conditions and criteria for a modified D1 dissection, submucosal GC, which is outside the criteria of a modified D1 dissection, has long been believed to merit at least a D2 dissection [14]. However, if the submucosal GC could be evaluated as preoperatively early (cT1) and node negative (cN0), the authors' research group has very recently noted the following two characteristics of positive node locations: (1) node positivity was up to N1 nodes among the intestinal type with a maximum diameter ≤1.5 cm, or a diffuse type with maximum diameter ≤1.0 cm, and (2) node positivity was N1 or up to the selective three stations of N2 nodes [stations around left gastric (station no. 7), common hepatic (station no. 8a), and celiac (station no. 9) arteries] if the maximum diameter exceeded the above cutoff diameter [47]. These findings suggest that removal of a N1 node as well as of the lymphatic chains along the left gastric, common hepatic, and celiac arteries is sufficient and can achieve a complete clearance of cancer-bearing nodes. In fact, retrospective analyses from the author's institute have elucidated identical survivals between cT1cN0 submucosal GC patients undergoing a modified D2 dissection and those receiving a wider dissection [47]. In this regard, a preferential N2 node dissection is termed as a modified D2 dissection to differentiate it from the newly defined "complete" D2 dissection. A modified D2 dissection is distinct from a complete D2 dissection in terms of leaving an intact spleen and pancreas, which leads to reduced morbidity and mortality rates, one goal of less invasive surgery [26,27]. From these results, it can be concluded that the essentially sufficient scope of lymphadenectomy for cT1cN0 submucosal gastric cancer is a modified D1 for those within the above cutoff diameter and a modified D2 for those exceeding it. A modified D2 dissection is also recommended in the JGCA guidelines [13].

Until the introduction of the JGCA guidelines, each study group proposed their own indications and the proposed amount of resections for submucosal GC as a less invasive treatment option [48–51]. These indications seem to be complicated, and the JGCA guidelines authorize the nation-wide performance of a modified D2 dissection as a less invasive surgery for submucosal GC.

However, the rationale for a modified D2 dissection for submucosal GC warrants further investigation because its performance has just started. In the authors' series (44 patients), a prospective audit has revealed 18% morbidity and 0% mortality (unpublished data), which are encouraging when compared with those from a series of a radical D2 lymphadenectomy [31–35]. Although underestimation occurred in 7% of patients undergoing a modified D2 dissection, no patients have experienced recurrence within a median follow-up period of 10 months, suggesting promising benefits of a modified D2 lymphadenectomy (unpublished data). A sufficient number of patients and longer follow-up period are required to draw any final conclusions concerning its rationality.

Reduced Resection of the Stomach

Local Resection with Adjacent Lymphadenectomy

Postoperative patient quality of life depends mostly on the amount of resection of the stomach [52]. In this regard, endoscopic mucosal resection (EMR) provides patients with an excellent quality of life because it preserves the whole stomach after treatment. However, there are some limitations for the performance of EMR, as it should be performed for those having no risk of node involvement. The GC not fulfilling the criteria for EMR has thus far undergone over two-thirds gastrectomy as a standard resection amount. Taking into account that the amount of resected stomach differs considerably between EMR and a conventional "over two-thirds" gastrectomy, a local resection has come to receive special attention to retain as much residual stomach volume as possible to help patients enjoy a better postoperative quality of life. Because a local resection inevitably limits a lymphadenectomy, the indications for a local resec tion should carefully be established.

Increasing recognition for the potential benefit of a local resection have prompted several investigators to establish the indications based on each institutional experience [53–59] (Table 3). Some indications listed in Table 3, however, do overlap with those of EMR in Japan, which are mucosal gastric cancer of an intestinal-type histology of either <2 cm in diameter for the elevated type, or <1 cm in diameter for a depressed without ulceration type [60]. However, no limitations of histological type are one of the characteristics of the indications for a local resection, because an undifferentiated type of GC is outside the criteria for EMR. In addition, a local resection with an adjacent lymphadenectomy has been proposed [53] on the basis of findings that the estimated risk of adjacent node positivity is 2.2%. An adjacent lymphadenectomy and frozen section examination during surgery enables the selection of infrequent but surely existing node-positive patients [53]. Excluding them from candidates for local resection by these intraoperative surveillances makes the application of a local resection possible for a wider segment of patients [53].

Whether a local resection offers a better quality of life without reducing curability warrants further investigation. Furthermore, the number of patients is presently too small to draw any conclusions, although the currently available survival data are excel-

TABLE 3. Proposed indications for local resection: review of the literature

		Gross form[a]			
Authors [reference]	Cancer depth	Elevated	Depressed Ul(−)	Depressed Ul(+)	Histology
Shimoyama et al. [53]	Mucosal	≦4.0 cm	≦4.0 cm	No indication	Any
Ohgami et al. [54]	Mucosal	≦2.5 cm	≦1.5 cm	No indication	Any
Yokoyama et al. [58]	Mucosal	Any	≦2.0 cm	≦2.0 cm	Any
Yasutake et al. [59]	Mucosal	≦3.5 cm	≦2.5 cm	No indication	Any

[a] Ul(−), without ulceration; Ul(+), with ulceration

Table 4. Treatment results of local resection: review of the literature

	Number (%) of patients				
Authors [reference]	Total	Submucosal invasion[b]	Margin positivity	Follow-up in months, mean (range)	Recurrence
Shimoyama[a]	17	0	2 (12%)	24 (8–50)	0
Ohgami et al. [54]	44	2 (5%)	0	23 (4–65)	0
Yokoyama et al. [58]	26	7 (27%)	2 (8%)	17 (6–44)	0
Yasutake et al. [59]	14	1 (7%)	NA	NA	0

[a] Unpublished data
[b] Proved postoperatively

lent (Table 4). Accordingly, the JGCA guidelines recognize a local resection as an investigational treatment option. One recent report is promising, demonstrating that a local resection could offer the best quality of life [61]. Another problem of a local resection seems to be the necessity for further surgery for several reasons, such as a deeper invasion proved postoperatively and/or a positive resection margin. The incompleteness of treatment by a local resection occurs only at an incidence of 10%. These facts reinforce the need for a more accurate preoperative evaluation of cancer staging as well as the cancer margin.

Pylorus-Preserving Gastrectomy

A pylorus-preserving gastrectomy (PPG) was initially introduced for peptic ulcer surgery [62,63] and has subsequently come to be applied to gastric cancer [64–72]. In contrast to peptic ulcer surgery, gastric cancer surgery should generally accompany lymph node dissection; thus, the question of the extent of a lymphadenectomy with PPG has been a matter of debate (Table 5). Some investigators do not perform suprapyloric lymph node clearance by preservation of the pyloric branch of the vagal nerve and right gastric artery to preserve pyloric blood flow and motility [65–68]. This procedure results in an incomplete D1 dissection because suprapyloric lymph nodes are classified as a N1 node for gastric cancer located in the middle or lower third of the stomach. Therefore, the indications for PPG without suprapyloric lymph node clearance are limited and complicated [65–68]. On the other hand, evidence that the right gastric artery and pyloric branch of the vagal nerve can be safely divided without affecting blood flow and motility of the pylorus [69,73] has prompted other investigators to perform PPG with suprapyloric node clearance. PPG with this procedure can realize a modified D2 dissection; thus, the indications for this type of PPG can be extended to submucosal GC or even wider [74].

PPG has been reported to have many advantages over conventional Billroth I reconstruction by preserving the pyloric function. The advantages include the prevention of dumping syndromes [64,75,76], the preservation of a reservoir function of the residual stomach [67], a reduction in chances of alkaline fluid regurgitation [77,78], the preservation of gallbladder function [78], and the maintenance of a better postoperative nutritional status [64]. The disadvantages are, if any, stasis of the remnant stomach. In this regard, several researchers investigated the postoperative remnant stomach function in detail after PPG. Postoperative pyloric ring contraction pressure was increased more according to the greater increased length of the antral segment

TABLE 5. Proposed indications for pylorus-preserving gastrectomy (PPG) with or without suprapyloric lymph node dissection: review of the literature

Authors [reference]	Suprapyloric lymph node dissection	Cancer depth	Location	Limitations
Isozaki et al. [65]	No	M	Lo	<2 cm for elevated type or <1 cm for depressed or mixed type
		M	Mid	<4 cm for elevated type or <2 cm for depressed or mixed type
Nishikawa et al. [66]	No	M or SMsl	Lo or Mid	Any
Nakane et al. [67]	No	M or SMsl	Lo or Mid	<3 cm
		M		<3 cm
Imada et al. [68]	No	SM		<3 cm for intestinal type or <1 cm for diffuse type
Sasaki et al. [70]	Yes	M or SM	Lo or Mid	<2 cm for elevated type or <1 cm for depressed type
Fujioka et al. [71]	Yes	M or SM	Mid	Any
Nakatani et al. [72]	Yes	M	Mid	Any
Zhang et al. [64]	Yes	M or SM	Lo or Mid	Any

M, mucosal cancer; SM, submucosal cancer; SMsl, slight submucosal invasion; Lo, lower one-third; Mid, middle one-third

[79], and a 1.5 to 2.5-cm length of the pyloric cuff is now considered to be the most desirable [80]. Interestingly, a PPG with dissection of the pyloric branch of the vagal nerve exhibited similar gastropyloroduodenal motility profiles to those without it, suggesting that the nerve dissection is not responsible for the gastric stasis during the early postoperative period [81]. Very recently, long-term functional evaluations after PPG have been reported for the first time, and the results proved that at least the liquid phase of gastric emptying was controlled at 5 years postoperatively even if the pyloric branch of the vagal nerve was dissected [82]. These physiological findings suggest that the suprapyloric lymph node dissection had no negative impact on gastric motility and that the postoperative stasis after PPG is transient, whereas PPG can prevent the development of dumping syndromes [82].

Therefore, the scope of the lymphadenectomy can be theoretically a modified D1 or even extended to a modified D2 according to the criteria just discussed. Because its application has been too recent to obtain long-term survival outcomes, and the indications of PPG have not been conclusively determined, PPG is positioned at this moment as an investigational option in the JGCA guidelines. However, PPG can be a promising option for gastric cancer surgery with an increasing potential for a postoperative better quality of life.

Segmental Gastrectomy

Segmental or central resection of the stomach was initially developed as a surgical procedure for gastric ulcer and it has, similarly to PPG, subsequently come to be applied to gastric cancer. This procedure aims to preserve more of the residual antral

TABLE 6. Proposed indications for segmental resection

Authors [reference]	Cancer depth	Limitations
Koufuji et al. [83]	M	1.0 cm ≦ D ≦ 3.5 cm for elevated type, 1.0 cm ≦ D ≦ 2.0 cm for depressed Ul(−) type
Furukawa et al. [84]	M	D ≦ 2.0 cm for elevated or mixed type
Iseki et al. [85]	Up to PM	≦5.0 cm
Ohwada et al. [86]	M	Outside the criteria for endoscopic mucosal resection
	SM	D≦ 5.0 cm, and differentiated type

M, mucosal layer; SM, submucosal layer; PM, proper muscle layer; D, maximum tumor diameter; Ul(−), without ulceration

volume than PPG; however, the scope of lymphadenectomy is inarguably less than PPG. Thus, segmental gastrectomy (SG) was recommended for a relatively smaller size of mucosal GC, and the indications for SG are undoubtedly limited (Table 6). For this reason, these indications for SG inevitably overlap those of EMR or local resection because perigastric node negativity is a prerequisite condition for SG [83,84]. Recently, some investigators have argued for the application of SG on a wider segment of GC with the lymphadenectomy extending to the regional nodes by skeletonizing left gastric and common hepatic arteries [85,86].

Early satiety after eating and stomal ulcers are major problems after SG. Patients undergoing SG with regional lymphadenectomy seem to experience abdominal fullness although the gastric emptying time gradually improves with postoperative period [87]. More residual antral volume, which is on one hand a characteristic of SG, may on the other hand account for the gastric stasis because, as is demonstrated in the PPG section, a longer antral segment is associated with unexpected pyloric ring contraction. Pyloroplasty, which is expected to relieve the symptoms of stasis, does not seem to be justified however because it increases the incidence of dumping syndrome and alkaline fluid regurgitation [86]. Resection of the fundic gland area and preservation of the pyloric gland area have been found to result in a reduced gastric acid secretion that eventually stimulates gastrin secretion. Hypergastrinemia is one of the factors responsible for stomal ulcer. Earlier studies have already found no appreciable effect of pyloroplasty on ulcer development [88,89]. Selective proximal vagotomy, being performed with perigastric node dissection, may reduce the risks of stomal ulcer [86]. Therefore, the validity of SG should be investigated by comparing PPG with regard to postoperative gastric motility.

Proximal Gastrectomy (PG)

Several epidemiological studies have elucidated a gradual increase in the incidence of cardia cancer [90,91] but a steady decline in the overall incidence of gastric cancer itself [92]. The distributional shift from distal to proximal lesions has pointed to a need for investigations into the patterns of lymphatic spread and optimal treatment strategies currently not definitively established. The efforts for investigation include the establishment of an optimal extent of resection (total or proximal gastrectomy), an optimal scope of lymphadenectomy, and an optimal type of reconstruction (with or without duodenal continuity, or with or without a gastric substitute).

In consideration of the clinical and pathological characteristics of this tumor entity, Nishi et al. proposed a definition of cardia cancer as an adenocarcinoma arising between the points 2 cm proximally and distally of the esophagogastric junction [93]. Siewert and Stein [94] more recently classified cardia cancer into three types focusing on an adenocarcinoma arising at or close to the esophagogastric junction. In this regard, cardia cancer according to Nishi's definition is almost equivalent to the Siewert type II cancer.

Comparisons of clinicopathological characteristics of cardia cancer between the series in the West and in Japan elucidated some points of contrast. The Western series demonstrated an equal frequency of each type of cardia cancer [95–97], whereas type I cancer was extremely rare in Japan [98–100] (Table 7). Furthermore, early cardia cancer comprised a yet minor component among all EGC even in Japan (Table 8), although each incidence of early cardia cancer among each Siewert type is higher than those in the West [96–98,100]. For this reason, in the Western countries, major interest has been focused on the advanced cardia cancer. Therefore, whether a total or prox-

TABLE 7. Incidence of each type of cardia cancer

	Number (%) of patients			
Authors [reference]	Total	Type I	Type II	Type III
Mariette et al. [95]	126	56 (44%)	44 (35%)	26 (21%)
Fein et al. [96]	74	15 (20%)	30 (41%)	29 (39%)
Siewert et al. [97]	1002	361 (36%)	271 (27%)	370 (37%)
Shimoyama et al. [98]	140	0	46 (33%)	94 (67%)
Kodera et al. [99]	177	0	33 (19%)	144 (81%)
Ichikura et al. [100]	65	1 (2%)	31 (48%)	33 (51%)

TABLE 8. Incidence and node positivity of type II early cardia cancer: review of the literature from the Japanese investigations

	Early Siewert type II or Nishi's cardia cancer, number of patients			
Authors [reference][a]	Total[b]	Mucosal[c]	Submucosal[c]	Positive station (station number)
Kumagaya	15 (2.1%)	2 [NA]	13 [NA]	
Suzuki	41 (2.6%)	NA	NA	
Niou	83 (6.4%)	42 [NA]	41 [NA]	
Oota	8 (1.3%)	5 [0]	3 [1]	First-tier node
Takeshita	21 (4.4%)	8 [0]	13 [0]	
Aoki	16 (3.1%)	4 [0][d]	10 [0]	
Shimoyama et al. [98]	20 (3.0%)	5 [0]	15 [1]	Left paracardial (no. 2)
Manzoni et al. [102]	12 (NA)	12 [4][e]		Left paracardial (no. 2) Lesser curvature (no. 3) Lesser curvature (no. 3) Celiac trunk (no. 9)

[a] The articles are listed in Ref. 106 unless reference number is stated
[b] numbers in parentheses indicate incidences of early cardia cancer in each study population
[c] Numbers in brackets indicate numbers of node-positive patients
[d] Two endoscopic mucosal resection (EMR) cases were excluded from node positivity analyses
[e] Mucosal and submucosal subclassification not specified

imal gastrectomy is the superior procedure, and to what extent the lymphadenectomy should be performed, remain unknown because of the lack of well-controlled studies for a comparison of these two procedures; furthermore, there is a lack of precise knowledge of which lymph node stations are most likely to be involved among early cardia cancer [98,101,102].

Table 8 provides detailed information currently available concerning the true yield of nodal metastasis among early type II cardia cancer in the Japanese series because Western publications do not refer to anatomical site-specific node positivity. Noticeably, the mucosal type II cardia cancer exhibits no nodal involvement, suggesting that EMR or local resection could be appropriate if technically feasible [98]. With one exceptional report [102], submucosal type II cardia cancer involves, if any, only perigastric stations adjacent to the cancer, and it rarely spreads beyond these restricted stations [98,101]. Even for type III early cancer, no nodal involvement in the distal stations (suprapyloric and infrapyloric stations) as well as at the splenic hilum support the feasibility of a PG for early cardia cancer without residual diseases in the lymph nodes left in situ [103]. In addition, PG exhibits superiority over a total gastrectomy with regard to reducing postoperative complaints [104]. These findings suggest that early type II and III cancers do not need to undergo a total gastrectomy or elective splenectomy for hilar control [30]. In this sense, discriminations of mucosal, submucosal, and advanced cardia cancers are quite important [105].

General agreement on the most appropriate type of reconstruction has yet to be reached. Proponents of jejunal interposition with or without a pouch expect the prevention of reflux esophagitis and more food intake by introducing a pouch as a gastric substitute [106]. Alternatively, others propose an esophagogastrostomy with antireflux wrap procedures [107,108]. Results of postoperative functional analyses suggest that the choice of reconstruction depends, at least in part, on the volume of the residual stomach. A PG of more than two-thirds was found to inversely diminish the nutritional advantages that were maximized by less than two-thirds PG, presumably because too small a remnant stomach has only the function of a pipe [109]. Furthermore, animal experiments have demonstrated that denervation of the stomach, which accompanies systematic lymphadenectomy, may facilitate remnant gastric cancer development [110]. On the other hand, patients undergoing gastroesophagostomy with a PG over one-half experienced significant gastroesophageal reflux [111]. These findings suggest that the larger GC, for which more than one-half PG is required to guarantee the negative distal resection margin, is not suitable for PG with esophagogastrostomy.

Because the questions of the optimal surgical procedures for early cardia cancer remain unresolved, the JGCA guidelines have not yet listed this type of surgery as a recommended less invasive surgery. Whether PG with either interposition or esophagogastrostomy contributes to improve patient quality of life warrants further investigation.

Conclusions

Despite evidence that the results of a D2 dissection as reported in the literature by Japanese groups did not find any correspondence with the series of Western randomized trials, most Japanese surgeons believe that a D2 dissection is a standard surgery for GC. On the other hand, the paucity of extensive node involvement among EGC patients raises the concept that EGC patients not necessarily undergo a D2 dissection. The ability to balance the risk of a D2 dissection against potential benefits in Japan has subsequently realized diversed treatment strategies for GC according to each stage, namely, from a wider resection for advanced GC to a less invasive surgery for EGC. Such diverse treatment strategies have been authorized by the recent JGCA guidelines, and we infer from the data currently available concerning the treatment results that the indications and options of a less invasive surgery for EGC are rational.

With the help of the JGCA guidelines, a modified D1 and a modified D2 dissection have been rapidly adopted in Japan as recommended scopes of lymphadenectomies, and the reduced resection amount such as a local resection, PPG, and segmental resection may be allowed as an investigational option. Further patient accrual is expected. In the event of a less invasive surgery, careful patient selection is mandatory. Advances in diagnostic procedures including technical devices may improve diagnostic accuracy, but underestimation errors still persist. Thus, another important concern arises as to whether the "underestimation error" does not interfere with the treatment results. Every effort should be made to identify candidates for a less invasive surgery on an individual basis based on a strict TN staging performance. More detailed patient survival rates with a larger patient series and longer follow-up periods as well as long-term functional results are necessary to substantiate the rationality of a less invasive surgery.

References

1. Sawai K, Takahashi T, Suzuki H (1994) New trends in surgery for gastric cancer in Japan. J Surg Oncol 56:221–226
2. Maruyama K, Sasako M, Kinoshita T, et al (1999) Can sentinel node biopsy indicate rational extent of lymphadenectomy in gastric cancer surgery? Fundamental and new information on lymph node dissection. Langenbeck's Arch Surg 384:149–157
3. Habu H, Takeshita K, Sunagawa M, et al (1986) Lymph node metastasis in early gastric cancer. Int Surg 71:244–247
4. Sowa M, Kato Y, Nishimura M, et al (1989) Surgical approach to early gastric cancer with lymph node metastasis. World J Surg 13:630–636
5. Maehara Y, Orita H, Okuyama T, et al (1992) Predictors of lymph node metastasis in early gastric cancer. Br J Surg 79:245–247
6. Shimoyama S, Seto Y, Yasuda H, et al (2000) Wider indications for the local resection of gastric cancer by adjacent lymphadenectomy. J Surg Oncol 75:157–164
7. Gotoda T, Yanagisawa A, Sasako M, et al (2000) Incidence of lymph node metastasis from early gastric cancer: estimation with a large number of cases at two large centers. Gastric Cancer 3:219–225
8. Kunisaki C, Shimada H, Nomura M, et al (2001) Appropriate lymph node dissection for early gastric cancer based on lymph node metastases. Surgery (St. Louis) 129:153–157
9. Yamaguchi T, Sano T, Katai H, et al (2001) Node negative mucosal gastric cancer: a follow up study. Jpn J Clin Oncol 31:153–156
10. Folli S, Morgagni P, Roviello F, et al (2001) Risk factors for lymph node metastases and their prognostic significance in early gastric cancer (EGC) for the Italian Research Group for Gastric Cancer. Jpn J Clin Oncol 31:495–499
11. Seto Y, Shimoyama S, Kitayama J, et al (2001) Lymph node metastasis and preoperative diagnosis of depth of invasion in early gastric cancer. Gastric Cancer 4:34–38

12. Stabile BE, Passaro E Jr (1985) Sequelae of surgery for peptic ulcer. In: Berk JE, Haubrich WS, Kalser MH, Roth JLA, Schaffner F (eds) Bochus gastroenterology, vol 2. Saunders, Philadelphia, pp 1225–1254
13. Nakajima T (2002) Gastric cancer treatment guidelines in Japan. Gastric Cancer 5:1–5
14. Japanese Gastric Cancer Association (1998) Japanese classification of gastric carcinoma, 2nd English edn. Gastric Cancer 1:10–24
15. Dent DM, Madden MV, Price SK (1988) Randomized comparison of R1 and R2 gastrectomy for gastric carcinoma. Br J Surg 75:110–112
16. Robertson CS, Chung SCS, Woods SDS, et al (1994) A prospective randomized trial comparing R1 subtotal gastrectomy with R3 total gastrectomy for antral cancer. Ann Surg 220:176–182
17. Cuschieri A, Weeden S, Fielding J, et al (1999) Patient survival after D1 and D2 resection for gastric cancer: long-term results of the MRC randomized surgical trial. Br J Cancer 79:1522–1530
18. Bonenkamp JJ, Hermans J, Sasako M, et al (1999) Extended lymph node dissection for gastric cancer. N Engl J Med 340:908–914
19. Kasakura Y, Mochizuki F, Wakabayashi K, et al (2002) An evaluation of the effectiveness of extended lymph node dissection in patients with gastric cancer: a retrospective study of 1403 cases at a single institution. J Surg Res 103:252–259
20. Maruyama K, Okabayashi K, Kinoshita T (1987) Progress in gastric cancer surgery in Japan and its limits of radicality. World J Surg 11:418–425
21. Siewert JR, Bottcher K, Stein H, et al (1998) Relevant prognostic factors in gastric cancer. Ten-year results of the German Gastric Cancer Study. Ann Surg 228:449–461
22. Roukos DH, Paraschou P, Lorenz M (2000) Distal gastric cancer and extensive surgery: a new evaluation method based on the study of the status of residual lymph nodes after limited surgery. Ann Surg Oncol 7:719–726
23. Kooby DA, Suriawinata A, Klimstra DS, et al (2003) Biologic predictors of survival in node-negative gastric cancer. Ann Surg 237:828–837
24. Harrison LE, Karpeh MS, Brennan MF (1998) Extended lymphadenectomy is associated with a survival benefit for node negative gastric cancer. J Gastrointest Surg 2:126–131
25. Hartgrink HH, Van de Velde CJH (2001) Update of the Dutch D1 vs D2 gastric cancer trial. In: Abstracts, Fourth International Gastric Cancer Congress, Abstracts, New York, p 665
26. Bonenkamp JJ, Songun I, Hermans J, et al (1995) Randomized comparison of morbidity after D1 and D2 dissection for gastric cancer in 996 Dutch patients. Lancet 345:745–748
27. Cuschieri A, Fayers P, Fielding J, et al (1996) Postoperative morbidity and mortality after D1 and D2 resections for gastric cancer: preliminary results of the MRC randomized controlled surgical trial. Lancet 347:995–999
28. Fujita T, Yamsazaki Y (2002) Influence of surgeon's volume on early outcome after total gastrectomy. Eur J Surg 168:535–538
29. Griffith JP, Sue-Ling HM, Martin I, et al (1995) Preservation of the spleen improves survival after radical surgery for gastric cancer. Gut 36:684–690
30. Kodera Y, Yamamura Y, Shimizu Y, et al (1997) Lack of benefit of combined pancreaticosplenectomy in D2 resection for proximal third gastric cancer. World J Surg 21:622–628
31. Pacelli F, Doglietto GB, Bellantone R, et al (1993) Extensive versus limited lymph node dissection for gastric cancer. A comparative study of 320 patients. Br J Surg 80:1153–1156
32. Sierra A, Regueira FM, Hernandez-Lizoarin JL, et al (2003) Role of the extended lymphadenectomy in gastric cancer surgery: experience in a single institution. Ann Surg Oncol 10:219–226
33. Siewert JR, Bottcher K, Roder JD, et al (1993) Prognostic relevance of systematic lymph node dissection in gastric carcinoma. Br J Surg 80:1015–1018
34. Lewis WG, Edwards P, Jonathan DB, et al (2002) D2 or not D2? The gastrectomy question. Gastric Cancer 5:29–34

35. Smith JW, Shiu MH, Kelsey L, et al (1991) Morbidity of radical lymphadenectomy in the curative resection of gastric carcinoma. Arch Surg 126:1469–1473
36. Wu C-W, Hsieh M-C, Lo S-S, et al (1997) Quality of life of patients with gastric adenocarcinoma after curative gastrectomy. World J Surg 21:777–782
37. Thybusch-Bernhardt A, Schmidt C, Kuchler T, et al (1999) Quality of life following radical surgical treatment of gastric carcinoma. World J Surg 23:503–508
38. Liano AD, Martinez FO, Ciga MA, et al (2003) Impact of surgical procedure or gastric cancer on quality of life. Br J Surg 90:91–94
39. Degiuli M, Sasako M, Ponti A, et al (1998) Morbidity and mortality after D2 gastrectomy for gastric cancer: results of the Italian Gastric Cancer Study Group Prospective Multicenter Surgical Study. J Clin Oncol 16:1490–1493
40. Roviello F, Marrelli D, Morgagni P, et al (2002) Survival benefit of extended D2 lymphadenectomy in gastric cancer with involvement of second level lymph nodes: a longitudinal multicenter study. Ann Surg Oncol 9:894–900
41. Jentschura D, Heubner C, Manegold BC (1997) Surgery for early gastric cancer: a European one-center experience. World J Surg 21:845–849
42. Gretschel S, Christoph F, Bembenek A, et al (2003) Body mass index does not affect systematic D2 lymph node dissection and postoperative morbidity in gastric cancer patients. Ann Surg Oncol 10:363–368
43. Oohara T (1991) Rational view of reduced radical gastrectomy for early gastric cancers. Jpn J Gastroenterol Surg 24:167–171
44. Shimoyama S, Joujima Y, Yasuda H, et al (2000) Prospectively performed modified D1 lymphadenectomy for clinically diagnosed mucosal, node negative gastric cancer: findings over the past decade. Int Surg 85:202–208
45. Sano R (1971) Pathological analysis of 300 cases of early gastric cancer. With special reference to cancer associated with ulcers. Gann Monogr Cancer Res 11:81–89
46. Kubota T, Ootani Y, Oogami M, et al (1996) Indication, method, and result of distal gastrectomy with D1 lymph node dissection. J Clin Surg 51:1287–1290
47. Shimoyama S, Yasuda H, Mafune K, et al (2002) Indications of a minimized scope of lymphadenectomy for submucosal gastric cancer. Ann Surg Oncol 9:625–631
48. Kunisaki C, Shimada H, Nomura M, et al (2001) Appropriate lymph node dissection for early gastric cancer based on lymph node metastases. Surgery (St. Louis) 129:153–157
49. Takeno S, Noguchi T, Kikuchi R, et al (2001) Analysis of early (pT1) gastric cancer with submucosal invasion: surgical management and possibility to schedule less invasive surgery. Ann Surg Oncol 8:605–610
50. Yamada H, Nihei Z, Yamashita T, et al (2001) Is lymphadenectomy needed for all submucosal gastric cancers? Eur J Surg 167:199–203
51. Gotoda T, Sasako M, Ono H, et al (2001) Evaluation of the necessity for gastrectomy with lymph node dissection for patients with submucosal invasive gastric cancer. Br J Surg 88:44–449
52. Roukos DH (1999) Current advances and changes in treatment strategy may improve survival and quality of life in patients with potentially curable gastric cancer. Ann Surg Oncol 6:46–56
53. Shimoyama S, Seto Y, Yasuda H, et al (2000) Wider indications for the local resection of gastric cancer by adjacent lymphadenectomy. J Surg Oncol 75:157–164
54. Ohgami M, Otani Y, Kumai K, et al (1999) Curative laparoscopic surgery for early gastric cancer: five years experience. World J Surg 23:187–193
55. Kitamura K, Yamaguchi T, Taniguchi H, et al (1997) Analysis of lymph node metastasis in early gastric cancer: rationale of limited surgery. J Surg Oncol 64:42–47
56. Yokota T, Saito T, Teshima S, et al (1998) Lymph node metastasis in early gastric cancer: how can surgeons perform limited surgery? Int Surg 83:287–290
57. Tsujitani S, Oka S, Saito H, et al (1999) Less invasive surgery for early gastric cancer based on the low probability of lymph node metastasis. Surgery (St. Louis) 125:148–154

58. Yokoyama N, Takashima S (1997) Laparoscopic local resection of the stomach by lesion lifting method for early gastric cancer. Gastroenterol Surg 20:1493–1499
59. Yasutake T, Ayabe H, Miura T (1997) Laparoscopic partial gastrectomy for early gastric cancers. Gastroenterol Surg 20:1507–1511
60. Makuuchi H, Kise Y, Shimada H, et al (1999) Endoscopic mucosal resection for early gastric cancer. Semin Surg Oncol 17:108–116
61. Seto Y, Yamaguchi H, Shimoyama S, et al (2001) Results of local resection with regional lymphadenectomy for early gastric cancer. Am J Surg 182:498–501
62. Maki T, Shiratori T, Hatafuku T, et al (1967) Pylorus-preserving gastrectomy as an improved operation for gastric ulcer. Surgery (St. Louis) 61:838–845
63. Hennesy TPJ, Weir DG, D'Auria D (1972) Pylorus-preserving gastrectomy in the treatment of duodenal ulcer. Br J Surg 59:27–29
64. Zhang D, Shimoyama S, Kaminishi M (1998) Feasibility of pylorus-preserving gastrectomy with a wider scope of lymphadenectomy. Arch Surg 133:993–997
65. Isozaki H, Okajima K, Momura E, et al (1996) Postoperative evaluation of pylorus preserving gastrectomy for early gastric cancer. Br J Surg 83:266–269
66. Nishikawa K, Kawahara H, Yumiba T, et al (2002) Functional characteristics of the pylorus in patients undergoing pylorus-preserving gastrectomy for early gastric cancer. Surgery (St. Louis) 131:613–624
67. Nakane Y, Akehira K, Inoue K, et al (2000) Postoperative evaluation of pylorus-preserving gastrectomy for early gastric cancer. Hepatogastroenterology 47:590–595
68. Imada T, Rino Y, Takahashi M, et al (1998) Postoperative functional evaluation of pylorus-preserving gastrectomy for early gastric cancer compared with conventional distal gastrectomy. Surgery (St. Louis) 123:165–170
69. Sawai K, Takahashi T, Fujioka T, et al (1995) Pylorus-preserving gastrectomy with radical lymph node dissection based on anatomical variations of the infrapyloric artery. Am J Surg 170:285–288
70. Sasaki I, Shiiba K, Naito H, et al (1996) Pylorus preserving gastrectomy for early gastric cancer. J Jpn Surg Soc 97:291–296
71. Fujioka T, Sawai K, Ohara M, et al (1994) Range of lymph node dissection and postoperative course in pylorus preserving gastrectomy for early gastric cancer located in the middle third of the stomach. J Jpn Surg Assoc 55:1938–1942
72. Nakatani K, Watanabe A, Nakano H, et al (1991) Pylorus preserving gastrectomy for early gastric cancer. Shujutsu 45:1825–1829
73. Spencer MP, Sarr MG, Hakim NS, et al (1989) Interdigestive gastric motility patterns: the role of vagal and nonvagal extrinsic innervation. Surgery (St. Louis) 106:185–194
74. Shimoyama S, Mafune K, Kaminishi M (2003) Indications of a pylorus-preserving gastrectomy for gastric cancer with proper muscle invasion. Arch Surg 138:1235–1239
75. Nishikawa K, Kawahara H, Yumiba T, et al (2002) Functional characteristics of the pylorus in patients undergoing pylorus-preserving gastrectomy for early gastric cancer. Surgery (St. Louis) 131:613–624
76. Hotta T, Taniguchi K, Kobayashi Y, et al (2001) Postoperative evaluation of pylorus-preserving procedures compared with conventional distal gastrectomy for early gastric cancer. Surg Today 31:774–779
77. Imada T, Rino Y, Takahashi M, et al (1998) Postoperative functional evaluation of pylorus-preserving gastrectomy for early gastric cancer compared with conventional distal gastrectomy. Surgery (St. Louis) 123:165–170
78. Kodama M, Koyama K, Chida T, et al (1995) Postoperative evaluation of pylorus-preserving gastrectomy for gastric cancer. World J Surg 19:456–461
79. Shiratori T, Nakatani K (1984) Pylorus preserving nearly total gastrectomy with jejunal interposition. Surg Ther 51:727–735
80. Nakane Y, Michiura T, Inoue K, et al (2002) Length of the antral segment in pylorus-preserving gastrectomy. Br J Surg 89:220–224

81. Nakabayashi T, Mochiki E, Garcia M, et al (2002) Pyloric motility after pylorus-preserving gastrectomy with or without the pyloric branch of the vagus nerve. World J Surg 26:577–583
82. Tomita R, Fujisaki S, Tanjoh K (2003) Pathophysiological studies on the relationship between postgastrectomy syndrome and gastric emptying function at 5 years after pylorus preserving distal gastrectomy for early gastric cancer. World J Surg 27:725–733
83. Koufuji K, Takeda J, Kodama I, et al (1997) Segmental gastrectomy for early gastric cancer in the middle part of the stomach. Jpn J Cancer Clin 43:284–288
84. Furukawa H, Hiratsuka M, Imaoka S, et al (1999) Phase II study of limited surgery for early gastric cancer: segmental gastric resection. Ann Surg Oncol 6:166–170
85. Iseki J, Takagi M, Touyama K, et al (2003) Feasibility of central gastrectomy for gastric cancer. Surgery (St. Louis) 133:68–73
86. Ohwada S, Nakamura S, Ogawa T, et al (1999) Segmental gastrectomy for early cancer in the mid stomach. Hepatogastroenterology 46:1229–1233
87. Ohwada S, Sato Y, Oriuchi N, et al (1999) Gastric emptying after segmental gastrectomy for early cancer in the middle third part of the stomach. Hepatogastroenterology 46:2081–2085
88. Amdrup E, Nielsen J, Jensen H (1970) Treatment of benign gastric ulcer by segmental gastric resection with and without pyloroplasty. Surgery (St. Louis) 68:759–765
89. Sekine T, Tsukamoto M, Sato T, et al (1975) An evaluation of segmental gastrectomy for gastric ulcer. One to ten year follow-up. Surgery (St. Louis) 78:508–514
90. Botterweck AAM, Schouten LJ, Volovics A, et al (2000) Trends in incidence of adenocarcinoma of the oesophagus and gastric cardia in ten European countries. Int J Epidemiol 29:645–654
91. Blot WJ, Devesa SS, Kneller RW, et al (1991) Rising incidence of adenocarcinoma of the esophagus and gastric cardia. JAMA 265:1287–1289
92. Devesa SS, Blot WJ, Fraumeni JF (1998) Changing patterns in the incidence of esophageal and gastric carcinoma in the United States. Cancer (Phila) 83:2049–2053
93. Nishi M, Kajisa T, Akune T, et al (1973) Gastric cardia cancer. Geka Shinryo 32:1328–1338
94. Siewert JR, Stein HJ (1996) Carcinoma of the cardia: carcinoma of the gastroesophageal junction—classification, pathology and extent of resection. Dis Esophagus 9:173–182
95. Mariette C, Castel B, Toursel H, et al (2002) Surgical management of and long-term survival after adenocarcinoma of the cardia. Br J Surg 89:1156–1163
96. Fein M, Fuchs K-H, Ritter MP, et al (1998) Application of the new classification for cancer of the cardia. Surgery (St. Louis) 124:707–714
97. Siewert JR, Feith M, Werner M, et al (2000) Adenocarcinoma of the esophagogastric junction. Results of surgical therapy based on anatomical/topographic classification in 1002 consecutive patients. Ann Surg 232:353–361
98. Shimoyama S, Aoki F, Kaminishi M (2001) Low incidence of lymph node metastasis in early gastric cardia cancer. Int J Surg Invest 3:369–376
99. Kodera Y, Yamamura Y, Shimizu Y, et al (1999) Adenocarcinoma of the gastroesophageal junction in Japan; relevance of Siewert's classification applied to 177 cases resected at a single institute. J Am Coll Surg 189:594–601
100. Ichikura T, Ogawa T, Kawabata T, et al (2002) Is adenocarcinoma of the gastric cardia a distinct entity independent of subcardial carcinoma? World J Surg 27:334–338
101. Kitamura K, Nishida S, Yamamoto K, et al (1998) Lymph node metastasis in gastric cancer in the upper third of the stomach: surgical treatment on the basis of the anatomical distribution of positive node. Hepatogastroenterology 45:281–285
102. Manzoni G, Morgagni P, Roviello F, et al (1998) Nodal abdominal spread in adenocarcinoma of the cardia. Results of a multicenter prospective study. Gastric Cancer 1:146–151
103. Katai H, Sano T, Fukagawa T, et al (2003) Prospective study of proximal gastrectomy for early gastric cancer in the upper third of the stomach. Br J Surg 90:850–853

104. Furukawa H, Hiratsuka M, Imaoka S, et al (1998) Limited surgery for early gastric cancer in cardia. Ann Surg Oncol 5:338–341
105. Shimoyama S, Yasuda H, Hashimoto M, et al (2004) Accuracy of linear array EUS for preoperative staging of gastric cardia cancer. Gastrointest Endosc 59:1–6
106. Takeshita K, Saito N, Saeki I, et al (1997) Proximal gastrectomy and jejunal pouch interposition for the treatment of early cancer in the upper third of the stomach: surgical techniques and evaluation of postoperative function. Surgery (St. Louis) 121:278–286
107. Shimoyama S, Aoki F, Kubota K, et al (2001) Minimally invasive surgery for the treatment of early gastric cardia cancer. Stomach Intest 36:689–693
108. Ichikawa D, Ueshima Y, Shirono K, et al (2001) Esophagogastrostomy reconstruction after limited proximal gastrectomy. Hepatogastroenterology 48:1797–1801
109. Nomura E, Isozaki H, Fujii K, et al (2003) Postoperative evaluation of function-preserving gastrectomy for early gastric cancer. Hepatogastroenterology 50:2246–2250
110. Kaminishi M, Shimizu N, Shimoyama S, et al (1995) Etiology of gastric remnant cancer with special reference to the effects of denervation of the gastric mucosa. Cancer (Phila) 75:1490–1496
111. Hsu C-P, Chen C-Y, Hsieh Y-H, et al (1997) Esophageal reflux after total or proximal gastrectomy in patients with adenocarcinoma of the gastric cardia. Am J Gastroenterol 92:1347–1350

Surgery for Advanced Gastric Cancer

KEN-ICHI MAFUNE

Introduction

Ever since the first successful gastrectomy was performed by C. Billroth in 1881, surgery has been the only hope of cure for gastric cancer. Because gastric cancer is one of the most common types of cancers in Japan, a variety of surgical procedures have been developed to treat it, especially after the establishment of the Japanese Research Society for Gastric Cancer (JRSGC, recently renamed as the Japanese Gastric Cancer Association, JGCA) in 1962. The general rules for gastric cancer study in surgery and pathology of the JRSGC have been widely accepted, and this enabled evaluation of the treatment results of different institutions, accumulation of nation-wide data, and eventually the establishment of treatment standards for gastric cancer. The results of many studies according to the general rules have shown a consecutive increase in postgastrectomy 5-year survival rates from 41.2% to 63.8% in Japan [1]. One reason for the improvement appears to be the increase in the number of cancers detected in the early stage as a result of improvements in diagnostic modalities. Another reason may be the widespread use of surgical procedures such as D2 lymph node dissection. However, only a minimal increase in 5-year survival rate after resection has been reported in English-language publications (from 20.7% before 1970, to 28.4% from 1981 to 1990) [2]. Wanebo et al. [3] reported on gastric cancer in the United States from various standpoints based on data from the tumor registries of United States hospitals and cancer programs approved by the American College of Surgeons. A comparison of the United States data for 1987 with Japanese data from the tumor registries of the JGCA for 1991 [4] showed that gastric cancer was being detected at a much earlier stage in Japan than in the United States. (Fig. 1a). Diagnostic improvements in Japan, mainly the adoption of mass-screening systems that use upper gastrointestinal (GI) series and endoscopy, may be responsible for the earlier detection of gastric cancer in Japan, and the 5-year survival rates for same-stage tumors are also much better in Japan than in the United States (Fig. 1b). These differences may be explained in part by the higher incidences of proximal and diffuse-

Department of Gastrointestinal Surgery, The University of Tokyo Graduate School of Medicine, 7-3-1 Hongo, Bunkyo-ku, Tokyo 113-8655, Japan
e-mail: maf-tky@umin.ac.jp

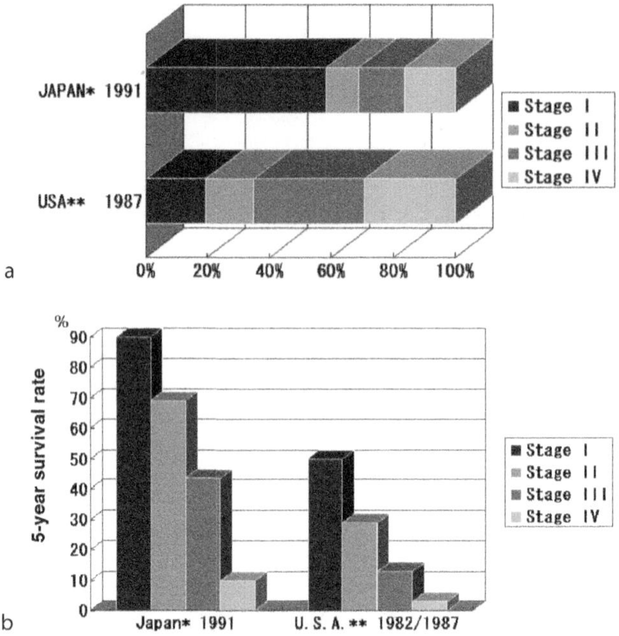

FIG. 1. Gastric cancer: comparison between Japan and the United States (USA). **a** Distribution according to UICC stage. **b** Five-year survival rates according to UICC stage. *JGCA Registration Committee; **Wanebo et al. [3]

type tumors in Western countries, and many Western surgeons have pointed out that any potential survival benefits associated with the D2 lymph node dissections performed in Japan may be due to stage migration rather than superior surgical technique [5]. Because N2 nodes cannot be diagnosed as positive unless they are resected and examined, many of the gastric cancer cases in the United States series may have been understaged. In any event, the large difference in the outcome between Japanese and United States patients can only be partially explained by these factors.

The most important factors affecting the outcome of patients with advanced cancer are whether the tumor is resectable and whether the tumor is curatively resected. The type of surgical procedure may also be important, but evaluating differences in outcome between surgical procedures is rather difficult. The results of several randomized trials comparing D2 dissection with D1 dissection in Western countries have produced results that are difficult for Japanese surgeons to interpret. Therefore, the intent of this chapter is to clarify the rationale for and discuss the results of surgical treatment for advanced gastric cancer.

Gastrectomy Plus D2 Lymph Node Dissection: A Standard Operation for Advanced Gastric Cancer

D2 Lymph Node Dissection

The stomach has numerous lymphatic drainage pathways, and although drainage is usually initially to lymph nodes along the lesser curvature and greater curvature of

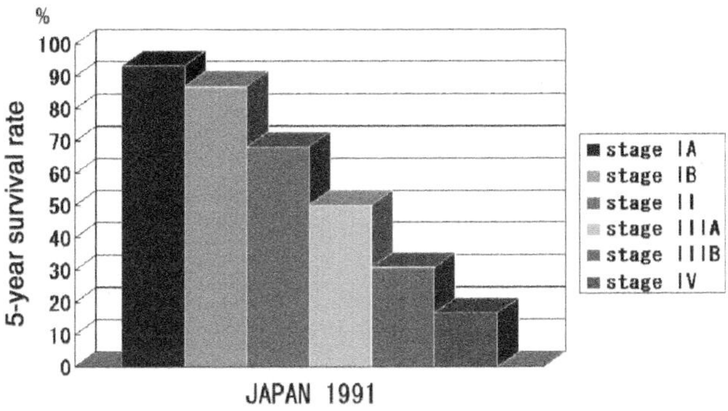

FIG. 2. Five-year survival rates after gastrectomy plus D2 dissection in Japan by stage

the stomach (perigastric or first-tier nodes), primary drainage nodes also include nodes along all three branches of the celiac axis (common hepatic, splenic, left gastric) and along the celiac artery itself (second-tier nodes). D2 dissection, in which the first- and second-tier nodes are dissected, has been a widely accepted, standard operation for advanced gastric cancer in Japan, and better 5-year survival rates after gastrectomy with D2 dissection have been reported by the JRSGC (Fig. 2). Therefore, general surgeons in Japan are trained to perform gastrectomy with D2 dissection, and a surgeon's ability to perform this procedure is a major requirement for becoming an established surgeon. The practice of D2 dissection in Western countries has long been hindered by the lower incidence of gastric cancer [6] and concern about serious complications in these countries [7,8], and the rate of D2 dissection in an overview of gastric cancer treatment in the United States was only 4.7% [3].

The rationale for performing D2 dissection in Japan is based on pathophysiological studies of lymph flow as well as retrospective analyses of survival data. However, no randomized trials comparing D2 and D1 lymph node dissection have been performed in Japan, because D2 dissection has long been regarded as a standard procedure that yields good results. Surgeons in Western countries, however, have questioned whether D2 dissection is actually superior to D1 dissection. Nevertheless, favorable patient survival after D2 gastrectomy has been reported in some non-Japanese retrospective nonrandomized trials [9,10], and at the end of the 1980s a randomized controlled trial of D1 versus D2 dissection (known as the Dutch trial) was started in the Netherlands under the supervision of a Japanese surgeon. Another randomized controlled trial of D1 versus D2 dissection (the Medical Research Council [MRC] trial) was initiated in the U.K., but these randomized trials comparing gastrectomy plus D1 dissection with gastrectomy plus D2 lymph node dissection have failed to demonstrate any survival advantages of D2 dissection [11,12], thus hindering worldwide acceptance of the procedure [13]. Sasako [14], however, has questioned the quality of the D2 dissections performed in these trials, because the series were characterized by very high postoperative mortality rates and extremely small hospital volumes. The Dutch and MRC trials included much lower numbers of patients treated per year and per hospital and much higher hospital mortality rates than in other studies.

Complications: Morbidity and Mortality After D2 Dissection

Bonenkamp et al. [15] reported morbidity and mortality in the Dutch trial. Among the 711 patients (380 D1, 331 D2) judged to have curable lesions in that trial, the D2 patients had a higher operative mortality rate than the D1 patients (10% versus 4%, $P = 0.004$) and experienced more complications (43% versus 25%, $P < 0.01$). Cuschieri et al. [16] reported morbidity and mortality in the MRC trial in the U.K. The D2 group in the MRC trial had a higher postoperative hospital mortality (13% versus 5.4%, $P = 0.04$) and a higher overall postoperative morbidity (46% versus 28%, $P < 0.001$). These high morbidity and mortality rates after D2 dissection are the major reasons why this procedure has not been accepted as standard worldwide.

Total or proximal gastrectomy for proximal tumors is more difficult to perform and is associated with a higher morbidity than distal gastrectomy. The incidence of proximal gastric tumors has been increasing in Western countries, but has been stable in Japan, and this phenomenon may in part explain the superior results in the Japanese studies. However, as pointed out by Sano et al. [17], there were no differences between the Dutch and Japanese studies in the distribution of the primary tumor sites or ratio of total gastrectomies to distal gastrectomies.

The postoperative complications of 273 patients who had undergone total or proximal gastrectomy at the University of Tokyo Hospital and the University of Tokyo Branch Hospital between 1991 to 2000 were retrospectively investigated to determine actual mortality and morbidity after total or proximal gastrectomy in the author's department (unpublished data). The postoperative morbidity rate in the author's department was 39.2%. Only 2 patients required a reoperation, and most of the other patients experienced mild complications requiring only intravenous antibiotics, short-term parental nutrition, or supportive care. The postoperative mortality rate was 0.72%. The primary cause of one of the two perioperative deaths was panperitonitis/sepsis secondary to perforation by the gastric cancer, and the cause of the other death was unknown (it was a sudden death and may have been caused by cerebral infarction). Neither of these patients had undergone a splenectomy or pancreatosplenectomy.

A comparison between our data with those of the Dutch and MRC trials revealed little difference in morbidity rates, but large differences in mortality rates. Both the Dutch and MRC trials reported a relatively high frequency of anastomotic leakage in the D2 dissection groups. Bonenkamp et al. [15] stated that the mortality rate after anastomotic leakage was about 10% in Japan, compared with 30% in their trial. Even in high-volume hospitals, major complications such as anastomotic leakage or intraabdominal abscesses have not been rare, and experience is needed to manage major adverse effects to avoid mortality. Cardiopulmonary complications are common in Western gastric cancer patients, and methods of treating leakage may also lead to treatment-related deaths. Moreover, additional abdominal complications are encountered less frequently in Japanese patients.

A review of reports on postgastrectomy morbidity revealed that the overall morbidity rates ranged from 13% to 44%, and increased morbidity was observed after pancreatosplenectomy (Table 1). Cuschieri et al. [16] claimed that the excess postoperative morbidity and mortality rates in the MRC trial could be accounted for by the inclusion of distal pancreatosplenectomies and splenectomies. Higher morbidity was

TABLE 1. Morbidity reports after gastrectomy

First author	Year published	n	Overall morbidity (%)	Morbidity (%) with splenectomy	Morbidity (%) with pancreatosplenectomy
Viste	1988	1010	28	42 (109/260)	NA
Gouzi	1989	169	34	NA	NA
Pacelli	1993	320	25	NA	NA
Siewert	1993	1654	30	NA	NA
Wu	1995	474	20	29 (65/226)	NA
Jatzko	1995	512	19	NA	NA
Bonenkamp	1995	711	44	41 (68/165)	55 (60/108)
Cuscheri	1996	400	37	54 (104/193)	56 (68/121)
Bozzetti	1999	624	13	19 (13/73)	37 (7/19)
Onate-Ocana	2000	208	20	42 (20/48)	47 (8/17)
Kasakura	2000	1938	22	40 (31/78)	75 (79/105)
Martin	2001	1283	31	29 (54/186)	37 (24/65)
Mafune	2005	272	39	22 (17/79)	48 (42/87)

NA, not available

also associated with distal pancreatectomies in a Japanese series. In the author's department, pancreatic fistulas were found in 38 of the 87 patients (44.0%) who had undergone pancreatosplenectomy and in 8 of the 79 patients (10.0%) who had undergone splenectomy, as opposed to in only 1 of 106 patients who had not undergone pancreatosplenectomy or a splenectomy (Mafune et al., unpublished data). This finding also suggested that pancreatosplenectomy should be avoided unless the pancreas is suspected to be involved by tumor.

A high body mass index may contribute to postoperative morbidity. The typical physical characteristics of Japanese patients, such as a shallow abdominal cavity and lower amounts of intraabdominal fatty tissue, enable a good intraoperative field of vision and easy access to the abdomen, leading to lower operative blood loss, and the body mass index is unassociated with the postoperative morbidity rate in Japan [18]. Even in Western countries, Gretshel et al. [19] reported that standard D2 dissection was justified for overweight patients and that there was no significant increase in morbidity. In our morbidity study, patients with pancreatic fistula (or leakage) had a significantly higher body mass index (BMI) ($P < 0.005$) than patients without pancreatic leakage. However, the mean BMI level of patients with pancreatic fistula in our study was still within normal BMI level in a Western report [19], and this may suggest that morbidity reports between Western countries and Japan cannot be directly compared because of difference of the BMI level.

Should D2 Lymph Node Dissection Be Continued in Japan?

The natural history of stomach cancer reveals a significant number of patients with positive second-tier lymph nodes (stations 7–12). Sasako et al. [20] reported metastatic rates for each lymph node station and 5-year survival rates after D2 dissection in patients with pathologically identified lymph node metastasis at each station. The second-tier lymph node stations had high rates of metastasis, and evidence of a benefit of lymph node dissection was seen in patients with metastasis to second-tier lymph nodes. These patients could not have been cured without a D2 dissection.

The German Gastric Cancer Group suggested that D2 lymph node dissection may benefit T2 and T3 node-negative subsets of patients by removing micrometastases [21], and thus D2 lymph node dissection may provide a stage-specific survival benefit without any increase in morbidity. A relatively greater survival advantage of ≥D2 dissection over <D2 for adequately staged T3N0 patients (5-year survival 60% versus 25%, $P = 0.03$) was demonstrated by a single specialized institution in the United States, even though it was a retrospective study of 1256 patients who had undergone R0 resection [22]. Therefore, gastrectomy plus D2 dissection has been advocated as a treatment modality for stage II and/or IIIA gastric cancer. This professional stance favoring D2 lymph node dissection in Japan [23,24] and some specialized Western institutions [21,25,26] is based on better stage-specific survival rates without any increase in adverse events [11,12,27,28]. Neither Japanese nor Western specialists have observed any difference between morbidity rates and mortality rates after a D2 dissection (22%–43%; 2%–6%) do not differ from those of a D1 dissection (28%–34%; 0%–7%) [11,12,24,27]. The operative mortality rates have been quite low even after D2 lymph node dissection.

Surgical experience is correlated with a lower morbidity rate [29,30]. The learning curve for performing a gastrectomy with a D2 dissection is steep [31], and Japanese general surgeons are taught this technique early during their surgical training [32]. Thus, the main criticism of the Dutch and the MRC trials has been the lack of experience of the surgeons participating in the study. Acceptable morbidity and mortality levels can be achieved in the hands of technically competent surgeons (Table 2). For

TABLE 2. Postoperative morbidity after total or proximal gastrectomy with D2 lymph node dissection

	University of Tokyo, Dept. of GI Surgery n = 272	Humboldt University, Dept. of Surgery & Surgical Oncology[a] n = 199	Cornell University, MSKCC, Dept. of Surgical Oncology n = 1283
Anastomotic leakage	21 (7.7%)	15 (7.5%)	80 (6.2%)
Anastomotic stenosis	8 (2.9%)	—	—
Pancreatic fistula	47 (17.0%)	15 (7.5%)	23 (1.8%)
Pancreatitis	1 (0.4%)	14 (7.0%)	—
Abscess	6 (2.2%)	8 (4.0%)	41 (2.2%)
Bleeding	1 (0.4%)	4 (2.0%)	22 (3.2%)
Cholecystitis	6 (2.6%)	—	—
Bile leakage	1 (2.2%)	—	—
Ileus	9 (0.4%)	2 (1/0%)	—
Pneumonia	7 (3.3%)	32 (16.1%)	85 (2.6%)
Sepsis	1 (0.4%)	—	19 (0.4%)
Cerebral	1 (0.4%)	1 (0.5%)	—
Cardiac	—	7 (3.5%)	88 (6.9%)
Thrombosis	—	4 (2.0%)	20 (1.6%)
Mortality	0.9%	3.5%	4%

MSKCC, Memorial Sloan-Kettering Cancer Center
[a] Total gastrectomy only

example, in an Italian study, a low morbidity rate and low mortality rate of 20.9% and 3.1%, respectively, were achieved for D2 dissections performed at specialized centers with a strict quality control system and without resecting the pancreatic tail, unless tumor involvement was suspected [33]. The Italian study also reported good survival data (overall 5-year survival rate, 55%), and a phase III randomized trial was started [34].

Conclusion

In conclusion, D2 dissection can be reasonably performed by experienced surgeons without significant additional surgical morbidity or mortality. Surgical experience, specific knowledge of the anatomy, and careful postoperative management by experienced teams are crucial to the success of D2 dissection.

Extended or Superextended Operations

Gastrectomy plus D2 dissection is known as "extended" surgery in Western countries, whereas Japanese surgeons employ D2 lymph node dissection as a standard technique and reserve the term "extended" for more aggressive procedures, such as gastrectomy plus D3 dissection. At a few Japanese institutions, wide, extensive resection with extended lymph node dissection has been performed in patients with advanced gastric cancer, and they have yielded good outcomes. As demonstrated in previous randomized D2 versus D1 trials, however, aggressive surgery may increase the risk of complications or treatment-related deaths.

D3 Dissection That Includes Paraaortic Lymph Node Dissection

Lymphatic drainage from the stomach flows to the perigastric nodes and/or the nodes around the celiac axis and its main branches, and then to the paraaortic nodes before entering the systemic circulation via the thoracic duct. Thus, the paraaortic nodes may be regarded as the final node station that can be dissected to remove the threat of systemic metastasis via the lymphatic system.

Microscopic metastasis in the paraaortic nodes has been reported in 20% to 30% of patients with advanced gastric cancer [35–38]. Although patients with paraaortic node involvement are generally not considered candidates for radical surgery, survival data in the Japanese literature have suggested improved survival after superextensive lymph node dissection in some long-term survivors [39,40]. D3 dissection consists of a D2 dissection plus removal of the nodes in the hepatoduodenal ligament, the nodes in the retropancreatic space, the nodes along the vessels of the transverse mesocolon, and the nodes around the abdominal aorta [41] (Fig. 3).

A large-scale prospective randomized controlled trial (the Japan Clinical Oncology Group [JCOG] study 9501) to compare D3 dissection and D2 dissection under strict quality control and data management was started in Japan in 1995. The extremely low hospital death rate of 0.8% after extended paraaortic lymph node dissections in a multiinstitutional study confirmed the findings in previous reports [42]. Several factors that explained the very low operative morbidity and mortality achieved in this JCOG trial were (a) only patients capable of tolerating paraaortic dissection were selected;

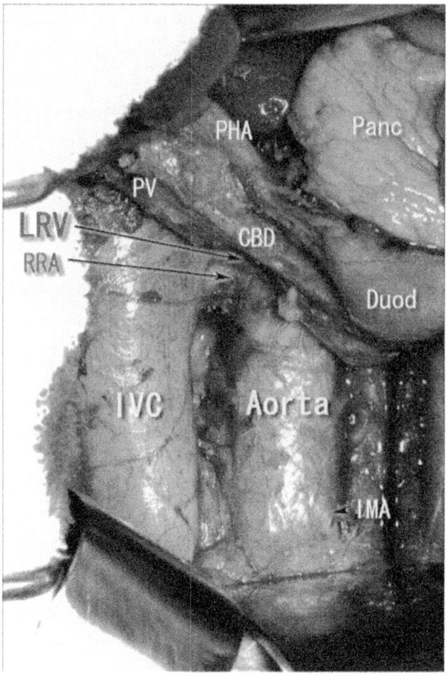

FIG. 3. Intraoperative finding after D3 dissection. *IVC*, inferior vena cava; *IMA*, inferior mesenteric artery; *LRV*, left renal vein; *RRA*, right renal artery; *CBD*, common bile duct, *PV*, portal vein; *PHA*, proper hepatic artery; *Panc*, pancreas; *Duod*, duodenum

(b) only specialist surgeons with an established track record of extended lymphadenectomy participated in the trial; (c) high-throughput centers were selected because of the skill of their surgeons and standardized postoperative management; and (d) pancreatectomy was avoided whenever possible, but splenectomy was performed with total gastrectomy in most cases. An analysis of patient survival in the JCOG trial is scheduled for August 2006, and the results should reveal whether D3 dissections can be expected to provide a survival benefit. However, the study did not exclude patients with paraaortic node metastasis, and that may reduce the expected survival rate.

Since 1997, the author's department has adopted a prospective node dissection strategy for third-tier lymph nodes, including those in the paraaortic area (D3 dissection), for clinically serosa-positive and/or ≧N2 disease patients. The criteria for D3 lymph node dissection were based on data from a retrospective study of D3 versus D2 lymph node dissection conducted from 1991 to 1996 in the author's department. D3 dissection that includes paraaortic lymph node dissection is a more invasive procedure than D2 dissection, but (a) it was not associated with any increase in postoperative mortality, and (b) there were few postoperative nutritional disadvantages [43]. The paraaortic node-positive patients in this study did not receive any therapeutic benefit from a D3 lymph node dissection, that is, their survival was identical to that of the D0 patients (Fig. 4a), nor did D3 dissection improve the survival of the T2 patients (Fig. 4b). The results of this prospective study indicated that D3 lymph node dissection may be beneficial for patients with ≧T3 and/or ≧N2 gastric cancer when the paraaortic nodes are cancer negative, although the difference in survival was not

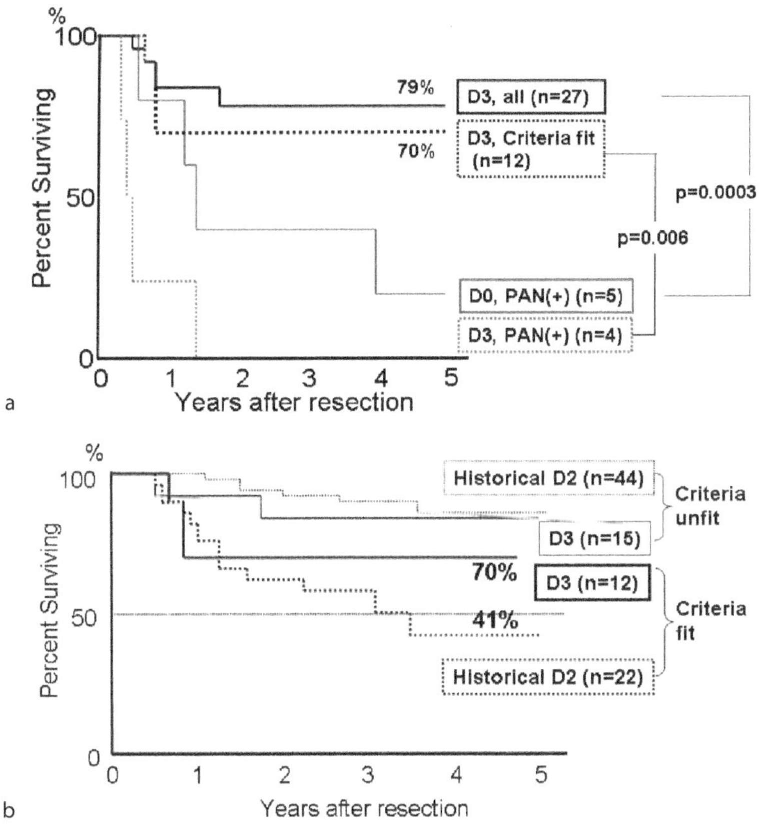

FIG. 4. Survivals after gastrectomy plus D3 dissection. **a** Overall/disease-specific survivals. The paraaortic node-positive patients did not receive any therapeutic benefit from a D3 dissection. **b** Benefit of prophylactic D3 dissection (disease-specific survivals). D3 dissection did not improve the survival of T2 patients (criteria unfit)

statistically significant. D3 dissection was demonstrated to have a favorable effect on survival only when the procedure was used for prophylaxis and not in paraaortic node-positive patients. The results of this study differed from those of other D3 studies regarding this point.

Extended D3 dissection may not only increase operative morbidity but may also affect the function of abdominal organs. Longer operating time and more intraoperative blood loss were usually indicated in the paraaortic lymph node dissection than those in the D2 dissection group [42–44], and the postoperative morbidity rate after paraaortic node dissection was higher, but the difference was not significant. Maeta et al. [44] reported prolonged retention of intraabdominal fluid and diarrhea as postoperative morbidity, and longer postoperative hospital stays, and Sano et al. [42] reported that paralytic ileus, abdominal and/or left pleural lymphorrhea requiring prolonged drainage, and severe diarrhea were specific to the extended paraaortic dissection group in their series. The incidence of these complications in the author's department, however, has been less than in other studies. Frequent ligation of lymph vessels or the use of hemoclips (or a vessel-sealing system) has prevented lymphorrhea or intraabdominal fluid collection, and preserving paraaortic ganglia has prevented paralysis of bowel movement or severe diarrhea. In any event, the morbidity after D3 dissection that includes paraaortic nodal dissection is not severe and is usually prevented by careful surgical maneuvers.

Appleby Procedure and Left Upper Abdominal Exenteration

In 1953, L.H. Appleby [45] reported a radical operation for gastric cancer. He described 13 gastric resections with removal of the entire celiac axis and its associated nodes en bloc for carcinoma of the stomach. Dividing the celiac axis and the peripheral part of the common hepatic artery enables the lymph nodes within the second tier, except the 12a and 14v stations, to be completely resected in an en bloc manner. The nodes at the 12a, 14v, and 16 stations can also be dissected during this procedure, but not en bloc. In 1968, T. Wada, a professor at the University of Tokyo, proposed the use of the Appleby method as an easy procedure for achieving a complete D2 lymph node dissection, and 81 patients have undergone the Appleby operation (in the author's department) in 1976 (Fig. 5a). The outcome of 60 patients who underwent curative resection in the Appleby group was significantly better than that of 64 patients in a historical control group ($P < 0.025$) (Fig. 5b). The survival of patients with lymph node metastasis, even in the second-tier nodes, was significantly better in the Appleby operation group than in the control group (Fig. 5c,d).

Based on these findings, the Appleby operation seemed to be a useful standard surgical protocol for advanced gastric cancer from this data. However, higher morbidity and mortality rates (30% and 6%, respectively) and Appleby operation-specific complications were encountered and prevented the procedure becoming popular. The decrease in blood flow in the proper hepatic artery led to frequent procedure-specific complications, such as temporary liver dysfunction, and 24% of the patients had serum glutamic oxaloacetie transaminase (GOT) levels above 200 KU on the first postoperative day. Partial liver necrosis (6%), cholecystitis (10%), or gallbladder necrosis (5%) were sometimes observed, and anastomotic leaks (12%), especially at the jejunoduodenal anastomosis (7%), were also caused by decreased blood flow. Pancreatic fistulas (7%) also occurred, but were much less frequent, with an incidence that was about the same as after conventional total gastrectomy with a distal pancreatosplenectomy. There was no operative mortality in the first 46 consecutive cases (in the author's department), but 5 surgery-related deaths occurred in the next 37 cases. They may have been mostly attributable to the surgeons' lack of skill and the lack of experience in postoperative care.

Left upper abdominal exenteration (LUAE) was proposed by T. Kajitani (Cancer Institute, Japan) as another procedure for en bloc resection for advanced gastric cancer. LUAE includes removal of the transverse colon, left adrenal gland, left kidney, and the lateral segment of the left lobe of the liver as well as the stomach, pancreatic tail, and spleen. This procedure enables complete bursaomentectomy (by continuous resection of the distal pancreas, spleen, and mesocolon) and lymph node dissection on the left side of the aorta. It has usually been performed to treat advanced cancers

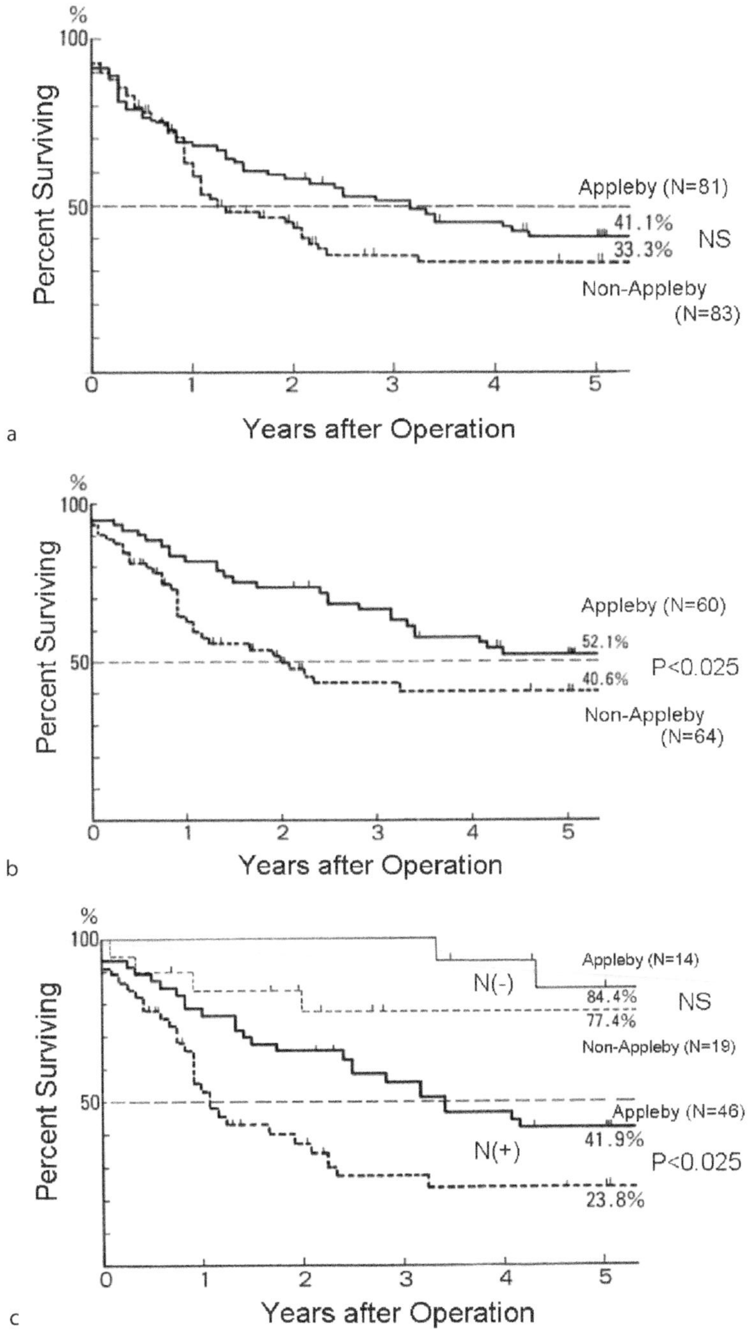

FIG. 5. Survival after Appleby operation: **a** all patients; **b** curative resection; **c** lymph node metastasis; **d** lymph node metastasis—N1 vs. N2

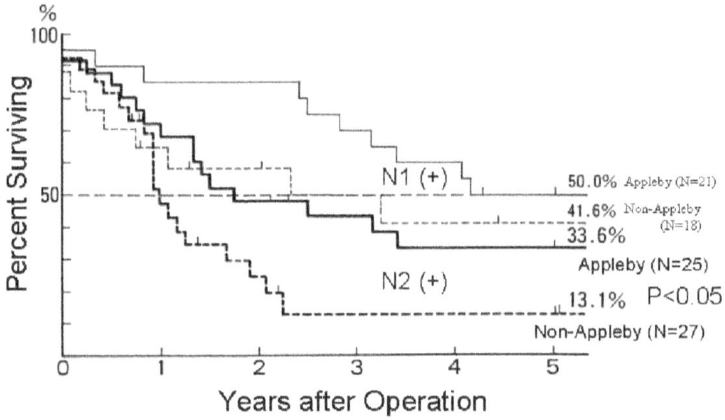

d

FIG. 5. *Continued*

with (a) extensive serosal invasion; (b) lymphatic permeation of surrounding tissues (in the early process of cancer invasion); (c) direct invasion of surrounding organs; or (d) a small degree of serosal or peritoneal cancer dissemination to the greater or lesser omentum or mesocolon. At the Cancer Institute in Japan, LUAE has mostly been performed for the invasive type of gastric cancers (85%, 71/91), 70% of which were Borrmann type 4 cancers [46]. The prognosis after surgery for type 4 gastric cancer, including linitis plastica, remains poor. Because the most frequent mode of recurrence is retroperitoneal involvement, LUAE was performed for patients with type 4 gastric carcinoma to remove the tumor and microinvasion surrounding the stomach. Hiratsuka and Furukawa [47] indicated by a histological study that prophylactic LUAE should be performed for the carcinoma fibrosum (linitis plastica) type in type 4 gastric cancer. However, the 5-year survival rate after the LUAE was about 10% [46]. Therefore, Furukawa et al. [48] proposed LUAE plus the Appleby method and reported that the procedure improved the survival of patients with stage III scirrhous cancer, but it was not effective for patients with stage IV cancer. Procedure-specific complications were also encountered; that is, one patient died of hepatic failure.

These operations were devised in an attempt to cure advanced gastric cancers with a very poor prognosis, and only several surgeons in specialized institution can perform them without any increase in adverse events.

Thoracoabdominal and Transhiatal Approach

A thoracoabdominal or transhiatal approach is usually selected for cardia cancer or for gastric cancer with esophageal invasion. The increasing incidence of cancers of the esophagogastric junction in Western countries has drawn attention to this tumor entity. There has been controversy as to whether the thoracoabdominal approach is superior to the abdominal and transhiatal approach to surgical treatment of the two subtypes of esophagogastric junction cancers, true cardia cancers, and subcardia cancers.

The results of a Dutch trial that compared right thoracotomy and the abdominal approach with the transhiatal approach for adenocarcinoma of the esophagus was reported in 2002 [49]. Mediastinal and abdominal lymph node dissection was performed in this trial, although mediastinal dissection by the transhiatal approach was limited to below the inferior pulmonary vein. Although the results indicated that the thoracotomy approach provided no significant survival benefit and that the morbidity rate was higher, it was concluded that the thoracotomy approach was superior in conclusion because of the wider lymph node dissection field. This study was performed on esophageal adenocarcinoma, mainly cardia cancer or lower esophageal cancer, that may arise around the esophagogastric junction. A randomized controlled trial in Japan revealed that left thoracoabdominal approach provided no survival benefit over the abdominal and transhiatal approach for true cardia or subcardia cancers with esophageal invasion of 3 cm or less (JCOG 9502) [50].

Gastric cancer invades the esophagus possibly because the tumor is in the advanced stage or behaves aggressively, and cardia cancer is different from gastric cancer with esophageal invasion in this respect. The survival benefit of extensive lymph node dissection in the mediastinum or additional lower esophagectomy for gastric cancer with esophageal invasion may be limited, because most patients die of peritoneal cancer dissemination, liver metastases, abdominal distant lymph node metastasis, and so on.

Pancreatoduodenectomy

Pancreatoduodenectomy is sometimes performed in patients with one of the following indications: (a) lymph node metastasis to third-tier lymph node stations; (b) duodenal invasion, usually more than 3 cm; (c) pancreatic invasion; (d) exposure of the tumor on the serosal surface of the duodenum; or (e) invasion of the mesocolon [46], and Oyama and Yamaguchi [51] reported that the reason for pancreatoduodenectomy in 202 surgical procedures for gastric cancer was direct invasion in 136 cases (67%), lymph node dissection in 48 cases (24%), and duodenal invasion in 6 cases (3%).

However, the survival benefits of pancreatoduodenectomy were limited because most patients died as a result of other causes, such as peritonitis carcinomatosa, liver metastasis, or distant lymph node metastasis. In the author's personal experience, only patients with direct tumor invasion of the pancreas with no lymph node metastasis have long postoperative survival times. Oyama and Yamaguchi [51] found that the outcome after pancreatoduodenectomy was poor if lymph node metastasis had occurred beyond the first-tier stations (≥N2) (5-year survival rate for ≥N2 2.7% versus 25%–27% for N1 of N0). Therefore, this procedure has not been accepted as a standard operation, and gastrojejunal anastomosis has usually been selected as an alternative procedure.

Conclusion

These extensive or superextensive surgical procedures for advanced cancer represent an attempt to increase the cure rate. The survival benefit, however, is limited, and the surgical procedure should be carefully selected for each patient. Adjuvant chemotherapy represents another attempt to treat advanced gastric cancer, and further investigation is required.

References

1. Maruyama K, Sasako M, Kinoshita T, et al (1993) Effectiveness of systematic lymph node dissection in gastric surgery. In: Nishi M, Ichikawa H, Nakajima T, Maruyama K, Tahara E (eds). Gastric cancer. Springer, Berlin, pp 293–305
2. Akoh JA, Macintyre IM (1992) Improving survival in gastric cancer review of 5-year survival rates in English publications from 1970. Br J Surg 79:293–299
3. Wanebo HJ, Kennedy BJ, Chmiel J, et al (1993) Cancer of the stomach: a patient care study by the American College of Surgeons. Ann Surg 218:583–592
4. Japanese Gastric Cancer Association, Registration Committee (2003) Gastric cancer treated in 1991 in Japan: data analysis of nationwide registry. Gastric Cancer 6(suppl): 1–14
5. Bunt A, Herman J, Smit V, et al (1995) Surgical/pathologic-stage migration confounds comparisons of gastric cancer survival rate between Japan and Western countries. J Clin Oncol 13:19–25
6. Fuchs CS, Mayer RJ (1995) Gastric carcinoma. N Engl J Med 333:32–41
7. Diggory MT, Cuschieri A (1985) R2/3 gastrectomy for gastric carcinoma: an audited experience of a consecutive series. Br J Surg 72:146–148
8. Dent DM, Madden MV, Price SK (1988) Randomized comparison of R1 and R2 gastrectomy for gastric carcinoma. Br J Surg 75:110–112
9. Pacelli F, Doglietto GB, Bellantone R, et al (1993) Extensive versus limited lymph node dissection for gastric cancer: a comparative study of 320 patients. Br J Surg 80:1153–1156
10. Siewert JR, Bottcher K, Roder JD, et al (1993) Prognostic relevance of systematic lymph node dissection in gastric carcinoma. German Gastric Carcinoma Study Group. Br J Surg 80: 1015–1018
11. Bonenkamp JJ, Hermans J, Sasako M, et al (1999) Extended lymph node dissection for gastric cancer. N Engl J Med 340:908–914
12. Cuschieri A, Weeden S, Fielding J, et al (1999) Patient survival after D1 and D2 resections for gastric cancer: long-term results of the MRC randomized surgical trial. Surgical Cooperative Group. Br J Cancer 79:1522–1530
13. Schmidt-Matthiesen A (1998) Should systematic lymph node dissection be recommended for gastric cancer? Contra. Eur J Cancer 34:1483–1486
14. Sasako M (2004) Role of surgery in multidisciplinary treatment for solid cancers. Int J Clin Oncol 9:346–351
15. Bonenkamp JJ, Songun I, Hermans J, et al (1995) Randomised comparison of morbidity after D1 and D2 dissection for gastric cancer in 996 Dutch patients. Lancet 345:745–748
16. Cuschieri A, Fayers P, Fielding J, et al (1996) Postoperative morbidity and mortality after D1 and D2 resections for gastric cancer: preliminary results of the MRC randomized controlled surgical trial. Lancet 347:995–999
17. Sano T, Sasako M, Yamamoto S, et al (2004) Gastric cancer surgery: morbidity and mortality results from a prospective randomized controlled trial comparing D2 and extended para-aortic lymphadenectomy—Japan Clinical Oncology Group study 9501. J Clin Oncol 22:2767–2773
18. Moriwaki Y, Kunisaki C, Kobayashi S, et al (2003) Does body mass index (BMI) influence morbidity and long-term survival in gastric cancer patients after gastrectomy? Hepatogastroenterology 50:284–288
19. Gretschel S, Christoph F, Bembenek A, et al (2003) Body mass index does not affect systematic D2 lymph node dissection and post operative morbidity in gastric cancer patients. Ann Surg Oncol 10:363–368
20. Sasako M, McCulloch P, Kinoshita T, et al (1995) New method to evaluate the therapeutic value of lymph node dissection for gastric cancer. Br J Surg 82:346–351
21. Siewert JR, Bottcher K, Stein HJ, et al (1998) Relevant prognostic factors in gastric cancer: ten-year results of the German Gastric Cancer Study. Ann Surg 228:449–461

22. Kooby DA, Suriawinata A, Klimstara DS, et al (2003) Biologic predictors of survival in node-negative gastric cancer. Ann Surg 237:828–837
23. Maruyama K, Sasako M, Kinishita T, et al (1998) Should systemic lymph node dissection be recommended for gastric cancer? pro. Eur J Cancer 34:1480–1483
24. Kasakura Y, Mochizuki F, Wakabayashi K, et al (2002) An evaluation of the effectiveness of extended lymph node dissection in patients with gastric cancer: a retrospective study of 1403 cases at a single institution. J Surg Res 103:252–259
25. Roukos DH, Lorenz M, Encke A (1998) Evidence of survival benefit of extended (D2) lymphadenectomy in Western patients with gastric cancer based on a new concept. A prospective long-term follow-up study. Surgery (St. Louis) 123:573–578
26. Harrison LE, Karpeh MS, Brennan MF (1998) Extended lymphadenectomy is associated with a survival benefit for node-negative gastric cancer. J Gastrointest Surg 2:126–131
27. Smith JW, Shiu MH, Kelsey L, et al (1991) Morbidity of radical lymphadenectomy in curative resection of gastric carcinoma. Arch Surg 126:1469–1473
28. Sue-Ling HM, Johnston D, Martin IG, et al (1993) Gastric cancer: a curable disease in Britain. Br J Surg 307:591–596
29. Birkmeyer JD, Stukel TA, Siewers AE, et al (2003) Surgeon volume and operative mortality in the United States. New Engl J Med 349:2117–2127
30. Fujita T, Yamazaki Y (2002) Influence of surgeon's volume on early outcome after total gastrectomy. Eur J Surg 168:535–538
31. Perikh D, Johnson M, Chagla L, et al (1996) D2 gastrectomy lessons from a prospective audit of the learning curve. Br J Surg 83:1595–1599
32. Moriwaki Y, Kobayashi S, Kunisaki C, et al (2001) Is D2 lymphadenectomy in gastrectomy safe with regard to the skill of the operator? Dig Surg 18:111–117
33. Degiuli M, Sasako M, Ponti A, et al (1998) Morbidity and mortality after D2 gastrectomy for gastric cancer: results of the Italian Gastric Cancer Study Group prospective multicenter surgical study. J Clin Oncol 16(4):1490–1493
34. Degiuli M, Sasako M, Ponti A, et al (2004) Survival results of a multicentre phase II study to evaluate D2 gastrectomy for gastric cancer. Br J Cancer 90(9):1727–1732
35. Takahashi S (1990) Study of para-aortic lymph node metastases of gastric cancer subjected to superextensive lymph node dissection (in Japanese with English abstract). J Jpn Surg Soc (Nippon Geka Gakkai Zasshi) 91:29–35
36. Kitamura M, Arai K, Iwasaki Y (1996) Clinicopathological studies and problems on para-aortic lymph node dissection: D4 dissection (in Japanese with English abstract). J Jpn Surg Soc (Nippon Geka Gakkai Zasshi) 97:302–307
37. Isozaki H, Okajima K, Fujii K, et al (1999) Effectiveness of paraaortic lymph node dissection for advanced gastric cancer. Hepatogastroenterology 46:549–554
38. Baba M, Hokita S, Natsugoe S, et al (1999) Paraaortic lymphadenectomy in patients with advanced carcinoma of the upper-third of the stomach. Hepatogastroenterology 47:893–896
39. Ohashi I, Takagi K, Konishi T, et al (1976) Five-year survival of patients with dissection of paraaortic lymph node metastases for gastric cancer (in Japanese with English abstract). Jpn J Gastroenterol Surg 9:112–116
40. Yonemura Y, Hashimoto T, Katayama K, et al (1985) Classification of paraaortic lymph nodes and significance of dissection of these nodes in gastric cancer (in Japanese with English abstract). Jpn J Gastroenterol Surg 18:1995–1999
41. Japanese Gastric Cancer Association (1998) Japanese classification of gastric carcinoma—2nd English edition. Gastric Cancer 1:10–24
42. Sano T, Sasako M, Yamamoto S, et al (2004) Gastric cancer surgery: morbidity and mortality results from a prospective randomized controlled trial comparing D2 and extended para-aortic lymphadenectomy—Japan Clinical Oncology Group Study 9501. J Clin Oncol 22: 2767–2773
43. Shimoyama S, Mafune K, Kaminishi M (2005) Safety of a paraaortic node dissection for selected advanced gastric cancer patients. Hepatogastnoenterology (in press)

44. Maeta M, Yamashiro H, Saito H, et al (1999) A prospective pilot study of extended (D3) and super extended para-aortic lymphadenectomy (D4) in patients with T3 or T4 gastric cancer managed by total gastrectomy. Surgery (St. Louis) 125:325–331
45. Appleby LH (1953) The celiac axis in the expansion of the operation for gastric carcinoma. Cancer (Phila) 6:704–707
46. Takagi K (1990) Extended operation (in Japanese). Gastroenterol Surg 13:789
47. Hiratsuka M, Furukawa H (2003) Application of left upper abdominal extentration. In: Arai K (ed) Knack and pitfalls of gastric surgery (in Japanese). Bunkodo, Tokyo, pp 109–111
48. Furukawa H, Hiratsuka M, Iwanaga T, et al (1997) Extended surgery—left upper abdominal extenteration plus Appleby's method—for type 4 gastric carcinoma. Ann Surg Oncol 4: 209–214
49. Hulscher JB, van Sandick JW, de Boer AG, et al (2002) Extended transthoracic resection compared with limited transhiatal resection for adenocarcinoma of the esophagus. N Engl J Med 347:1662–1669
50. Sasako M, Sano T, Sairenji M, et al (2004) Left thorac-abdomonal approach (LT) compared with abdominal and transhiatal approach (AT) for cardia or sub-cardia cancer. Results of a surgical randomized controlled trial (JCOG 9502). J Clin Oncol 22:314s
51. Oyama S, Yamaguchi T (2003) Application of pancreatoduodenectomy. In: Arai K (ed) Knack and pitfalls of gastric surgery (in Japanese). Bunkodo, Tokyo, pp 112–115

Laparoscopic Gastrectomy

Seigo Kitano, Tsuyoshi Etoh, and Norio Shiraishi

Introduction

The advantages of laparoscopic surgery for the treatment of gastrointestinal benign disease have been well demonstrated [1]. Although the operative time for laparoscopic procedures is generally longer than that for conventional open gastrectomy, laparoscopic gastrectomy is superior to open surgery by virtue of its reduced surgical invasiveness, less postoperative pain, earlier hospital discharge, lower hospital cost, better cosmesis, and a better quality of life as a result of smaller skin incisions and minimized trauma to the abdominal wall [2–6]. Since our first experience with laparoscopy-assisted distal gastrectomy (LADG) using the Billroth I reconstruction in a patient with early gastric carcinoma in 1991 [7], the use of laparoscopic gastrectomy for gastric carcinoma has increased worldwide. The application of laparoscopic surgery to cure gastric carcinoma, however, remains controversial. Thus far, several case-controlled studies have investigated different aspects of the laparoscopic technique for the treatment of gastric carcinoma, mainly in Japan [8–11]. While waiting for a large randomized trial to be conducted, a review of the literature can inform us of the status of laparoscopic gastrectomy.

Laparoscopic Treatment of Gastric Carcinoma

Current Status of Laparoscopic Gastric Resection

The goal of any curative surgical approach to gastric carcinoma should be a complete resection, leaving no residual neoplasm after the operation.

For the management of patients with early lesions, wide agreement exists about therapy by laparoscopic surgery. There are three options for the management of early gastric carcinoma: (1) laparoscopic wedge resection (LWR), (2) intragastric mucosal resection (IGMR), and (3) laparoscopic gastrectomy (totally laparoscopic, laparoscopy-assisted, and hand-assisted). Regional lymph nodes may be involved in

---

Department of Surgery I, Oita University Faculty of Medicine, Hasama-machi, Oita 879-5593, Japan
e-mail: kitano@oita-med.ac.jp

early gastric carcinoma, but this is much less common in lesions limited to the mucosa only (2%–3%) than in submucosal lesions (15–20%) [12,13]. Lymphatic vessel invasion, histological tumor ulceration, and tumor diameter (>30 mm) are independent factors predicting regional lymph node metastasis [14]. These data suggest that most early carcinomas are located only in the gastric wall and that local resection of the gastric wall is adequate for complete clearance. Theoretically, laparoscopic local resection, such as LWR or IGMR, can be applied to treat early gastric carcinoma without risk factors for lymph node metastasis. On the other hand, laparoscopic gastrectomy, such as LADG, was developed to treat early gastric carcinoma in which there is some risk of lymph node metastasis at the perigastric portion (n1). The Guidelines for Gastric Cancer Treatment of the Japanese Gastric Cancer Association present two indications for LADG: (1) mucosal carcinoma without preoperatively diagnosed lymph node metastasis, and (2) carcinoma with submucosal invasion and without preoperatively diagnosed lymph node metastasis [15]. However, it is sometimes difficult to diagnose lymph node metastasis preoperatively, and the diagnostic accuracy rate is very low. Therefore, indications of LWR, IGMR, and LADG are generally determined by tumor size, depth of cancer invasion, the presence of ulceration, and histological type.

To treat advanced gastric carcinoma, D1 dissection of only perigastric lymph nodes is considered inadequate by most Japanese and some Western surgeons. In Japan, D2 lymph node dissection is routine practice. Japanese surgeons established the techniques of D2 lymphadenectomy in which the lymph nodes in the first (perigastric) and second (along the celiac artery and its branches) tier are systematically dissected. By this surgical therapy, 30%–40% of patients with metastasis in even second-tier lymph nodes have survived more than 5 years [16]. However, surgeons in the United States and other Western countries rarely perform extensive prophylactic lymphadenectomy. Based on two European randomized trials (RCT) that in comparing D1 and D2 showed high operative mortality, exceeding 10% in the D2 group, the British NHS Cancer Guidance officially discourages the use of D2 in clinical practice [17,18].

D1 gastrectomy is eminently feasible through the laparoscopic or laparoscopy-assisted approach. Because laparoscopic gastrectomy has improved the outcome of D1 lymph node dissection for early gastric carcinoma, laparoscopic procedures with D2 lymph node dissection have been recently tried for advanced gastric carcinoma in Japan. Some investigators reported low mortality and morbidity in laparoscopic gastrectomy with D2 lymph node dissection [8,19,20]. However, it seems technically difficult to dissect extragastric lymph nodes (group 2 nodes, based on the 13th Japanese edition of the Japanese Classification of Gastric Carcinoma) using the laparoscopic approach [21]. D2 lymphadenectomy using the laparoscopic approach requires a learning curve, as does conventional open surgery. So far, it is difficult to draw any conclusions from these limited early reports. To establish the acceptability of laparoscopic gastrectomy with D2 lymph node dissection against advanced gastric carcinoma, a safe technique and a new instrument must be developed.

Technical Aspects of Laparoscopic Gastric Resection

The techniques of laparoscopic gastric resection, including laparoscopic wedge resection (LWR), intragastric mucosal resection (IGMR), and laparoscopy-assisted distal gastrectomy (LADG), are described next.

Laparoscopic Wedge Resection (LWR)

LWR is performed by the lesion-lifting method developed by Ohgami et al. [22] as shown in Fig. 1.

1. The cancerous lesion and the gastric wall around it are exposed endoscopically and laparoscopically.
2. The abdominal wall and gastric wall near the lesions are pierced with a 12-G sheathed needle.
3. A small metal rod with a fine wire is inserted into the stomach through the outer sheath, and the sheath is removed.
4. The lesion is lifted by retracting the metal rod and resected with a wedge-shaped part of the stomach with the use of an endoscopic stapler.
5. After the resected specimen is removed, the abdomen is closed.

The lesion must be removed with an adequately clear margin. To resect the lesion successfully, Altorjay et al. modified the lesion-lifting technique to create a "double-lifting" method [23].

Intragastric Mucosal Resection (IGMR)

IGMR is performed by techniques developed by Ohashi et al. [24] as shown in Fig. 2.

1. Three trocars are placed in the gastric lumen, penetrating both the abdomen and the stomach walls, under endoscopic and laparoscopic observation.
2. These trocars fix the gastric wall to the abdominal wall with a balloon.
3. After the laparoscope and two forceps are inserted into the stomach through the trocars, dots are placed around the lesion to indicate the removal margin, and a mucosal resection is performed.
4. Hemostasis is achieved by electrocautery and laser.
5. The resected specimen is extracted by endoscope.
6. Each balloon is then deflated, and the trocars are pulled out.
7. Each port in the stomach is sutured laparoscopically, and the abdomen is closed.

For IGMR, it is important to access the gastric lumen easily and to obtain an optimal operative field. Several new devices, such as the expandable sleeve, can be used instead of forceps with a balloon to provide the necessary easy access.

Laparoscopy-Assisted Distal Gastretomy (LADG)

The essentials for LADG with D1 lymph node dissection for gastric carcinoma are listed here.

1. Under general anesthesia with tracheal intubation, a 10 mmHg pneumoperitoneum is created and a laparoscope is inserted through the subumbilical incision.
2. Four cannulas for grasping and dissecting instruments are placed in the upper abdomen (Fig. 3).
3. The greater omentum and gastrocolic ligament are dissected laparoscopically outside the epigastric arcade (Fig. 4).
4. The right gastroepiploic vessels are cut to facilitate dissection of lymph nodes at the subpyloric portion (Fig. 5).

5. The lesser omentum is opened and the suprapyloric lymph nodes are dissected after the right gastric artery and vein are divided between clips.
6. The stomach is fully mobilized, and the left gastric artery and vein are divided using clips and ligatures (Fig. 6).
7. The left cardiac and superior gastric lymph nodes are dissected down to the distal portion of the stomach (Fig. 7).
8. A 5-cm-long upper midskin incision is made just below the xiphoid, and the mobilized stomach is pulled out through this minilaparotomy wound. The distal two-thirds of the stomach is resected using staplers (Fig. 8).
9. The perigastric lymph nodes are completely dissected along with the distal portion of the stomach.
10. Billroth I gastroduodenostomy is carried out through the minilaparotomy wound, with the same handsewn technique as used for conventional open surgery (Fig. 9).

Other Types of Laparoscopic Gastrectomy

Given the tools available today, laparoscopic proximal and total gastrectomies are still challenging [25–28]. In both these procedures, esophageal anastomosis is performed laparoscopically [26]. Even with the use of a circular stapler, however, this part of the surgery is technically complicated. The totally laparoscopic approach may become easier with the development of improved staplers for transoral application. Hand-assisted laparoscopy, using one of the currently available devices, may simplify the performance of these highly complex procedures. More recently, to preserve the function of the gastric remnant after gastrectomy, some surgeons have performed a laparoscopic pylorus-preserving gastrectomy without injuring vegal nerves such as the pyloric or hepatic branch [10].

Short-Term Outcome

Several case-controlled studies have evaluated the short-term outcome of laparoscopic surgery for early gastric carcinoma. The advantages of laparoscopic gastric resection compared with open gastric resection are summarized in Table 1. Prospective and retrospective analyses by a single institution showed bowel function recovery between 1 and 3 days after laparoscopic gastric resection. In several case-controlled studies, bowel function recovered significantly faster after laparoscopic gastrectomy than after open gastrectomy. In addition, patient quality of life has been assessed by several studies, focusing mainly on postoperative pain and analgesic requirements. In several studies, pain after laparoscopic surgery was also significantly less than that after open surgery [2,5,6].

Other short-term advantages of the laparoscopic procedures were demonstrated by a randomized trial at a single institution, which revealed better postoperative pulmonary function in 14 patients who underwent LADG compared to 14 patients who underwent open distal gastrectomy [29]. Patients after laparoscopic surgery had a significantly faster recovery in forced respiratory volume per second and in forced vital capacity.

Regarding the cost, a case-controlled study showed that LADG is less expensive than conventional open gastrectomy (total hospital charge, ¥1336 $\times$ 10^3 vs. ¥1411 $\times$ 10^3)

TABLE 1. Short-term benefits of laparoscopic gastrectomy compared with open gastrectomy

Clinical course after operation:
Less blood loss
Reduced analgesic request
Earlier first eating
Earlier first flatus
Earlier first walking
Earlier hospital discharge
Lower hospital cost
Better cosmesis
Pulmonary function
Better forced capacity at post operative day (POD) 3
Better forced expiratory volume in 1 at POD 3
Inflammation
Lower peak of number of white blood cells (WBC)
Lower peak of C-reactive protein (CRP)
Lower peak of inter leukin (IL-6)

because both the postoperative recovery period and the hospital stay are shorter (16.1 vs. 20.5 days) [30]. However, Rosin et al. noted problems with LADG, including the complexity of the procedure and long operating time [31].

Follow-Up Evaluation

With regard to operative curability, the surgical margins and the number of dissected lymph nodes in laparoscopic gastrectomy are equivalent to those in conventional open gastrectomy. Table 2 lists several noncomparative or comparative studies of short-term follow-up evaluation of laparoscopic gastrectomy [4,27,29,32–35]. However, the issues regarding the recurrence rates and the long-term survival rate remain unclear. Most retrospective published studies were composed of a small number of patients and showed short-term follow-up. In addition, no long-term results have been recorded after laparoscopic gastrectomy. In the near future, a multicenter randomized controlled trial is needed to confirm the advantages in the long-term outcome of laparoscopic gastric resection for early gastric carcinoma.

Morbidity Related to Laparoscopic Gastric Resection

A survey conducted by the Japan Society for Endoscopic Surgery showed the incidences of intraoperative and postoperative complications to be 2.1% and 4.6% after LWR and 4.2% and 6.5% after IGWR, respectively [36]. The major intraoperative and postoperative complications are bleeding and gastric dysemptying, respectively, for both LWR and IGMR. After LADG, the incidences of intraoperative and postoperative complications are 1.4% and 9.7%, respectively. The major intraoperative complication after LADG is bleeding and the major postoperative complications are gastric dysemptying, anastomotic leakage, and wound infection. Recently, a randomized controlled trial of a small number of cases demonstrated no significant difference in the incidence of complications, such as anastomotic leakage, anastomotic

Table 2. Follow-up evaluation of laparoscopic gastrectomy

Authors	Year	Study design	*N*	Candidate	Lymph node disssection	Follow-up (months)	Recurrence (cases)
Azagra et al. [1]	1999	RNC	Lap 13	T2–T3	D1 or D2	Mean, 27.5	2
Hüscher et al. [33]	2000	RNC	Lap 45	T2–T4	D1 or D2 or D3	Mean, 43	1
Ballesta-Lopez et al. [34]	2002	RNC	Lap 25	T1–T2	D1	7–63	0
Kitano et al. [29]	2002	RNC	Lap 116	T1	D1	Mean, 45	0
Tanimura et al. [27]	2003	RNC	Lap 28	T1	D1 or D2	1–36	0
Reyes et al. [4]	2001	RC	Lap 9 Open 12	Stage I–IV	Not described	1–36	0
Kitano et al. [35]	2002	PR	Lap 14 Open 14	T1	D1	Mean, 21.5	0

RNC, retrospective noncomparative study; RC, retrospective comparative study; PR, prospective randomized controlled study; Lap, laparoscopic gastrectomy; Open, open gastrectomy

stenosis, bleeding, and wound infection, between an LADG group and a conventional open gastrectomy group [29]. However, laparoscopic gastric resection for gastric carcinoma is still under development. Under laparoscopic surgery, some adverse events occur that are technically associated with laparoscopic gastrectomy.

Bleeding

Bleeding related to lymph node dissection is the most frequent complication during laparoscopic gastrectomy. It is important to recognize the anatomy as seen in a limited, two-dimensional monitor and to maintain a perspective that allows the prevention of accidental bleeding.

Injury of the Gastrointestinal Tract

When the walls of the stomach, transverse colon, or duodenum are strongly grasped by forceps to extend them, they can be accidentally injured. If these injuries happen, they should be repaired carefully by an intraabdominal suturing technique or automatic suturing.

Injury of Solid Organs

When the lymph node is dissected superior to the pancreas, parenchyma of the pancreas can be injured accidentally by forceps or by an ultrasonically activated device. The liver and spleen also can be injured when they are strongly retracted. All procedures should be done gently and carefully under laparoscopic surgery because of the limited operative view and the mobility of each instrument.

Port Site Metastasis

The issues of port site metastasis are still unresolved. Therefore, a understanding of physiology and the development of correct measures are needed to prevent it. Although recent papers in a clinical setting have demonstrated that laparoscopic colectomy in patients with advanced colorectal cancer has a long-term survival rate equivalent to that of open surgery and does not increase port site metastases [37–39], it is dangerous to apply these results for colorectal cancer to advanced gastric carcinoma. The few reported cases regarding port site metastasis in gastric carcinoma were all related to advanced tumors or diffuse carcinomatosis [33]. The presence of serosal penetration may be associated with this phenomenon.

Conclusion

Laparoscopic surgery for gastric carcinoma has been shown to be potentially superior to traditional laparotomy with regard to short-term benefits. The technique seems safe and capable of fulfilling oncological criteria for cancer surgery. However, questions regarding recurrence rates and long-term survival have not yet been satisfactorily answered. Further follow-up and a review of large, multicenter randomized trials are needed before widespread acceptance of the technique can be recommended. Finally, surgeons with sufficient expertise and ongoing peer-reviewed data collection may currently offer this therapy to appropriately selected patients.

References

1. Azagra JS, Goergen M, De Simone P, et al (1999) The current role of laparoscopic surgery in the treatment of benign gastroduodenal diseases. Hepatogastroenterology 46:1522–1526
2. Schwenk W, Bohm B, Muller JM (1998) Postoperative pain and fatigue after laparoscopic or conventional colorectal resections. A prospective randomized trial. Surg Endosc 12: 1131–1136
3. Adachi Y, Suematsu T, Shiraishi N, et al (1999) Quality of life after laparoscopy-assisted Billroth I gastrectomy. Ann Surg 229:49–54
4. Reyes CD, Weber KJ, Gagner M, et al (2001) Laparoscopic vs. open gastrectomy. A retrospective review. Surg Endosc 15:928–931
5. Yano H, Monden T, Kinuta M, et al (2001) The usefulness of laparoscopy-assisted distal gastrectomy in comparison with that of open distal gastrectomy for early gastric cancer. Gastric Cancer 4:93–97
6. Shimizu S, Noshiro H, Nagai E, et al (2003) Laparoscopic gastric surgery in a Japanese institution: analysis of the initial 100 procedures. J Am Coll Surg 197:372–378
7. Kitano S, Iso Y, Moriyama M, et al (1994) Laparoscopy-assisted Billroth I gastrectomy. Surg Laparosc Endosc 4:146–148
8. Tanimura S, Higashino M, Fukunaga Y, et al (2001) Hand-assisted laparoscopic distal gastrectomy with regional lymph node dissection for gastric cancer. Surg Laparosc Endosc Percutan Tech 11:155–160
9. Asao T, Hosouchi Y, Nakabayashi T, et al (2001) Laparoscopically assisted total or distal gastrectomy with lymph node dissection for early gastric cancer. Br J Surg 88:128–132
10. Horiuchi T, Shimomatsuya T, Chiba Y (2001) Laparoscopically assisted pylorus-preserving gastrectomy. Surg Endosc 15:325–328
11. Avital S, Brasesco O, Szomstein S, et al (2003) Technical considerations in laparoscopic resection of gastric neoplasms. Surg Endosc 17:763–765
12. Sano T, Kobori O, Muto T (1992) Lymph node metastasis from early gastric cancer: endoscopic resection of tumour. Br J Surg 79:241–244
13. Yasuda K, Shiraishi N, Suematsu T, et al (1999) Rate of detection of lymph node metastasis is correlated with the depth of submucosal invasion in early stage gastric carcinoma. Cancer (Phila) 85:2119–2123
14. Yamao T, Shirao K, Ono H, et al (1996) Risk factors for lymph node metastasis from intramucosal gastric carcinoma. Cancer (Phila) 77:602–606
15. Nakajima T (2002) Gastric cancer treatment guidelines in Japan. Gastric Cancer 5:1–5
16. Sasako M, McCulloch P, Kinoshita T, et al (1995) New method to evaluate the therapeutic value of lymph node dissection for gastric cancer. Br J Surg 82:346–351
17. Bonenkamp JJ, Songun I, Hermans J, et al (1995) Randomised comparison of morbidity after D1 and D2 dissection for gastric cancer in 996 Dutch patients. Lancet 345:745–748
18. Cuschieri A, Fayers P, Fielding J, et al (1996) Postoperative morbidity and mortality after D1 and D2 resections for gastric cancer: preliminary results of the MRC randomised controlled surgical trial. The Surgical Cooperative Group. Lancet 347:995–999
19. Uyama I, Sugioka A, Matsui H, et al (2000) Laparoscopic D2 lymph node dissection for advanced gastric cancer located in the middle or lower third portion of the stomach. Gastric Cancer 3:50–55
20. Goh PM, Khan AZ, So JB, et al (2001) Early experience with laparoscopic radical gastrectomy for advanced gastric cancer. Surg Laparosc Endosc Percutan Tech 11:83–87
21. Japanese Gastric Cancer Association (1998) Japanese Classification of Gastric Carcinoma, 2nd English edn. Gastric Cancer 1:10–24
22. Ohgami M, Otani Y, Kumai K, et al (1999) Curative laparoscopic surgery for early gastric cancer: five years experience. World J Surg 23:187–192
23. Altorjay A, Szanto I, Garcia J, et al (1996) Endoscope-assisted laparoscopic resection of the gastric wall. Orv Hetil 137:2743–2745

24. Ohashi S (1995) Laparoscopic intraluminal (intragastric) surgery for early gastric cancer. A new concept in laparoscopic surgery. Surg Endosc 9:169–171
25. Ikeda Y, Sasaki Y, Niimi M, et al (2002) Hand-assisted laparoscopic proximal gastrectomy with jejunal interposition and lymphadenectomy. J Am Coll Surg 195:578–581
26. Mochiki E, Nakabayashi T, Kamimura H, et al (2002) Gastrointestinal recovery and outcome after laparoscopy-assisted versus conventional open distal gastrectomy for early gastric cancer. World J Surg 26:1145–1149
27. Tanimura S, Higashino M, Fukunaga Y, et al (2003) Laparoscopic gastrectomy with regional lymph node dissection for upper gastric cancer. Gastric Cancer 6:64–68
28. Kim YW, Han HS, Fleischer GD (2003) Hand-assisted laparoscopic total gastrectomy. Surg Laparosc Endosc Percutan Tech 13:26–30
29. Kitano S, Shiraishi N, Fujii K, et al (2002) A randomized controlled trial comparing open vs. laparoscopy-assisted distal gastrectomy for the treatment of early gastric cancer: an interim report. Surgery (St. Louis) 131:S306–S311
30. Adachi Y, Shiraishi N, Ikebe K, et al (2001) Evaluation of the cost for laparoscopy-assisted Billroth I gastrectomy. Surg Endosc 15:932–936
31. Rosin D, Brasesco O, Rosenthal RJ (2001) Laparoscopy for gastric tumors. Surg Oncol Clin N Am 10:511–529
32. Azagra JS, Goergen M, De Simone P, et al (1999) Minimally invasive surgery for gastric cancer. Surg Endosc 13:351–357
33. Huscher CG, Anastasi A, Crafa F, et al (2000) Laparoscopic gastric resections. Semin Laparosc Surg 7:26–54
34. Ballesta-Lopez C, Ruggiero R, Poves I, et al (2002) The contribution of laparoscopy to the treatment of gastric cancer. Surg Endosc 16:616–619
35. Kitano S, Shiraishi N, Kakisako K, et al (2002) Laparoscopy-assisted Billroth-I gastrectomy (LADG) for cancer: our 10 years' experience. Surg Laparosc Endosc Percutan Tech 12: 204–207
36. Kitano S, Bandoh T, Kawano K (2001) Endoscopic surgery in Japan. Minim Invasive Ther Allied Technol 12:215–219
37. Franklin ME, Kazantsev GB, Abrego D, et al (2000) Laparoscopic surgery for stage III colon cancer: long-term follow-up. Surg Endosc 14:612–616
38. Lujan HJ, Plasencia G, Jacobs M, et al (2002) Long-term survival after laparoscopic colon resection for cancer: complete five-year follow-up. Dis Colon Rectum 45:491–501
39. Lacy AM, Garcia-Valdecasas JC, Delgado S, et al (2002) Laparoscopy-assisted colectomy versus open colectomy for treatment of non-metastatic colon cancer: a randomised trial. Lancet 359:2224–2229

Color Plates

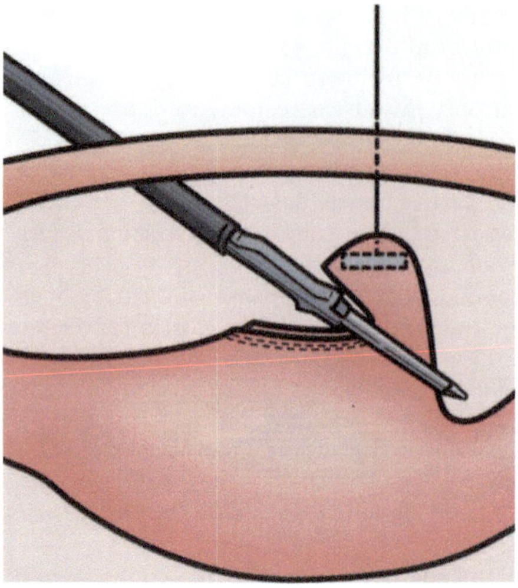

Fig. 1. Local wedge resection (LWR) by the lesion-lifting method

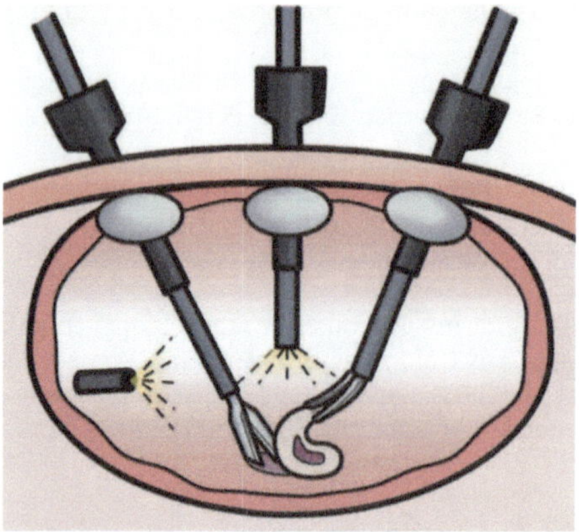

Fig. 2. Intragastric mucosal resection (IGMR)

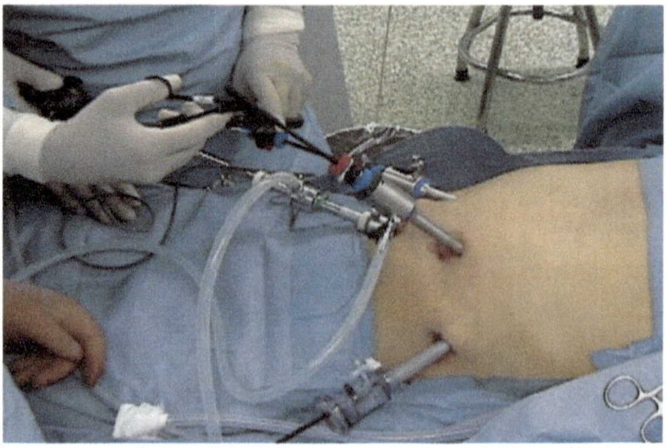

Fig. 3. Placement of four cannulas

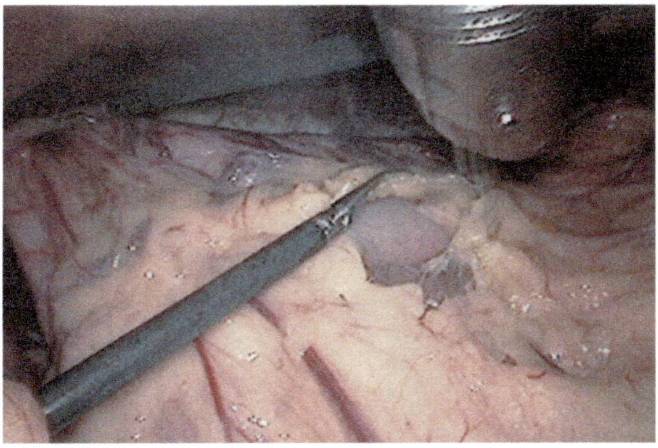

FIG. 4. Dissection of the greater omentum and gastrocolic ligament outside the epigastric arcade

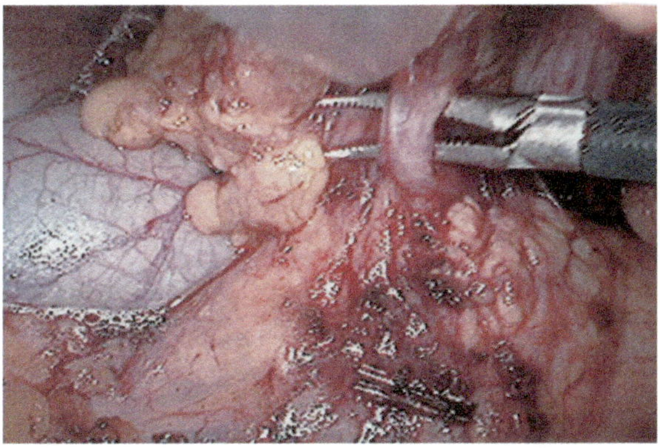

FIG. 5. Cutting the right gastroepiploic vessels

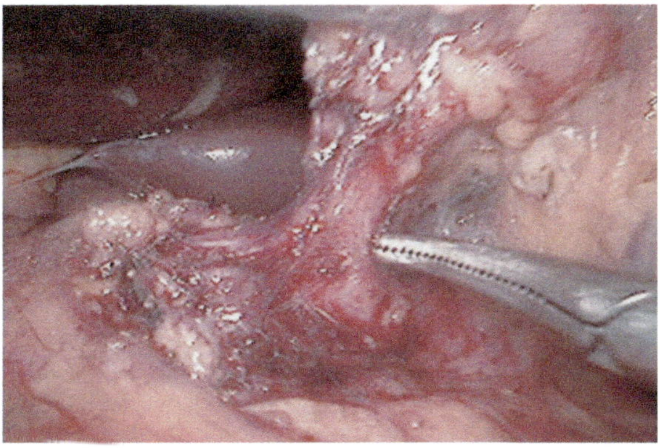

FIG. 6. Cutting the left gastric vessels

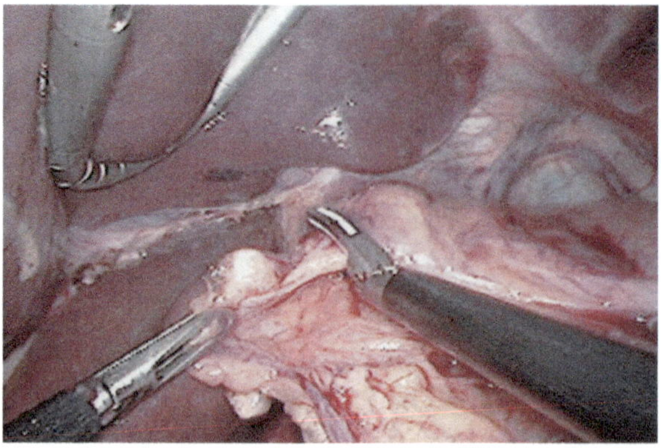

Fig. 7. Dissection of the left cardiac and superior gastric lymph nodes

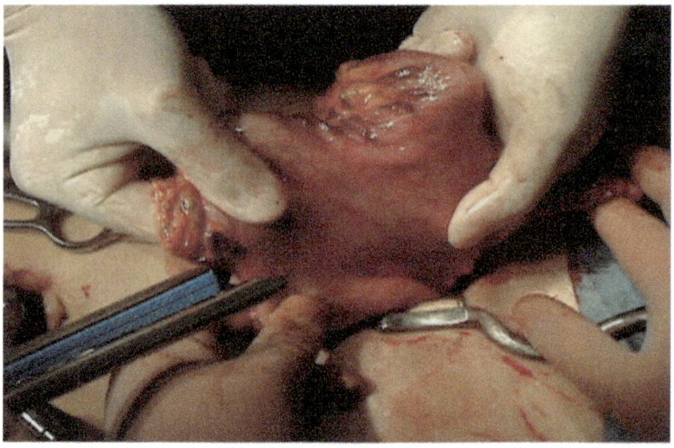

Fig. 8. Resection of the distal two-thirds of the stomach through a minilaparotomy wound

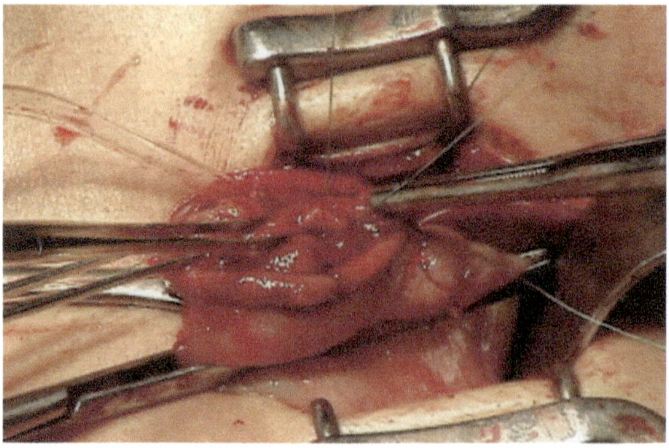

Fig. 9. Anastomosis by Billroth I method

Chemotherapy for Advanced Unresectable Gastric Cancer

Atsushi Ohtsu

Introduction

Gastric cancer is a major health problem in many regions of the world. Despite remarkable improvement in survival as a result of early detection and curative surgery, approximately 50 000 deaths were observed in Japan in 2001 [1]. Unresectable advanced or recurrent gastric cancer still has a poor prognosis, with a median survival of less than 9 months. Randomized trials have demonstrated that the 5-fluorouracil (5-FU)-based regimen provides superior survival and quality of life in patients with advanced gastric cancer when compared to best supportive care [2–4]. However, this survival advantage appears to be marginal, and no standard regimens worldwide have yet been established, although various challenges have been conducted.

Recently developed new agents, such as irinotecan, S-1, and taxanes, may have potential to break through this status. Newer-generation regimens with these agents are being investigated in randomized trials worldwide. A molecular targeting agent is another new topic in the field of chemotherapy and is also under development for gastric cancer. This review focuses on the results of newer-generation regimens, particularly in Japan, after a brief summary of older-generation regimens.

Overview of the Older-Generation Regimens

Results from Randomized Controlled Trials

During the past two decades, various randomized trials (Table 1) have been carried out. In Europe, a combination of flurorouracil, doxorubicin, and high-dose methotrexate (FAMTX) used to be a standard regimen based on the European Organization for Research and Treatment of Cancer (EORTC) trials [5]. However, this regimen failed to demonstrate any superiority to other combination regimens, 5-FU plus cisplatin or etoposide plus 5-FU/leucovorin, in the subsequent EORTC randomized study [6].

Division of Gastrointestinal Oncology/Digestive Endoscopy, National Cancer Center Hospital East, 6-5-1 Kashiwanoha, Kashiwa, Chiba 277-8577, Japan
e-mail: aohtsu@east.ncc.go.jp

TABLE 1. Results of randomized trials using older-generation regimens

Study	Treatment	No. of patients	Response rate (%)	Median survival (months)	*P* value
Wils et al.	5-FU + ADM + MMC	103	7	6.7	0.004
(1991) [5]	5-FU + ADM + MTX	105	33	9.6	
Kim et al.	5-FU	94	26	6.9	ns
(1993) [9]	5-FU + ADM + MMC	98	25	6.6	
	5-FU + CDDP	103	51	8.5	
Webb et al.	5-FU + ADM + MTX	130	21	5.7	0.0009
(1997) [7]	Epirubicin + CDDP + 5-FU	126	45	8.9	
Vanhoefer et al.	5-FU + CDDP	134	20	7.2	ns
(2000) [6]	Etoposide + LV/5-FU	132	9	7.2	
	5-FU + ADM + MTX	133	12	6.7	
Ohtsu et al.	5-FU	106	11	7.1	ns
(2003) [10]	5-FU + CDDP	104	34	7.3	
	UFT + MMC	70	9	6.0	

5-FU, 5-fluorouracil; ADM, adriamycin; MMC, mitomycin C; MTX, methotrexate; CDDP, cisplatin; LV, leucovorin; UFT, ftorafur and uracil

Another randomized study in the United Kingdom revealed the superiority of a combination of epirubicin, cisplatin (CDDP), and 5-FU (ECF) to FAMTX in terms of survival [7], although survival results of these studies were limited, with a median survival time (MST) ranging from 6 to 8 months. Other trials including 5-FU alone as a control arm and in comparision with FU-based regimens also failed to demonstrate survival prolongation of combination regimens [8,9].

The Japan Clinical Oncology Group (JCOG) has carried out a randomized controlled trial comparing 5-FU alone with UFT (ftorafur and uraeil) + mitomycin C (UFTM) and with 5-FU + CDDP (FP) for advanced gastric cancer (JCOG 9205) [10]. A total of 280 patients with advanced gastric cancer were randomly allocated and analyzed for survival, response, and toxicity. At the interim analysis, the UFTM arm showed a significantly inferior survival with higher incidences of hematological toxicities than control arm 5-FU alone, and the registration to UFTM was terminated. Both investigational regimens, FP and UFTM, had a significantly higher incidence of hematological toxicities than 5-FU alone, although they were feasible. The overall response rates of 5-FU alone, FP, and UFTM arms were 11%, 34%, and 9%, respectively. The median progression-free survival was 1.9 months with 5-FU alone, 3.9 months with FP, and 2.4 months with UFTM, respectively. Although FP demonstrated a higher response rate ($P < 0.001$) and longer progression-free survival than 5-FU alone ($P < 0.001$), no differences in overall survival were observed between the arms; the median survival times and 1-year survival rates were 7.1 months and 28% with 5-FU, 7.3 months and 29% with FP, and 6.0 months and 16% with UFTM, respectively. This study concluded that both investigational regimens, FP and UFTM, showed no survival advantages as compared to 5-FU alone, and 5-FU alone still remains a reference arm in future trials for advanced gastric cancer.

Based on the results of these randomized trials, no regimens have exceeded 5-FU alone, and there still remain limitations on efficacy results in older-generation regimens: the results ranged from 10% to 35% in response rate, from 6 to 8 months in MST, and around 10% in 2-year survival.

Results in Patients with Peritoneal Metastasis

Peritoneal metastasis is the major site developing from gastric cancer. However, these patients usually have poor general condition, impairment of oral intake, and complications such as bowel obstruction and hydronephrosis, which may prolong elimination of the agents. These patients with peritoneal dissemination are excluded from the phase II study because these studies usually require response evaluation as a primary endpoint whereas these patients usually have no measurable lesions. Thus, a specifically targeted study should be conducted. A phase II study of sequential combination of methotrexate (MTX) plus 5-FU (JCOG 9603) has been carried out in patients with malignant ascites [11]. A total of 37 patients were registered: remarkable decreases of ascites were observed in 13 (35%) patients, including 4 (11%) with disappearance of ascites, whereas 2 (5%) patients died of treatment-related toxicity. Results from retrospective analysis also showed similar efficacy for this population. Based on the results, a phase III study comparing 5-FU alone with MTX/5-FU (JCOG 0106) in patients with peritoneal dissemination has been initiated in the JCOG.

Results in Patients with Bone Metastasis

Bone metastasis is a rare mode of cancer metastasis in patients with gastric cancer. However, if it occurs, it is usually associated with diffuse involvement and occasionally complicated with disseminated intravascular coagulation (DIC). Thus, the prognosis is very dismal. For such cases, we attempted palliative chemotherapy with sequential MTX/5-FU and have reported a retrospective analysis of 18 gastric cancer patients with bone metastasis who underwent this treatment [12]. Of the 18, 9 patients (50%) had the complication of DIC before initiation of chemotherapy, and 8 of them (89%) recovered from it. The median survival times for all patients and for the 9 with DIC were 186 and 113 days, respectively, and 2 patients (11%) survived longer than 1 year. Although grade 4 leukopenia was observed in 3 patients (17%), no treatment-related deaths occurred. Based on these results, this combination therapy may have palliative potential and be a feasible treatment for gastric cancer patients with bone metastasis, with or without DIC.

Multivariate Analysis for Prognosis and Long-Term Results

Between 1985 and 1997, a total of 497 patients with advanced gastric cancer were enrolled onto four phase II studies and one phase III study in the Japan Clinical Oncology Group. Univariate and multivariate analysis for prognosis were carried out by log-rank test and by Cox's proportional hazard model, respectively [13]. Baseline patient background was median age of 61 years; 176, 238, and 86 patients with PS 0, 1, and 2, respectively; 84 patients with prior gastrectomy; and 315, 148, and 34 patients with one, two, or more metastatic sites, respectively. Thirty-nine (8%) and 11(2%) patients have survived longer than 2 and 5 years. Univariate analysis revealed that the 315 patients with a single metastatic site have survived longer than the remaining 182 patients ($P < 0.01$), and the 77 patients with only abdominal lymph node involvement

TABLE 2. Univariate and multivariate analysis for prognosis by each variable

		Univariate analysis			Multivariate analysis	
Variable	*n*	MST (months)	2-year Survival (%)	*P* value	Relative risk	95% CI
Age						
<60 years	219	7.8	10.5	0.04	—	
>60 years	278	6.8	5.8		1.16	0.97–1.40
Sex						
Male	364	7.2	8.2	0.9	—	
Female	133	7.2	6.8		0.93	0.75–1.14
PS						
0	175	9.9	11.0	<0.01	—	
1	236	6.8	8.5		1.16	1.08–1.25
2	86	5.1	0			
Histological types						
Intestinal	228	7.8	9.2	0.3	—	
Diffuse	266	6.5	6.8		1.13	0.97–1.30
Macroscopic types						
Scirrhous	137	6	4.4	0.04	—	
Nonscirrhous	360	7.6	9.2		1.27	1.02–1.25
History of gastrectomy						
Yes	84	8.3	14.3	0.02	—	
No	413	6.8	6.5		1.01	0.92–1.10
No. of metastatic sites						
1	315	8.3	9.5	<0.01	—	
2	148	5.9	5.4		1.32	1.14–1.53
≥3	34	5.4	2.9			

Multivariate analysis includes all the variables listed in the table
MST, mean survival time; CI, confidence interval; PS, performance status

have also survived longer than 117 patients with only liver metastasis ($P = 0.03$). In the multivariate analysis, better PS, small number of metastatic sites, and macroscopically nonscirrhous type were significantly associated with better prognosis (Table 2).

Characteristics of the 11 five-year survivors are summarized in Table 3. The 11 patients consisted of 8 with paraaortic node metastases alone as an "unresectable factor," 1 with paraaortic and cervical node metastases, and the remaining 2 patients with only liver metastasis. Ten of the 11 patients achieved overall responses to the initial chemotherapy: 5 patients achieved complete response (CR) at the initial chemotherapy, and 1 patient achieved CR by the second-line chemotherapy. One patient, who had not achieved an objective response to the initial chemotherapy (FP), achieved CR in the third-line chemotherapy, consisting of 5-fluorouracil + doxorubicin + mitomycin C. Of the 11, 8 patients have received surgical resections: 4 patients had undergone gastrectomy before initiating the chemotherapy and the other 4 patients underwent surgical resection after achieving downstaging by the initial chemotherapy, including 2 with pathological CR in the surgically resected specimen. The remaining 3 patients have not received surgical resection during the follow-up

TABLE 3. Characteristics of 11 five-year survivors

Age	Sex	PS	Macroscopy	Histology	Metastatic site	Gastrectomy	Initial regimen	Response, 1st/2nd	Survival (months)	Alive/dead
75	M	0	N	Diffuse	Liver	—	5Fuci	CR/–	60	D
65	M	0	N	Intestinal	Abdominal LN	B	5Fuci	PR/PR	61	A
46	M	0	N	Diffuse	Abdominal LN	B	5Fuci	PR/–	63	A
55	M	1	N	Intestinal	Liver	—	UFTM	PR/CR	65	A
47	M	0	N	Intestinal	Abdominal LN	B	FP	CR/–	85	A
52	M	1	N	Intestinal	Abdominal LN	—	5′FP	CR/–	86	D
57	M	1	N	Diffuse	Abdominal LN	A	EAP	PR/–	87	D
53	M	0	N	Diffuse	Abdominal LN	A	EAP	CR/–	88	A
49	F	0	N	Diffuse	Abdominal LN	B	FP	NC/CR	90	A
58	M	0	N	Intestinal	Abdominal and Cervical LN	A	EAP	CR/–	103	A
62	M	1	N	Intestinal	Abdominal LN	A	5′FP	PR/–	108	A

N, nonscirrhous type; LN, lymph node; A, after initial chemotherapy; B, before initial chemotherapy; UFTM, UFT+MMC; FP, 5-FU+CDDP; 5′FP, 5′FUDR+CDDP; EAP, etoposide+ADM+CDDP; CR, complete response; PR, partial response

period. Ten of the 11 5-year survivors presented no evidence of disease at 5 years, whereas 2 patients died after 5 years of recurrence of primary disease.

These results indicated that better PS, small number of metastatic sites, and macroscopically nonscirrhous type are independent favorable factors for survival. There was a small population of long-term survivors, particularly in patients with only paraaortic node metastasis as the "unresectable factor."

New-Generation Regimens

Single-Agent and Combination Studies in Japan

Recently, four promising agents, irinotecan (CPT-11), S-1, docetaxel, and paclitaxel, have become commercially available for treatment of gastric cancer in Japan. Results from single-agent registration studies for approval and their combinations are shown in Table 4.

CPT-11 is an inhibitor of DNA-topoisomerase I, which is a crucial enzyme involved in DNA replication and transcription. In the single-agent study, moderate activity of this agent was confirmed with a response rate of approximately 20% [14]. This agent was then investigated in combination with CDDP [15,16]. A phase II study of this combination achieved high response rate of 48% with MST of 9 months in all patients and of 59% with MST of 11 months in chemo-naive patients. The major toxicities were neutropenia and diarrhea: grade 4 neutropenia was observed in 57% and grade 3 or 4 diarrhea in 20% of the patients. This agent was then combined with MMC; the phase I/II study of this combination revealed similar efficacy results and less toxicity than the CPT-11 + CDDP regimen [17]. This regimen was evaluated in the phase II study as a second-line setting after failure of FU-based regimens [18]. Of the 45 patients registered, 13 patients achieved partial response (PR) with a response rate of 29%. Median progression-free survival was 4 months. Toxicities were moderate; grade 4 neutropenia was observed in 29% and grade 3 anorexia in 24% of the patients. This study concluded that this regimen could be a treatment option in patients resistant to FU-based regimen.

S-1 is a new oral fluoropyrimidine that consists of three components: tegafur; which is a prodrug of 5-FU, CDHP, which competes with dihydropyrimidine dehydrogenase, and oxonic acid, which suppresses the gastrointestinal toxicity of tegafur. This agent is highly active with a response rate of 45% (45/101) in the two registration phase II studies and is widely used in Japan [19,20]. Various attempts in combination with other agents such as CDDP, CPT-11, and taxanes have been conducted. First, this agent

TABLE 4. Results of the single-agent study in Japan

Agents	No. of patients	Response rate	MST (months)
CPT-11	76 (20)	18% (25%)	NS (NS)
S-1	101 (101)	45% (45%)	8.3 (8.3)
Docetaxel	129 (51)	17% (18%)	7.5 (NS)
Paclitaxel	60 (28)	23% (21%)	11.5 (11.4)

Numbers in parentheses are results in chemonaive patients
CPT-11, irinotecan; NS, not stated

was combined with CDDP. This combination phase I/II study was scheduled as S-1 40 mg/m^2 twice daily for consecutive 21 days and 2-h infusion of CDDP at 60–70 mg/m^2 on day 8, which was repeated every 5 weeks [21]. This study revealed an excellent response rate of 76% with MST of 12.6 months. Toxicities were moderate but easily manageable; grade 3 or 4 hematological and nonhematological toxicities were 15.8% and 26.3%, respectively. Another combination, S-1 + CPT-11, is also promising. A phase I/II study of this combination revealed similar response rates of around 50% with a MST of 14 months [22].

The taxanes docetaxel and paclitaxel inhibit microtubule depolymerization and have moderate activity for gastric cancer with a response rate of around 20% in their single-agent studies [23–26]. Taxanes also have promising activity as a second-line treatment, and their combinations are now being investigated as a frontline treatment. The Swiss Group for Clinical Cancer Research has reported a phase II study of docetaxel 85 mg/m^2 with CDDP 75 mg/m^2 administered once every 3 weeks for advanced gastric cancer and observed a response rate of 52% and median time to progression of 6.6 months [27].

Randomized Controlled Trials Including Newer-Generation Regimens

There are three randomized trials under investigation including the above new-generation regimens in Japan. In JCOG, three-arm randomizations were designed. This study (JCOG 9912) compares 5-FU alone, as a control arm based on the results from the previous study (JCOG 9205), with a combination of CPT-11 + CDDP and with S-1 alone. This study requires a sample size of 450, and final accrual will be completed in 2005. The second study is a randomized trial comparing S-1 alone with S-1 + CDDP (sponsored by Taiho) with a sample size of 300, and the third study (sponsored by Wyeth) is comparing S-1 alone with 5-FU/leucovorin with a sample size of 200. Final results of the JCOG 9912 and the Taiho study will appear in 2006–2007.

An international randomized controlled trial (V-325) comparing CDDP + 5-FU (CF) with docetaxel + CDDP + 5-FU (DCF) was conducted outside of Japan, and the interim results were reported at the Annual Meeting of the American Society of Clinical Oncology in 2003 [28]. The doses and schedule of the DCF arm were docetaxel 75 mg/m^2 on day 1, CDDP 75 mg/m^2 on day 1, and 5-FU 750 mg/m^2/day as continuous infusion on days 1–5, repeated every 3 weeks; the dose and schedule of CF arm were CDDP 100 mg/m^2 on day 1 and 5-FU 1000 mg/m^2/day as continuous infusion on days 1–5 given every 4 weeks. At the interim analysis on 232 patients, time to progression was superior ($P = 0.0008$) for DCF (5.2 months compared to 3.7 months for CF). MST was also longer for patients receiving DCF (10.2 months) than those receiving CF (8.5 months, $P = 0.0064$). Neutropenic fever, infections, diarrhea, and mucositis were also higher for DCF than CF. These results indicated the superiority of DCF to CF for advanced gastric cancer.

To date, the interpretation of V-325 study results appears to be controversial. Although this study confirmed the superiority of DCF compared to CF in terms of efficacy, MST of the DCF arm was 10.2 months, which does not seem to be a definite improvement. The latest combination studies in Japan, although the numbers of the patients were small, yielded 12 months or longer MST (Table 5). According to the ret-

TABLE 5. Treatment results of newer-generation regimens in Japan and V325 study

Regimen	Phase	No. of patients	Response rate	MST (months)
CPT-11 + CDDP	II	44 (29)	48% (59%)	9.0 (10.8)
CPT-11 + MMC	I/II	30 (16)	50% (63%)	8.5 (NS)
S-1 + CDDP	I/II	25 (25)	75% (76%)	12.5 (12.5%)
S-1 + CPT-11	I/II	40 (40)	55% (55%)	14.0 (14.0)
Docetaxel + CDDP + 5-FU (V325 study)s	III	111 (111)	39% (39%)	10.2 (10.2)

Number in parentheses are results in chemonaive patients; NS, not stated

rospective analysis of National Cancer Center Hospital East, the MST of 111 patients treated with chemotherapy for advanced unresectable gastric cancer in daily practice was improved to 11 months after application of the newer-generation regimens. Whether the superiority of DCF can be accepted should await obtaining the results of ongoing randomized trials in Japan.

Molecular Targeting Agents Under Investigation

Recently developed molecular targeting agents may provide a significant impact in this field, as successful results of bevacizumab and cetuximab have been observed in colorectal cancer [29,30].

Gefitinib is an orally active epidermal growth factor receptor tyrosine kinase inhibitor (EGFR-TKI) that has shown single-agent activity against non-small cell lung cancer. A Japan–Europe joint phase II study was conducted to investigate the efficacy, tolerability, and pharmacokinetics of gefitinib in patients with metastatic gastric adenocarcinoma [31]. Seventy-five patients (32 Japanese, 43 non-Japanese) were randomized to receive 250 mg/day or 500 mg/day gefitinib orally. Disease control was achieved in 13 patients: 1 (250 mg/day) had a partial response and 12 had stable disease (4 at 250 mg/day, 8 at 500 mg/day), with a disease control rate of 18%. The most common drug-related adverse events were diarrhea (45.9%), rash (35.1%), and anorexia (12.2%). Drug-related grade 3/4 adverse events were experienced by 11.1% and 23.7% of patients given 250 mg/day and 500 mg/day gefitinib, respectively. Gefitinib exposure appeared to be unaffected by ethnicity or previous gastric surgery. Furthermore, there was no marked difference in plasma concentration in patients with disease control (partial response plus stable disease) versus progressive disease. In conclusion, gefitinib monotherapy was generally well tolerated, but its activity seemed to be limited.

Investigations of two other molecular targeting agents are now being planned. EMD72000 is a 95% humanized monoclonal antibody against EGFR that showed promising activity for colorectal adenocarcinoma in the phase I study [32]. This agent has less toxicity, particularly in allergic reaction and skin rash, than cetuximub, which is a chimeric antibody against EGFR. The single-agent phase II study is going to begin in patients with EGFR-positive gastric tumors. Another planned agent is trastuzumab, a monoclonal antibody to Her2 protein, which is widely used in patients with Her2-overexpressing breast cancer. We have evaluated the frequency of Her2 overexpression and the concordance between protein expression and gene amplification in 200 surgical and endoscopic biopsy specimens using two commercial immunohistochemical (IHC) kits and fluorescence in situ hybridization (FISH) [33]. Among these 200 cases, 46 (23%) of the patients were found to exhibit Her2 protein overexpression. The following IHC scores were obtained: 0, 126 (63%); 1+, 28 (14%); 2+, 12 (6%); and 3+, 34 (17%). Gene amplification examined with FISH was observed in 54 cases (27.1%). Among the 200 biopsy specimens, Her2 protein overexpression was observed in 21.5% of the specimens (2+, 7.5%, and 3+, 14%). The concordance rate between the surgically resected materials and the biopsy specimens was 88.7%. From these background results, trastuzumab can be applied for clinical trial in patients with Her 2 overexpressed gastric cancer.

Conclusions

Older-generation regimens against advanced gastric cancer have limited efficacy. No standard regimens worldwide, as well as in Japan, have been established yet, and a limited number of patients have achieved objective response and long-term survival. However, some of the new-generation regimens improved response rate more than 50% and suggested survival prolongation in the preliminary studies. These treatments are being investigated in ongoing randomized studies in Japan, and we should wait for the results to confirm these improvements. Recent development of molecular technology has produced various types of molecular targeting agents. These agents are the other new hopes for improving efficacy results with less toxicity than classic cytotoxic agents. Understanding the biology of gastric cancer may result in better targets or cellular pathways to be modified or blocked by therapeutic interventions. Additionally, improvement of the clinical trial design and molecular surrogate in clinical research will lead to the development of better treatments. Both clinical and biology research will be more important.

References

1. "Cancer Statistics in Japan" Editorial Board (2003) Cancer statistics in Japan. Foundation for Promotion of Cancer Research, Tokyo
2. Murad AM, Santiago FF, Petroianu A, et al (1993) Modified therapy with 5-fluorouracil, doxorubicin, and methotrexate in advanced gastric cancer. Cancer (Phila) 72:37–41
3. Glimelius B, Hotfmann K, Haglund U, et al (1994) Initial or delayed chemotherapy with best supportive care in advanced gastric cancer. Ann Oncol 5:189–190
4. Pyrhonen S, Kuitumen T, Nyandoto P, et al (1995) Randomized comparison of fluorouracil, epidoxorubicin and methotrexate (FEMTX) plus best supportive care alone in patients with non-resectable gastric cancer. Br J Cancer 71:587–591
5. Wils JA, Klein HO, Wagener JT, et al (1991) Sequential high-dose methotrexate and fluorouracil combined with doxorubicin: a step ahead in the treatment of advanced gastric cancer: a trial of the European Organization for Research and Treatment of Cancer Gastrointestinal Tract Cooperative Group. J Clin Oncol 9:827–831
6. Vanhoefer U, Rouger P, Wilke H, et al (2000) Final result of a randomized phase III trial of sequential high-dose methotrexate, fluorouracil, and doxorubicin, versus etoposide, leucovorin, and fluorouracil versus infusional fluorouracil and cisplatin in advanced gastric cancer: a trial of the European Organization for Research and Treatment of Cancer Gastrointestinal Tract Cooperative Group. J Clin Oncol 81:2648–2657

7. Webb A, Cunningham D, Scarffe H, et al (1997) Randomized trial comparing epirubicin, cisplatin and fluorouracil, versus fluorouracil, doxorubicin, and methotrexate in advanced esophagogastric cancer. J Clin Oncol 15:261–267
8. Cullinan SA, Moertel CG, Wieland HS, et al (1994) Controlled evaluation of three drug combination regimens versus fluorouracil alone for the therapy of advanced gastric cancer. J Clin Oncol 12:412–416
9. Kim NK, Park YS, Heo DS, et al (1993) A phase III randomized study of 5-fluorouracil and cisplatin versus 5-fluorouracil, doxorubicin, and mitomycin C versus 5-fluorouracil alone in the treatment of advanced gastric cancer. Cancer (Phila) 71:3813–3818
10. Ohtsu A, Shimada Y, Shirao K, et al (2003) Randomized phase III trial of 5-fluorouracil alone versus 5-fluorouracil plus cisplatin versus uracil and tegafur plus mitomycin C in patients with unresectable advanced gastric cancer: the Japan Clinical Oncology Group Study (JCOG 9205). J Clin Oncol 21:54–59
11. Yamao T, Shirao K, Shimada Y, et al (2004) Phase II study of sequential methotrexate and 5-fluorouracil for advanced gastric cancer with malignant ascites. Jpn J Clin Oncol 34:316–322
12. Hironaka S, Boku N, Ohtsu A, et al (2000) Sequential methotrexate and 5-fluorouracil therapy for gastric cancer patients with bone metastasis. Gastric Cancer 3:19–23
13. Yoshida M, Ohtsu A, Boku N, et al (2004) Long-term Survival and Prognostic Factors in Patients with Metastatic Gastric Cancer Treated with Chemotherapy in the Japan Clinical Oncology Group (JCOG) Study. Jpn J Clin Oncol 34:654–659
14. Kambe M, Wakui A, Nakano I, et al (1993) A late phase II study of irinotecan (CPT-11) in patients with advanced gastric cancer. Proc Am Soc Clin Oncol 12:198
15. Shirao K, Shimada Y, Kondo H, et al (1997) Phase I-II study of irinotecan hydrochloride combined with cisplatin in patients with advanced gastric cancer. J Clin Oncol 15:921–927
16. Boku N, Ohtsu A, Shimada Y, et al (1999) Phase II study of a combination of irinotecan and cisplatin against metastatic gastric cancer. J Clin Oncol 17:319–323
17. Yamao T, Shirao K, Matsumura Y, et al (2001) Phase I-II study of irinotecan combined with mitomycin C in patients with advanced gastric cancer. Ann Oncol 12:1729–1735
18. Hamaguchi T, Ohtsu A, Hyodo I, et al (2004) A phase II study of irinotecan and mitomycin C combination therapy in patients with fluoropyrimidine-resistant advanced gastric cancer: The Japan Clinical Oncology Group trial (JCOG 0109). Proc Am Soc Clin Oncol 23:330
19. Sakata Y, Ohtsu A, Horikoshi N, et al (1998) Late phase II study of novel oral fluoropyrimidine anticancer drug S-1 (1 M tegafur-0.4 M gimestat 1 M otastat potassium) in advanced gastric cancer patients. Eur J Cancer 34:1715–1720
20. Koizumi W, Kurihara M, Nakano S, et al (2000) Phase II study of S-1, a novel oral derivative of fluorouracil, in advanced gastric cancer. Oncology 58:191–197
21. Koizumi W, Tanabe S, Saigenji K, et al (2003) A phase I-II study of S-1 combined with cisplatin in patients with advanced gastric cancer. Br J Cancer 89:2207–2212
22. Narahara H, Takiuchi H, Tsujinaka T, et al (2002) Phase I study of CPT-11 plus S-1 in patients with metastatic gastric cancer. Proc Am Soc Clin Oncol 21:170
23. Taguchi T, Sakata Y, Kanamaru R, et al (1998) Late phase II study of RP56976 (docetaxel) in patients with advanced/recurrent gastric cancer: a Japanese Co-operative Study Group trial (group A). Jpn J Cancer Chemother 25:1915–1924
24. Mai M, Sakata Y, Kanamaru R, et al (1998) Late phase II study of RP56976 (docetaxel) in patients with advanced/recurrent gastric cancer: a Japanese Co-operative Study Group trial (group B). Jpn J Cancer Chemother 25:1933–1937
25. Ohtsu A, Boku N, Tamura F, et al (1998) An early phase II study of three-hour infusional paclitaxel for advanced gastric cancer. Am J Clin Oncol 21:416–419
26. Yamada Y, Shirao K, Ohtsu A, et al (2001) Phase II trial of paclitaxel by three-hour infusion for advanced gastric cancer with short premedication for prophylaxis against paclitaxel-associated hypersensitivity reactions. Ann Oncol 12:1133–1137
27. Roth AD, Maibach R, Martinelli G, et al (2000) Docetaxel (taxotere)-cisplatin (TC): an effective drug combination in gastric carcinoma. Ann Oncol 11:301–306

28. Ajani JA, Van Cutsem E, Moiseyenko V, et al (2003) Docetaxel (D) cisplatin, 5-fluorouracil compare to cisplatin (C) and 5-fluorouracil (F) for chemotherapy-naive patients with metastatic or locally recurrent unresectable gastric carcinoma (MGC): interim results of a randomized phase III trial (V325). Proc Am Soc Clin Oncol 22:249
29. Hurwitz H, Fehrenbacher L, Novotny W, et al (2004) Bevacitumab plus irinotecan, fluorouracil, and leucovorin for metastatic colorectal cancer. N Engl J Med 350:2235–2242
30. Cunningham D, Humblet Y, Siena S, et al (2003) Cetuximab (C225) alone or in combination with irinotecan (CPT-11) in patients with epidermal growth factor receptor (EGFR)-positive irinotecan-refractory metastatic colorectal cancer (MCRC). Proc Am Soc Cin Oncol 22:252
31. Doi T, Koizumi W, Siena S, et al (2003) Efficacy, tolerability and pharmacokinetics of gefitinib (ZD1839) in pretreated patients with metastatic gastric cancer. Proc Am Soc Clin Oncol 22:258
32. Vanhoefer U, Tewes M, Rojo F, et al (2004) Phase I study of the humanized antiepidermal growth factor receptor monoclonal antibody EMD72000 in patients with advanced solid tumors that express the epidermal growth factor receptor. J Clin Oncol 22:175–184
33. Yano T, Ochiai A, Doi T, et al (2004) Expression of Her 2 in gastric cancer: comparison between protein expression and gene amplification using a new commercial kit. Proc Am Soc Clin Oncol 23:325

Adjuvant or Neoadjuvant Chemotherapy Against Advanced Gastric Carcinoma

Kenji Omura

Introduction

Gastric carcinoma is one of the most common malignancies in the world. Furthermore, the cure rate of gastric carcinoma with surgery is not satisfactory, at 20%–30% in Western countries and 60% in Japan. For developing countries, the curability of gastric carcinoma is far lower. There exist two ways to improve the outcome of gastric carcinoma treatment other than improving surgical procedures. One is to locate the lesion and make the diagnosis of gastric carcinoma when it is still in an early stage. For a tumor with invasion limited within the mucosal layer, diagnosed as a differentiated carcinoma, and a diameter within 2 cm, it can be cured even by endoscopic mucosal resection (EMR). For cases when the invasion depth has reached the submucosal layer, the patient should undergo gastrectomy, resulting in an expected 5-year survival rate of 90%. However, it is difficult to make the diagnosis of gastric carcinoma in the early stages in many countries. Almost all patients with early gastric carcinoma have no complaints. Consequently, it is necessary to perform studies on a large number of people with no complaints to find an early gastric carcinoma, and this is quite cost-ineffective.

Another way to improve the prognosis of gastric carcinoma is to kill the carcinoma cells with anticancer drugs. In the past two decades, several anticancer drugs have been found to have considerable cytotoxic effects against gastric carcinoma and thus have been introduced in clinical settings. In this chapter, anticancer drugs used for adjuvant chemotherapy are presented with specific emphasis on their cytotoxic mechanisms. Efforts to determime valuable regimens for neoadjuvant chemotherapy against advanced gastric carcinoma with noncurative factor(s) are also described, and evidence is also presented regarding the efficacy of adjuvant chemotherapy after curative surgery for advanced gastric carcinoma.

General and Cardiovascular Surgery, Kanazawa University School of Medicine, 13-1 Takaramachi, Kanazawa 920-8641, Japan
e-mail: omura@med.kanazawa-u.ac.jp

Drugs Used for Adjuvant or Neoadjuvant Chemotherapy Against Advanced Gastric Carcinoma

5-Fluorouracil

5-Fluorouracil (5-FU) is the most frequently prescribed anticancer drug for the treatment of gastric carcinoma. The metabolic pathway and the mechanism responsible for the cytocidal effect of 5-FU have been almost fully elucidated. 5-FU is converted to an active form, 5-fluorodeoxyuridine monophosphate (FdUMP), after glucosylation (Fig. 1). 5-FU is glucosylated through three pathways. Each pathway is catalyzed by orotate phosphoribosyltransferase (OPRT [EC 2.4.2.10]) (pathway 1), uridine phosphorylase [EC 2.4.2.3] (pathway 2), or thymidine phosphorylase [EC 2.4.2.4] (pathway 3) (Fig. 2). Among these, the one catalyzed by OPRT is considered to be the main pathway. Dihydropyrimidine dehydrogenase (DPD [EC 1.3.1.2]) acts as a rate-limiting enzyme in the degradation pathway of 5-FU (Fig. 3). Thymidylate synthase (TS [EC 2.1.1.45]) is a rate-limiting enzyme associated with de novo synthesis of pyrimidine nucleotides and is also the target enzyme of 5-FU. Inhibition of TS by 5-FU is accomplished by occupying its active site with FdUMP and methylenetetrahydrofolate (CH_2H_4PteGlu) (Fig. 4) to form an inactive ternary complex (TC) (Fig. 5). Theoretically, 1 mole of FdUMP and CH_2H_4PteGlu is necessary to inhibit 1 mole of TS when occupying its active site. The rate of thymidylate synthase inhibition (TSIR) for gastric carcinoma tissue extraction in the presence of sufficient FdUMP decreases as TS expression increases (Fig. 6) [1].

CH_2H_4PteGlu deficiency should occur in rapid-growth tissue because it is consumed during the synthesis of pyrimidine nucleotide. CH_2H_4PteGlu is necessary not

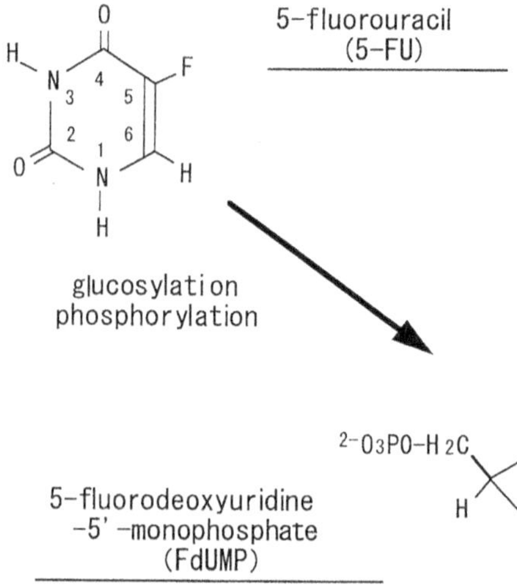

Fig. 1. Structural formulas of *5-fluorouracil* (*5-FU*) and its active form, 5-fluorodeoxyuridine-5′-monophosphate (FdUMP)

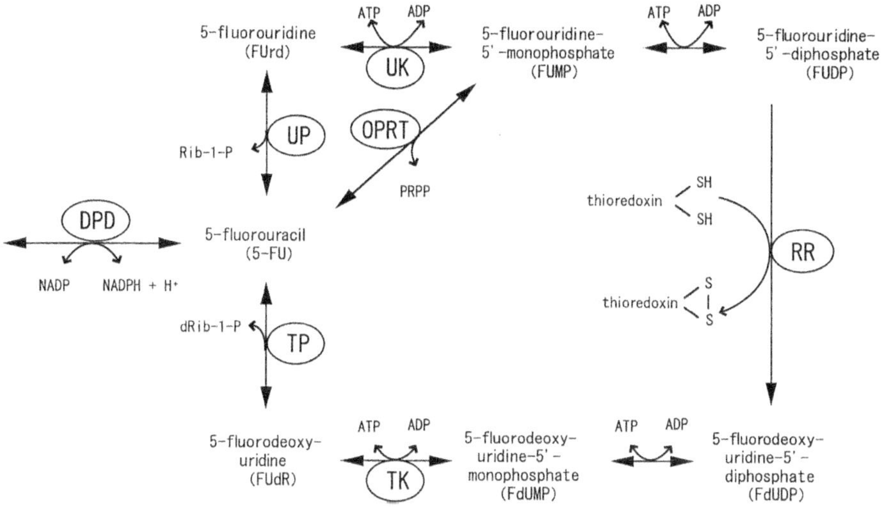

FIG. 2. Glucosylation pathways of *5-FU*

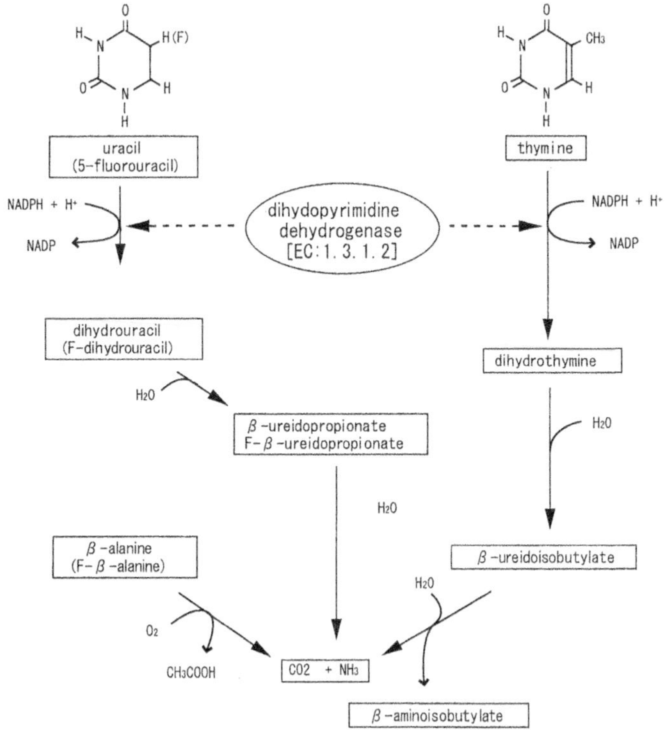

FIG. 3. Degradation pathways of pyrimidine bases

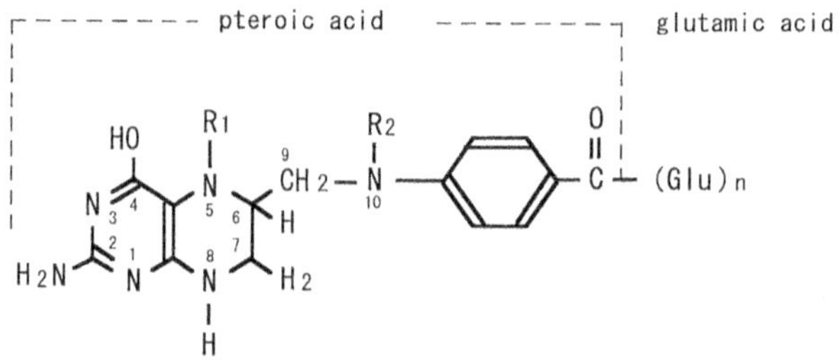

FIG. 4. Structural formula of reduced folate

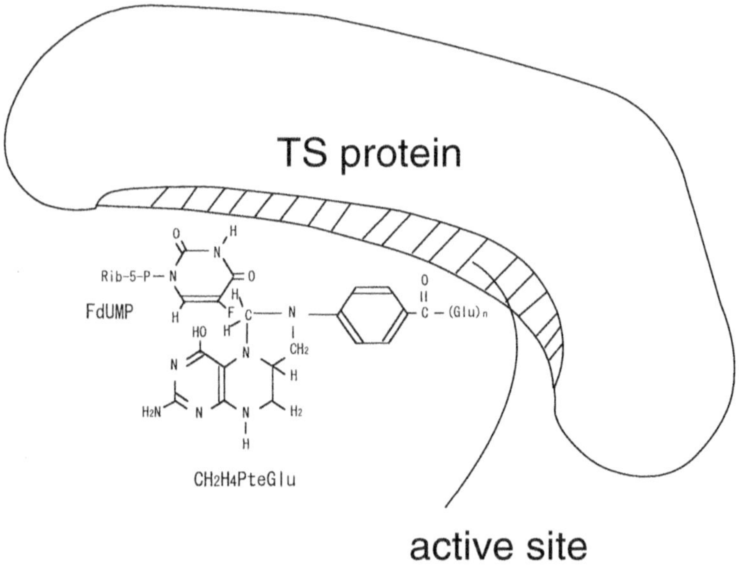

FIG. 5. Inhibition of thymidylate synthase (*TS*) by *FdUMP* through the formation of an inactive ternary complex with methylenetetrahydrofolate (*$CH_2H_4PteGlu$*)

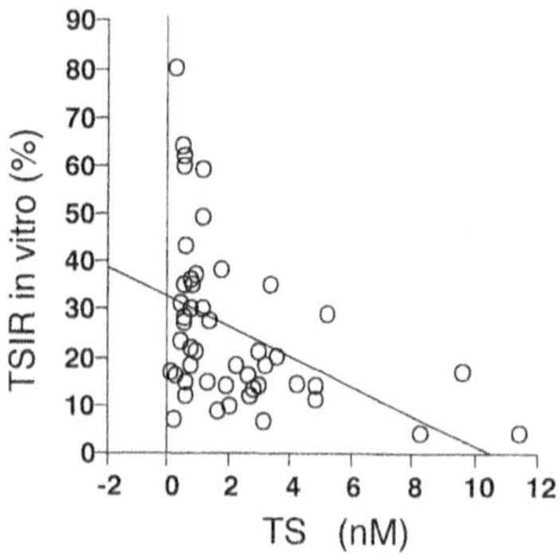

FIG. 6. Correlation between thymidylate synthase inhibition (*TSIR*) and *TS* expression in vitro

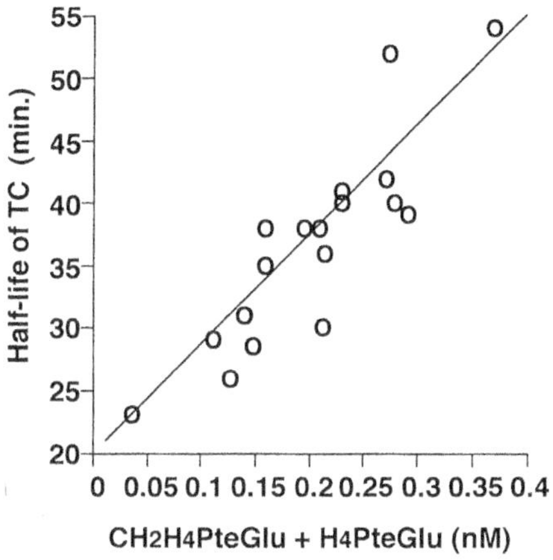

FIG. 7. Correlation between the half-life of TC and concentration of reduced folate in vitro

TABLE 1. Enzyme activity of glucosylation and degradation pathways in gastric carcinoma patients (nmol/g tissue per minute)

	Glucosylation (phosphorylation pathway)			
	OPRT	UP and UK	TP and TK	DPD
Gastric carcinoma (n = 22)	0.5 ± 0.7	4.5 ± 3.9	9.0 ± 4.7	1.4 ± 1.0
Metastatic lymph node (n = 5)	0.2 ± 0.2	1.6 ± 0.5	8.3 ± 4.8	1.1 ± 0.8
Normal gastric mucosa (n = 14)	0.2 ± 0.2	2.6 ± 3.2	4.4 ± 3.3	1.8 ± 0.7

OPRT, orotate phosphoribosyltransferase; UP, uridine phosphorylase; UK, uridine kinase; TP, thymidine phosphorylase; TK, thymidine kinase; DPD, dihydropyrimidine dehydrogenase

only for forming TC but also for stabilizing it (Fig. 7). Consequently, the administration of folinate calcium (leucovorin, LV), which is a precursor of CH_2H_4PteGlu, enhances the anticancer effect of 5-FU. For example, LV clinically enhances the anticancer effect of 5-FU in colorectal carcinoma. A meta-analysis of 18 randomized clinical trials (RCTs) comparing 5-FU to LV/5-FU confirmed a twofold increase in tumor response and a statistically significant survival benefit [2].

5-FU-resistant tumors possess high levels of DPD activity [3,4]. Conversely, tumors expressing low levels of DPD show a significantly better response to 5-FU than those with a high mRNA level and DPD activity [3,5]. The activity of DPD is three times higher than that of OPRT in gastric carcinoma (Table 1) [1]. Consequently, more than 80% of administered 5-FU is detoxified and excreted as F-β-alanine in urine [6]. To obtain satisfactory 5-FU antitumor activity, it is necessary to inhibit DPD or otherwise circumvent DPD-induced inactivation.

Two oral fluorinated pyrimidines containing DPD inhibitor have been introduced for clinical use. These drugs, referred to as DPD inhibitory fluoropyrimidines (DIF), include S-1, which is composed of tegafur, 5-chloro-2,4-dihydroxypyridine (CDHP), and potassium oxonate (Oxo) in a molar ratio of 1:0.4:1 (Fig. 8) [7]. CDHP compet-

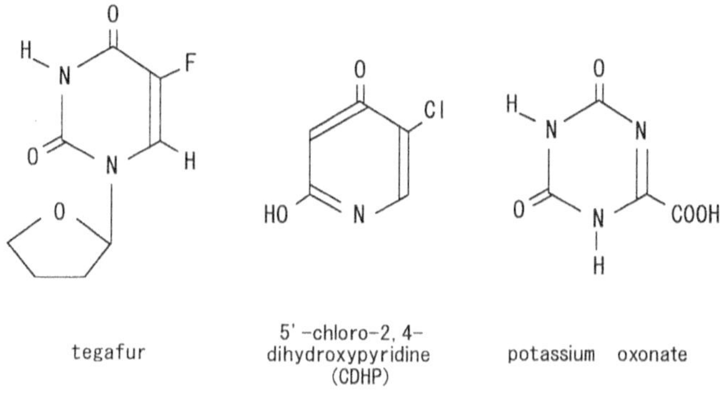

Fig. 8. Constituents of S-1

itively inhibits DPD 200 times more effectively than uracil, which is a mild and competitive inhibitor of DPD in vitro. Oxo is a potential inhibitor of OPRT and mainly distributes in the gastrointestinal mucosa after oral administration. Consequently, Oxo selectively ameliorates gastrointestinal tegafur toxicity by decreasing FdUMP production in the gastrointestinal mucosa. S-1 is now recognized as the most promising anticancer drug for treating gastric carcinoma.

In a phase II study of S-1 for advanced or recurrent gastric carcinoma, the response rate was 46.5% (60/129) with a 90% confidence interval of 37.7%–55.5% [7]. Gastrointestinal (GI) S-1 toxicity was markedly decreased compared with tegafur and uracil (UFT) or 5′-deoxy-5-fluoro-uridine (5′DFUR), but bone marrow suppression after S-1 administration was increased. This finding indicates that the cytotoxicity of tegafur except for GI toxicity is enhanced by CDHP. Conversely, GI toxicity was diminished by oral administration of Oxo. S-1 resulted in a high response rate against advanced or metastatic gastric carcinoma even when administered alone. The combination effect of S-1 and other anticancer drugs including CDDP is described in another chapter.

The toxicity profile of DIF shows that it is tolerable, with typical fluoropyrimidine toxicities (e.g., nausea and anorexia) seen at the maximum tolerated dose. Of note is the paucity of other toxicities, in particular hand–foot syndrome, neurological sequelaec, and cardiotoxicity, [8]. Although not well understood, these toxicities may be secondary to 5-FU catabolites including F-β-alanine. Such catabolites are less likely to be formed from S-1, and therefore these toxicities are not typically observed after S-1 treatment [9].

Cisplatin

Cisplatin (*cis*-dichloro-diamine platinum (II), CDDP) is frequently used during adjuvant chemotherapy against gastric carcinoma. The structure of CDDP is simple (Fig. 9); CDDP forms an intrastrand or interstrand G-G adduct or G-A adduct that disturbs the replication of DNA. The mechanisms of resistance to CDDP are complex and not completely understood. One of these may occur by the loss of the mismatch repair complex, which may explain the observation that oxaliplatin [(*trans*-

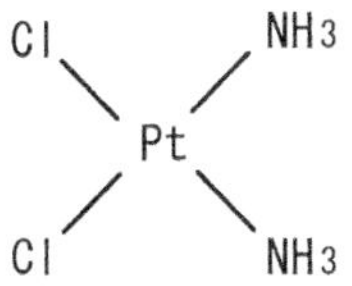

FIG. 9. Structural formula of cisplatin

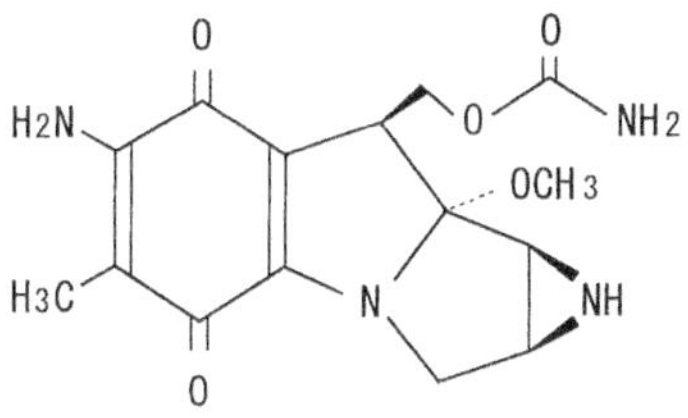

FIG. 10. Structural formula of mitomycin C

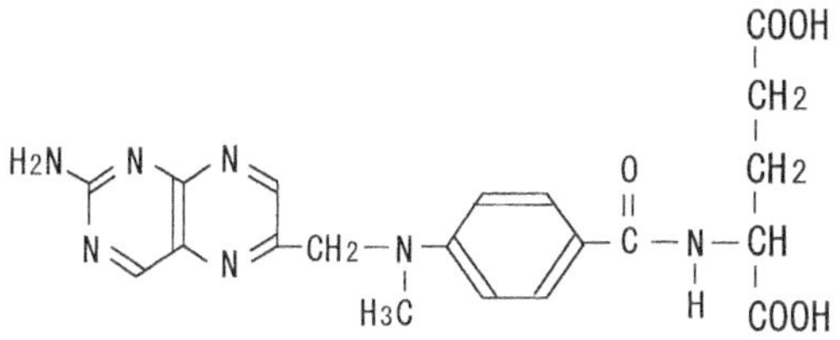

FIG. 11. Structural formula of methotrexate

R,*R*)diaminocyclohexane-oxalatoplatinum (II)] shows antitumor effects in CDDP-resistant tumors [10].

Mitomycin C

Mitomycin C (MMC) is an antitumoral antibiotic substance (Fig. 10). It is used in the clinical treatment of several malignancies including gastric carcinoma. MMC exhibits its cytotoxic activity mainly by making cross-links between complementary strands of DNA [11] because DNA interstrand cross-links represent highly lethal damage to the cell [12]. MMC was a primary drug used in chemotherapy against gastric carcinoma 20–30 years ago. However, it is now only a supportive drug and exhibits no obvious clinical effects in well-designed RCTs [13].

Methotrexate

Methotrexate (4-amino-4-deoxy-10-methyl pteroylglutamic acid, MTX) is a folate antagonist (Fig. 11). It is a powerful inhibitor of dihydrofolate reductase (DHFR), which catalyzes the reductive formation of tetrahydrofolate (H_4PteGlu) from dihydrofolate (H_2PteGlu) and H_4PteGlu formatin from folate (PteGlu). H_4PteGlu plays a role as a shuttle of 1-carbon units, including methyl and methylene residues. CH_2H_4PteGlu, which is formed from H4PteGlu after receiving a CH_2 group from serine

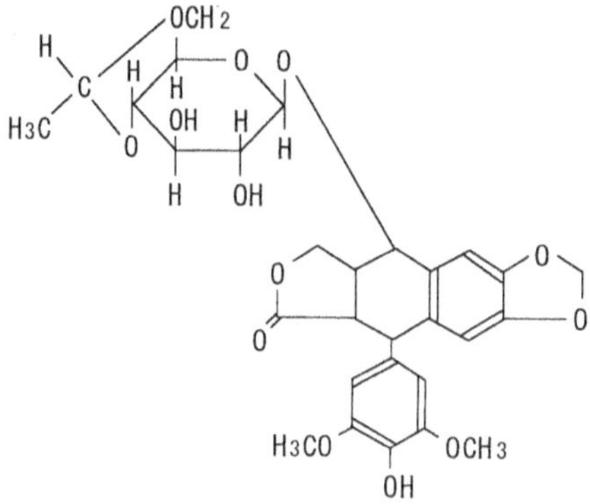

FIG. 12. Structural formula of etoposide

or glycine, is converted to H_2PteGlu during de novo synthesis of pyrimidine nucleotides. Consequently, the inhibition of DHFR results in fatal metabolic abnormalities and finally cell death.

MTX remains one of the anticancer drugs most commonly used during chemotherapy against gastric carcinoma. When concomitantly used with 5-FU, MTX may affect 5-FU as an enhancer. However, MTX is used at doses for which its own anticancer effects are exerted in such situations. Hence, the enhancer effect of MTX on 5-FU is uncertain.

Etoposide

Etoposide (ETO) is a semisynthetic epipodophylloxin (Fig. 12) and a inhibitor of topoisomerase II, which exists as a homodimer in 170-kDa (topo-IIα) and 180-kDa (topo-IIβ) forms. Topoisomerase II regulates the topology of DNA, and the inhibitory action of ETO results from the formation of a ternary complex with topo-II and DNA, thereby inhibiting the relegation of broken DNA strands. This action causes DNA damage and ultimately results in apoptotic cell death. ETO now plays a supporting role in adjuvant chemotherapy against gastric carcinoma.

Neoadjuvant Chemotherapy Against Advanced Gastric Carcinoma

Even in Japan, many patients are diagnosed with gastric carcinoma at a moderate or more advanced stage, and their prognosis is poorer than that of early or slightly advanced gastric carcinoma if curative surgery is carried out. The survival of advanced gastric cancer patients who do not undergo surgery is poor. However, the prognosis of patients who do undergo noncurative surgery is also quite poor. Their median survival time (MST) is shorter than 1 year, which is comparable to that of patients who do not undergo surgery, whose median survival time is also shorter than 1 year. Neoadjuvant chemotherapy (NAC) is a preoperative treatment involving anticancer drug(s) mainly intended to bring about stage reduction. NAC attempts to induce tumor reduction, resolve invasion into adjacent organ(s), or melt away lymph node metastases. After such treatment, it is easy and/or less invasive to remove diseased tissue in patients who showed a good response. Thus, the primary purpose of NAC for advanced gastric carcinoma is to increase the ratio of complete resection.

The definition of "unresectable gastric carcinoma" has not reached consensus around the world. The main reason for this is that its definition varies between many countries, where different surgical procedures are performed. As D2 lymph node dissection is routinely performed on advanced gastric carcinoma in Japan, N2 does not force the surgeon to abandon curative surgery for gastric carcinoma. However, D2 lymph node dissection, which is concomitantly performed with gastrectomy, is still not a standard surgical procedure in other countries. Several reports from Western countries suggest that D2 lymph node dissection increases the surgical morbidity and mortality rate to an unacceptable extent. Consequently, D0 or D1 lymph node dissection is carried out during surgery for gastric carcinoma in many countries. Thus, the factor that brings about an incomplete resection varies. D0 surgery is insufficient for the patients with lymph node metastases. Therefore, only gastric carcinomas without lymph node metastasis are good candidates for gastrectomy without preoperative chemotherapy in countries where D0 surgery is mainly performed. In another words, lymph node-positive gastric carcinoma should be considered to obtain stage reduction.

Although complete resection is the ideal therapy for gastric carcinoma by which absolute cure is expected, a considerable number of the advanced gastric cancer patients who undergo curative surgery suffer from recurrent disease. The secondary purpose of NAC is to ensure the curability of surgery for moderately advanced gastric carcinoma, which has a considerable recurrence rate even if curative surgery is performed. Such recurrent disease develops because of remnant micrometastases, whereby NAC is applied to melt away this type of tissue.

Indications and Results for Neoadjuvant Chemotherapy Against Advanced Gastric Carcinoma

For cases of incomplete resection when a tumor is expected upon preoperative examination, including computed tomography (CT) scanning and magnetic resonance imaging (MRI), surgery must be avoided. Considering the noncurative factor(s), performance status, and possibility for stage reduction, NAC should be performed before surgery for complete tumor resection, including metastatic lymph nodes and adjacent organ(s) that have been invaded. Highly advanced gastric carcinoma is a good indication of NAC, such as cT3, cT4, and/or N+. M1 gastric carcinomas are also an indication for NAC, because incomplete resection provides no benefit to these patients. However, the factor that makes the patient unable to undergo complete resection of the disease differs between countries and institutes. Palliative surgery without preoperative treatment or emergency surgery is acceptable in cases of massive bleeding from the tumor or tumor obstruction.

Stage II–IIIb gastric carcinomas may be an indication for NAC. These cancers can be cured if the patient undergoes D2 lymph node dissection, but there is a considerable risk of recurrence after surgery. A few phase II studies on NAC for resectable gastric carcinoma have been reported [14,15]. However, NAC for resectable gastric carcinoma should still be considered as a trial treatment.

There is no RCT for NAC against advanced gastric carcinoma. Consequently, there is no quality evidence regarding the benefit of NAC for advanced gastric carcinoma. A few phase II studies reported that NAC for highly advanced gastric carcinoma that were unresectable enabled some patients to undergo surgery (Table 2) [14–19]. The survival rate of resected patients or responders was better than that of unresected patients or nonresponders, respectively. However, the efficacy of NAC for advanced but resectable gastric carcinoma has not been proven [14,15,20].

Postoperative Adjuvant Chemotherapy Against Advanced Gastric Carcinoma

For cases of gastric carcinoma without distant metastasis and no invasion to adjacent organ(s), curative surgery with sufficient lymph node dissection is usually performed without preoperative treatment. However, diagnostic tools including CT scanning, ultrasonography, and fluorodeoxy glucose-positron emission tomography (FDG-PET) are not completely reliable in ruling out the existence of metastatic lesions. Consequently, it is necessary to perform postoperative adjuvant chemotherapy. Chemotherapy is beneficial for patients who have occult residual disease.

Indication and Results of Postoperative Adjuvant Chemotherapy Against Advanced Gastric Carcinomas

Patients with advanced gastric carcinoma who undergo surgery are indicated for postoperative adjuvant chemotherapy, whereby performance status and the possibility of recurrence should considered. pT1pN0 or pT2pN0 is excluded from postoperative adjuvant chemotherapy.

Many clinical trials involving postoperative adjuvant chemotherapy against gastric carcimona have been performed. However, no apparent benefit of postoperative adjuvant chemotherapy has been proven for gastric carcinoma [13,21–26]. Several meta-analyses of RCTs involving postoperative adjuvant chemotherapy have been reported (Table 3) [27–32]. From these, a significant survival benefit of postoperative adjuvant chemotherapy against advanced gastric carcinoma was observed. However, chemotherapy and the quality of surgery varied for RCTs analyzed in these reports. Well-designed RCTs are mandatory to estimate the efficacy of postoperative adjuvant chemotherapy.

Adjuvant Chemoradiotherapy Against Advanced Gastric Carcinoma

Macdonald et al. [33] reported the results of an RCT to evaluate the efficacy of postoperative adjuvant chemoradiotherapy against gastric carcinoma (Intergroup 0116). The regimen of this study is shown in Fig. 13. The medial overall survival for the

TABLE 2. Reports of neoadjuvant chemotherapy against gastric carcinoma

Reference	Patient stage	No. of patients	Regimen	Results
Nakajima et al. [18]	Incurable GC	30	LV/5-FU/CDDP/ETO	MST was 12.7 months for responders and 4.7 months for nonresponders.
Cascinu et al. [17]	Unresectable and/or metastatic GC	105	CDDP/LV/5-FU/EPI	Overall RR was 65%; MST was 11 months and 1-year survival rate was 42%.
Gallardo-Rincon et al. [16]	Unresectable GC, details not described	60	CDDP/LV/5-FU/ETO	NAC permitted a 17.5% resection rate.
Takahashi et al. [15]	Resectable schirrous GC	20	MTX/LV/5-FU/ADM	NAC improved the curative resection rate but not the survival rate.
Yano et al. [19]	Unresectable GC: any of peritoneal seeding, T4 to unresectable lesion, paraaortic LN matastases, etc.	34	5-FU/EPI/MTX/CDDP ($n = 13$) THP/5-FU/LV/CDDP/MMC ($n = 20$)	Patients able to undergo salvage surgery showed better prognosis.
Schuhmacher et al. [20]	Locally advanced GC: stages III A, III B, or IV	42	ETO/ADM/CDDP	MST was 19.1 months for all patients. Only patients who underwent a compete resection experienced a survival benefit.
Ott et al. [14]	Locally advanced GC cT3 or cT4, N^+, M0	49	CDDP/5-FU/LV	Overall RR was 26%. The 5-year survival rate of the responders was 90%.

NAC, neoadjuvant chemotherapy; RR, response rate; MST, median survival time; GC, gastric cancer; 5-FU, 5-fluorouracil, LV, leucovorin; CDDP, cisplatin; ETO, etoposide; EPI, epirubicin; ADM, adriacin; MTX, methotrexate; THP, therarubicin; LN, lymph node; MMC, mitomycin C

TABLE 3. Reports of meta-analyses of adjuvant chemotherapy against gastric carcinoma

Author (year)	No. of trials	No. of patients	Odds ratio (95% CI)	*P*
Hermans et al. (1993) [32]	11	2096	0.88 (0.78–1.08)	NR
Earle and Maroun (1999) [31]	13	1990	0.80 (0.68–0.97)	$P = 0.012$
Mari et al. (2000) [30]	21	3658	0.82 (0.75–0.89)	$P < 0.001$
Janunger et al. (2002) [29]	21	3962	0.84 (0.74–0.96)	NR
Panzini et al. (2002) [27]	17	3118	0.72 (0.62–0.84)	NR
Hu et al. (2002) [28]	14	4543	0.81 (0.70–0.94)	$P = 0.0008$

NR, not reported

chemoradiation group was 36 months, which was significantly longer than that of the surgery-alone group ($P = 0.005$). Following this report, adjuvant chemoradiation was recommended in North America. However, this study has one important problem associated with it. The quality of surgery performed on patients enrolled in it was poor. In spite of recommendations made regarding D2 lymph node dissection, only 10% underwent this type of surgery. Furthermore, more than half the patients (54%) underwent D0 dissection. Such quality of surgery is far from acceptable in Japan. Thus, the local control obtained by surgery in this study is deemed to be crude. Furthermore, the 3-year survival rate of the chemoradiation group was only 50%. Radiation provides local control during cancer treatment and should have compensated for poor lymph node dissection in this study. A high-quality RCT including strict D2 dissection is necessary to confirm the clinical benefit of chemoradiotherapy after curative surgery for gastric carcinoma. Macdonald and colleagues immediately reported that their study was partially incomplete [34].

Conclusion

An update regarding the significance of adjuvant chemotherapy for the treatment of gastric cancer has been described. The structure and anticancer mechanism of drugs used during adjuvant chemotherapy against gastric carcinoma are also described. Recent advances in cancer chemotherapy and molecular targeting therapy are promising, and it is believed that these advances will provide improvements in the prognosis of advanced gastric carcinoma. Well-designed RCTs are mandatory to obtain quality evidence for adjuvant chemotherapy against gastric carcinoma.

Patients

Resected adenocarcinoma of the stomach (any stage) n = 556

Lymph node dissection; D0 303 (54%), D1 199 (36%), D2 54 (10%)

Methods

Randomization was performed to designate the patients for surgery alone or postoperative chemoradiation.

Surgery-alone group (n = 275)

Adjuvant chemoradiation group (n = 281)

① 5-FU 425 mg/m^2		days 1–5
leucovorin 20 mg/m^2		days 1–5
② 4,500 cGy of radiation	180 cGy/day, 5 days/week, for 5 weeks starting on day 29.	
③ 5-FU 400 mg/m^2	On the first four and the last three days of radiation.	
leucovorin 20 mg/m^2	On the first four and the last three days of radiation.	
④ 5-FU 425 mg/m^2		days 1–5
leucovorin 20 mg/m^2		days 1–5
	Starting after one month after completion of chemoradiotherapy, q 4 weeks, 2 cycles.	

FIG. 13. Study design of Intergroup 0116

References

1. Dohden K, Ohmura K, Watanabe Y (1993) Ternary complex formation and reduced folate in surgical specimens of human adenocarcinoma tissues. Cancer (Phila) 15:471–480
2. Piedbois P, Michiels S (2003) Survival benefit of 5FU/LV over 5FU bolus in patients with advanced colorectal cancer: an updated meta-analysis based on 2751 patients. Proc Am Soc Clin Oncol 22:294
3. Salonga D, Danenberg KD, Johnson M, et al (2000) Gene expression levels of dihydropyrimidine dehydrogenase and thymidylate synthase together identify a high percentage of colorectal tumors responding to 5-fluorouracil. Clin Cancer Res 6:1322–1327
4. Jiang W, Lu Z, He Y, et al (1997) Dihydropyrimdine dehydrogenase activity in hepatocellular carcinoma: implication for 5-fluorouracil-based chemotherapy. Clin Cancer Res 3:395–339
5. Ishikawa Y, Kubota T, Otani Y, et al (1999) Dihydropyrimidine dehydrogenase activity and messenger RNA level may be related to the antitumor effect of 5-fluorouracil on human tumor xenografts in nude mice. Clin Cancer Res 5:883–889
6. Heggie GD, Sommadossi JP, Cross DS, et al (1987) Clinical pharmacokinetics of 5-fluorouracil and its metabolites in plasma, urine, and bile. Cancer Res 47:2203–2206
7. Sugimachi K, Maehara Y, Horikoshi N, et al (1999) An early phase II study of oral S-1, a newly developed 5-fluorouracil derivative for advanced and recurrent gastrointestinal cancers. Oncology 57:202–210
8. Pazdur R, Lassere Y, Diaz-Canton E, et al (1996) Phase I trials of uracil-tegafur (UFT) using 5- and 28-day administration schedules: Demonstration of schedule-dependent toxicities. Anticancer Drugs 7:728–733
9. Diasio B (2001) Clinical implication of dihydropyrimidine dehydrogenase on 5-FU pharmacology. Oncology 15:21–26

10. Iyer VN, Szybalski W (1963) A molecular mechanism of mitomycin action: linking of complementary DNA strands. Proc Natl Acad Sci USA 50:335–362
11. Vaisman A, Varchenko M, Umar A, et al (1998) The role of hMLH1, hMSH3, and hMSH6 defects in cisplatin and oxaliplatin resistance: correlation with replication bypass of platinum-DNA adducts. Cancer Res 58:3579–3585
12. Brendel M, Ruhland A (1984) A relationship between functionality and genetic toxicology of selected DNA-damaging agents. Mutat Res 133:51–85
13. Nashimoto A, Nakajima T, Furukawa H, et al (2003) Randomized trial of adjuvant chemotherapy with mitomycin, fluorouracil, and cytosine arabinoside followed by oral fluorouracil in serosa-negative gastric cancer: Japan Clinical Oncology Group 9206-1. J Clin Oncol 21:2282–2287
14. Ott K, Sendler A, Becker K, et al (2003) Neoadjuvant chemotherapy with cisplatin, 5-FU, and leucovorin (PLF) in locally advanced gastric cancer: a prospective phase II study. Gastric Cancer 6:159–167
15. Takahashi S, Kinoshita T, Konishi M, et al (2001) Phase II study of sequential high-dose methotrexate and fluorouracil combined with doxorubicin as a neoadjuvant chemotherapy for scirrhous gastric cancer. Gastric Cancer 4:192–197
16. Gallardo-Rincon D, Onate-Ocana LF, Calderillo-Ruiz G, et al (2000) Neoadjuvant chemotherapy with P-ELF (cisplatin, etoposide, leucovorin, 5-fluorouracil) followed by radical resection in patients with initially unresectable gastric adenocarcinoma: a phase II study. Ann Surg Oncol 7:45–50
17. Cascinu S, Labianca R, Alessandroni P, et al (1997) Intensive weekly chemotherapy for advanced gastric cancer using fluorouracil, cisplatin, epi-doxorubicin, 6S-leucovorin, glutathione, and filgrastim: a report from the Italian Group for the Study of Digestive Tract Cancer. J Clin Oncol 15:3313–3319
18. Nakajima T, Ota K, Ishihara S, et al (1997) Combined intensive chemotherapy and radical surgery for incurable gastric cancer. Ann Surg Oncol 4:203–208
19. Yano M, Shiozaki H, Inoue M, et al (2002) Neoadjuvant chemotherapy followed by salvage surgery: effect on survival of patients with primary noncurative gastric cancer. World J Surg 26:1155–1159
20. Schuhmacher CP, Fink U, Becker K, et al (2001) Neoadjuvant therapy for patients with locally advanced gastric carcinoma with etoposide, doxorubicin, and cisplatinum. Closing results after 5 years of follow-up. Cancer (Phila) 91:918–927
21. Chipponi J, Huguier M, Pezet D, et al (2004) Randomized trial of adjuvant chemotherapy after curative resection for gastric cancer. Am J Surg 187:440–445
22. Takiguchi N, Fujimoto S, Koda K, et al (2002) Postoperative adjuvant chemotherapy is effective in gastric cancer with serosal invasion: significance in patients chosen for multivariate analysis. Oncol Rep 9:801–806
23. Bajetta E, Buzzoni R, Mariani L, et al (2002) Adjuvant chemotherapy in gastric cancer: 5-year results of a randomised study by the Italian Trials in Medical Oncology (ITMO) Group. Ann Oncol 13:299–307
24. Chang HM, Jung KH, Kim TY, et al (2002) A phase III randomized trial of 5-fluorouracil, doxorubicin, and mitomycin C versus 5-fluorouracil and mitomycin C versus 5-fluorouracil alone in curatively resected gastric cancer. Ann Oncol 13:1779–1785
25. Neri B, Cini G, Andreoli F, et al (2001) Randomized trial of adjuvant chemotherapy versus control after curative resection for gastric cancer: 5-year follow-up. Br J Cancer 84:878–880
26. Nakajima T, Nashimoto A, Kitamura M, et al (1999) Adjuvant mitomycin and fluorouracil followed by oral uracil plus tegafur in serosa-negative gastric cancer: a randomized trial. Gastric Cancer Surgical Study Group. Lancet 354:273–277
27. Panzini I, Gianni L, Fattori PP, et al (2002) Adjuvant chemotherapy in gastric cancer: a meta-analysis of randomized trials and a comparison with previous meta-analyses. Tumori 88:21–27
28. Hu JK, Chen ZX, Zhou ZG, et al (2002) Intravenous chemotherapy for resected gastric cancer: meta-analysis of randomized controlled trials. World J Gastroenterol 8:1023–1028

29. Janunger KG, Hafstrom L, Glimelius B (2002) Chemotherapy in gastric cancer: a review and update meta-analysis. Eur J Surg 168:597–608
30. Mari E, Floriani I, Tinazzi A, et al (2000) Efficacy of adjuvant chemotherapy after curative resection for gastric cancer: a meta-analysis of published randomized trials. Ann Oncol 11:837–843
31. Earle CC, Maroun JA (1999) Adjuvant chemotherapy after curative resection for gastric cancer in non-Asian patients: revisiting a meta-analysis of randomized trials. Eur J Cancer 35:1059–1064
32. Hermans J, Bonenkamp JJ, Boon MC, et al (1993) Adjuvant therapy after curative resection for gastric cancer: meta-analysis of randomized trials J Clin Oncol 11:1441–1447
33. Macdonald JS, Smalley SR, Benedetti J, et al (2001) Chemoradiotherapy after surgery compared with surgery alone for adenocarcinoma of the stomach or gastroesophageal junction. N Engl J Med 345:725–730
34. Hundahl SA, Macdonald JS, Benedetti J, et al (2002) Surgical treatment variation in a prospective, randomized trial of chemoradiotherapy in gastric cancer: the effect of undertreatment. Ann Surg Oncol 9:278–286

Part 6

Recent Topics in Gastric Carcinoma Research

Micrometastasis of Gastric Cancer

SHOJI NATSUGOE, MASATAKA MATSUMOTO, HIROSHI OKUMURA, AKIHIRO NAKAJO, KOKI TOKUDA, FUTOSHI MIYAZONO, SUMIYA ISHIGAMI, SHUICHI HOKITA, SONSHIN TAKAO, and TAKASHI AIKOU

Introduction

Even patients with gastric cancer who undergo complete resection and have no histological evidence of lymph node metastasis sometimes experience recurrence after operation [1–3]. Why do cancers recur despite the performance of macroscopically and histologically radical resections? This recurrence is probably caused by micrometastasis to the lymph nodes, circulating blood, and abdominal cavity [4,5]. It is known that occult lymph node micrometastases have been identified by detailed histological examination in additional sections [6,7]. In recent years, the development of sensitive immunohistochemical technique and reverse transcription-polymerase chain reaction (RT-PCR) has led to the detection of micrometastases [4,5]. The concept of isolated tumor cells (ITC) has been introduced in the TNM classification [8]. In this issue, ITC was defined as single tumor cells or small clusters of cells not more than 0.2 mm in greatest dimension that are usually detected by immunohistochemistry or molecular methods, but which may be verified with hematoxylin and eosin (H&E) stains. The clinical significance of ITC or micrometastasis is still unknown in gastric cancer patients.

Since 1996, our laboratory has pursued gene diagnosis to detect lymph node micrometastasis, free cancer cells in the circulating blood, and disseminated cancer cells in the abdominal cavity in patients with gastric cancer. In the present chapter, we demonstrate the current results of micrometastasis, including ours, and discuss the role, significance, and problem of perioperative gene diagnosis in gastric cancer surgery.

Lymph Node Micrometastasis

Immunohistochemical Detection of Micrometastasis

We examined lymph node micrometastasis by immunohistochemistry using AE1/AE3 (Dako, Carpinteria, CA, USA) in 1761 lymph nodes obtained from 67 gastric cancer patients who were diagnosed as free of lymph node metastasis by routine histologi-

Department of Surgical Oncology and Digestive Surgery, Kagoshima University School of Medicine, 8-35-1 Sakuragaoka, Kagoshima 890-8520, Japan
e-mail: natsugoe@m2.kufm.kagoshima-u.ac.jp

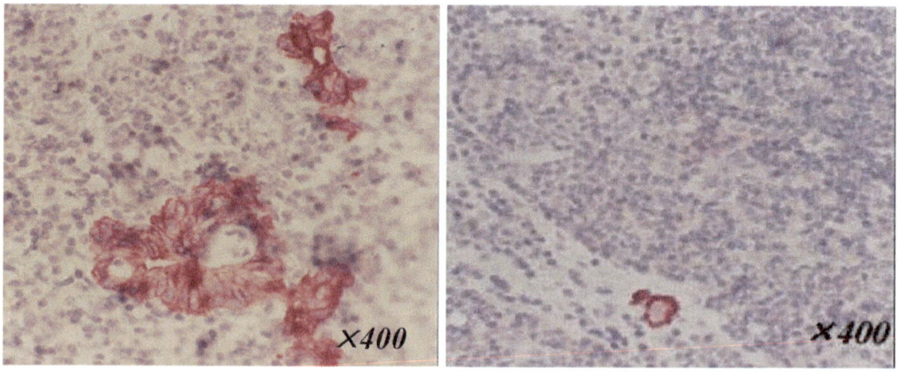

Fig. 1. **a** Micrometastasis in a lymph node as detected by immunohistochemical staining with anticytokeratin AE1/AE3. Micrometastasis was defined as metastasis consisting of tumor cells or a small cluster of carcinoma cells with surrounding stromal change. **b** Tumor cell microinvolvement (TCM) in a lymph node. Microinvolvement was defined as carcinoma cells without surrounding stromal change

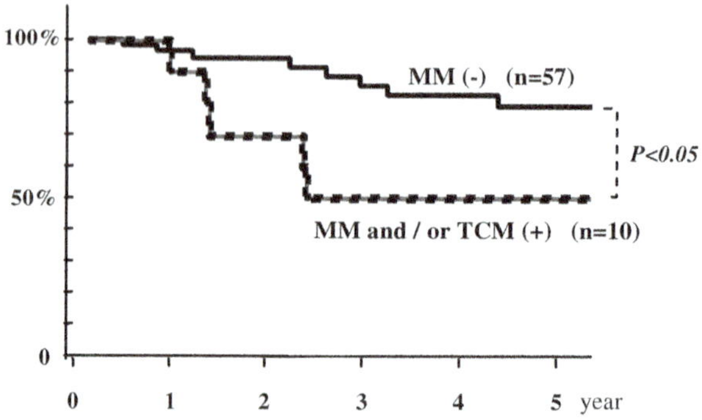

Fig. 2. Survival curve of patients who did or did not have micrometastasis in one or more lymph nodes. *MM*, micrometastasis; *TCM*, tumor cell microinvolvement

cal examination [9]. Tumor involvement of lymph nodes was divided into two categories: tumor cell microinvolvement (TCM), individual tumor cells without a change in the stroma and micrometastasis; and cluster formation of tumor cells with stromal reaction (Fig. 1) [5,10]. Thirty (1.5%) of the 1761 lymph nodes showed micrometastasis and/or TCM. Micrometastasis with or without TCM was found in 10 patients, and TCM alone was found in 4 patients; 6 (18.2%) of the 33 patients with T1 tumor and 8 (23.5%) of the 34 patients with T2 tumor had occult lymph node metastasis. The 5-year survival rate was worse among those with micrometastasis with or without TCM than among those without micrometastasis (Fig. 2) [10–19]. Some authors have reported the detection rate and clinical outcome in patients with micrometastasis (Table 1). The rate of micrometastasis ranged from 8% to 90%. There were some problems regarding the difference of antibody used, identification between micrometastasis and immune cells, and estimation of micrometastasis, especially in single cells. It is important to apply such methods in the clinical field. Recently, we have introduced

TABLE 1. Reports of lymph node micrometastasis detected by immunostaining

Author [Reference]	Antibody	Case	Patients	Positivity	Prognosis
Siewert et al. 1996 [10]	AE1/AE3,Ber-EP4	100	T1–T3	90	(+)
Ishida et al. 1997 [11]	CK,CEA	109	St.I–IV	18	(+)
Harrison et al. 2000 [12]	CAM5.2	25	T1–T4N0	36	(+)
Nakajo et al. 2001 [9]	AE1/AE3	67	T1,T2,N0	21	(+)
Yasuda et al. 2002 [13]	CAM5.2	64	T2T3N0	32	(+)
Lee et al. 2002 [14]	AE1/AE3	153	T1–T4	49	(+)
Stachura et al. 1998 [15]	CK18	40	T1	8	(−)
Kikuchi et al. 1999 [16]	AE1/AE3	51	T2T3N0	43	(−)
Saragoni et al. 2000 [17]	CK	139	T1N0	17	(−)
Choi et al. 2002 [19]	CK8	88	T1(SM)	32	(−)
Fukagawa et al. 2001 [18]	CK	107	T2N0	36	(−)

(+), significant; (−), not significant

rapid immunohistochemical detection of lymph node micrometastasis during operation, which took 30 min to complete [20]. Such a method is useful for determining distant lymphadenectomy by examination of regional nodes for advanced cancer and examining the presence or absence of nodal involvement in sentinel node navigation surgery for early cancer.

Micrometastasis Detected by RT-PCR

We examined 312 lymph nodes obtained from 50 patients (pT1, 41; pT2, 5; pT3, 3; and pT4, 1) with node-negative gastric cancer [21]. The clinical characteristics of micrometastasis were investigated after RT-PCR using carcinoembryonic antigen (CEA) as a primer and immunohistochemistry using anticytokeratin antibody (AE1/AE3) were performed. The number of patients and micrometastases detected by RT-PCR was 14 and 17 and by immunohistochemistry was 7 and 8, respectively. RT-PCR was a more sensitive method than immunohistochemistry. Micrometastasis by RT-PCR correlated with depth of tumor invasion and lymphatic invasion. Regarding pT1 tumor, 9 patients with micrometastasis had tumors that were of the macroscopically depressed type and 2 cm or more in diameter. These results supported the indication of endoscopic mucosal resection.

There were some reports of micrometastasis detected by RT-PCR (Table 2) [21–24]. The detection rate of micrometastasis was different because of various stages of the patients in each report. The RT-PCR method is actually more sensitive than the other methods. However, there are some problems for RT-PCR technique as follow: (1) some complicated procedures for management of specimens, (2) contamination of other specimens, (3) selection of primer, (4) presence of pseudogene, and (5) suitable setup of sensitivity for amplification. The relationship between micrometastasis detected by RT-PCR and clinical outcome is still unknown. In the near future, we should analyze a large number of patients with micrometastasis under certain conditions such as the same primer and the same stage.

The question arises whether occult micrometastasis implant and proliferate in the lymph node. Izbicki and Hosch reported that implantation and proliferation of

TABLE 2. Reports of lymph node micrometastasis detected by reverse transcription-polymerase chain reaction (RT-PCR)

Author [Reference]	Primer	LN	Patients	Positivity	Prognosis
Noguchi et al. 1996 [22]	CK19	100	12	15	Unknown
Mori et al. 1995 [23]	CEA	87	13	54	Unknown
Okada et al. 2001 [24]	CEA,CK20,MAGE3	414	28	12	Unknown
Matsumoto et al. 2002 [21]	CEA	312	50	5	Unknown

LN, lymph node

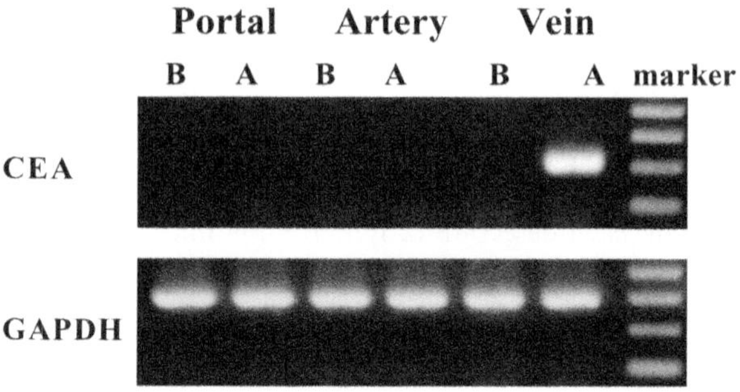

FIG. 3. Example of expression of carcinoembryonic antigen (*CEA*) mRNA. CEA mRNA was positive in the portal vein after resection. *GAPDH*, glyceraldehyde phosphate dehydrogenase. *B*, before resection; *A*, after resection

micrometastasized cancer cells in the lymph nodes were confirmed by an experiment of transplantation metastasis using nude mice [25,26]. Further study should be required in the relationship between proliferation of micrometastasis and autoimmune system.

Free Cancer Cells in the Circulating Blood

Circulating cancer cells recently have been detectable with RT-PCR. We examined the relationship between molecular detection of circulation cancer cells according to the time course during surgical procedure and blood-borne metastases [27]. Blood samples from 57 patients with gastric cancer were obtained from the portal vein, peripheral artery and superior vena cava before and after tumor dissection. After total RNA was extracted from each blood sample, CEA-specific RT-PCR was performed (Fig. 3). CEA mRNA was detected in the blood of 21 (36.8%) of 57 patients. CEA mRNA expression was not detected in the blood obtained from 15 healthy volunteers and 15 patients with benign disease. The positive rate increased in proportion to the depth of tumor. The incidence of positive CEA mRNA did not differ among the various sites of blood sampling. The appearance of circulating cancer cells was related to the surgical maneuver. A significant relationship was found between the detection of CEA mRNA and blood-borne metastases (Table 3). These results suggested that surgical

TABLE 3. Expression of carcinoembryonic antigen (CEA) mRNA (CEA mRNA) and blood-borne metastases after surgery

	Expression of CEA mRNA		
	Negative	Positive	*P* value
No recurrence	36	17	0.029
Recurrence	0	4	
Number of patients	36	21	

TABLE 4. Reports of free cancer cells in blood detected by RT-PCR

Author [Reference]	Primer	Case	Positivity	Recurrence
Yeh et al. 1998 [28]	CK19	34	21	(+)
Majima et al. 2000 [29]	CEA,CK20	52	10, 10	Unknown
Nishida et al. 2000 [30]	CAM5.2	36	22	Unknown
Piva et al. 2000 [31]	CEA	30	37	Unknown
Miyazono et al. 2001 [27]	CEA	57	37	(+)
Ikeguchi et al. 2003 [32]	CK20	55	27	Unknown

(+), significant

maneuvers were a possible cause of hematogeneous metastasis, and patients with positive CEA mRNA had a high risk of blood-borne metastasis even after curative resection.

The frequency of free cancer cells in blood detected by RT-PCR reportedly ranged from 10% to 37% (Table 4) [27–32]. Epithelial markers such as cytokeratin and CEA were generally used as primers. To date, as the clinical significance is still unclear because of the small number of patients, we should clarify clinical outcome by long-term follow-up in patients with disseminated tumor cells in blood in a large number of patients.

Although the frequency of hematogeneous metastasis differed depending on the animal species or cancer cell lines, an animal experiment revealed that cancer metastasis developed only when more than a certain number of cancer cells was injected intravenously [33–35]. However, the mechanism of cancer metastasis still remains unclear as to whether most free cancer cells die or are unable to adhere to the vascular endothelium. Basically, it is necessary to clarify the characteristics of the cancer cells that are considered to establish a metastatic lesion. These cells possess the ability to adhere and infiltrate to the vascular endothelium, proliferate outside the blood vessel, and subsequently induce vascularization [36,37].

Free Cancer Cells in the Peritoneal Cavity

Peritoneal dissemination is one of the most common modes of gastric cancer recurrence, even after curative resection [38]. Cytological examination of peritoneal lavage is a useful means of detecting free cancer cells in the peritoneal cavity and predicting recurrence [39–41]. However, some patients with negative cytological findings

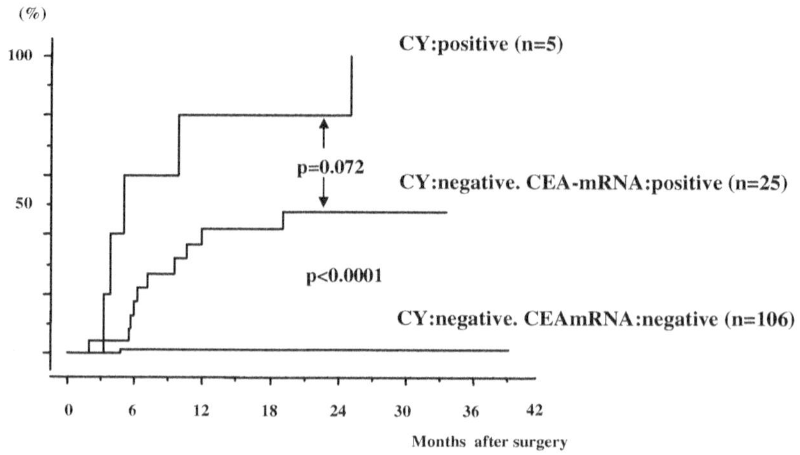

FIG. 4. Cumulative rate of peritoneal recurrence according to cytology results and CEA mRNA expression by reverse transcription-polymerase chain reaction (RT-PCR). *CY*, cytology

have been diagnosed later with peritoneal metastasis. We investigated free cancer cells in the peritoneal lavage fluid by both conventional cytological examination (Papanicolaou and Giemsa staining) and CEA-specific RT-PCR. Peritoneal lavage was performed in 136 patients who underwent curative gastrectomy [42]. After laparotomy, the left subphrenic and Douglas cavities were filled with 200 ml isotonic sodium chloride and peritoneal lavage fluid was collected. Among 136 patients, 5 patients (3.6%) were positive for free cancer cells by cytological examination and 30 (22.1%) were positive by RT-PCR. The frequency of RT-PCR results increased according to lymph node metastases, lymphatic invasion, tumor depth, and stage grouping. The incidence of peritoneal recurrence was significantly higher in patients with positivity than those with negativity by RT-PCR. Among cytologically negative patients, survival was significantly shorter in patients with positive than in those with negative CEA mRNA expression (see Fig. 3). Therefore, the technique of RT-PCR was more sensitive than cytological examination in the detection of free cancer cells and prediction of peritoneal recurrence.

There have been several reports regarding the detection of free cancer cells in the peritoneal cavity by the immunohistochemical or RT-PCR method (Table 5) [42–47]. According to these reports, the detection rate was higher in immunostaining than in RT-PCR. It is necessary to compare the sensitivity of both methods using peritoneal fluid obtained from same patients. In all reports, interestingly, the presence of free cancer cells detected by such methods correlated well with peritoneal recurrence. Therefore, it should be considered that patients with positive finding by molecular diagnosis are at a risk of developing peritoneal recurrence.

It is difficult to make a decision of intraperitoneal chemotherapy for these cases when disseminated metastasis is not macroscopically observed. Early detection and eradication of free cancer cells before the development of metastases could help to improve the outcome of patients after tumor resection. The development of useful

TABLE 5. Reports of free cancer cells in peritoneal lavage fluid detected by immunostaining and RT-PCR

Author [Reference]	Antibody/Primer	Case	Positivity	Prognosis
Immunostaining				
Benevolo et al. 1998 [43]	B72.3,AR3,BD5	144	35	(+)
Vogel et al. 1999 [44]	HEA-125	111	49	(+)
RT-PCR				
Yonemura et al. 2001 [45]	CEA	230	17	(+)
Yonemura et al. 2001 [46]	MMP-7	152	18	(+)
Kodera et al. 1998 [47]	CEA	189	21	(+)
Tokuda et al. 2003 [42]	CEA	131	22	(+)

(+), significant

tactics for disseminated micrometastasis in the peritoneal cavity is expected in the near future.

Conclusions

Owing the development of biological and genetic techniques, the presence of micrometastasis in the lymph node, circulating blood, and abdominal cavity has been confirmed. The mechanism of implantation and proliferation of micrometastasis should be basically clarified. Furthermore, we should also investigate the relationship between micrometastasis and the autoimmune system. Clinically, the significance of micrometastasis should be surveyed in a large number of patients with the same stage and surgery. Because it may take a long time for occult micrometatsasis to form recurrent disease, long-term follow-up data are required to elucidate the clinical significance.

Although surgery is performed to primarily treat many gastric cancer patients, it is inversely the final chance for survival of cancer cells. Therefore, the perioperative prevention of micrometastasis is important when curative surgery is performed. Patients with micrometastasis seem to have a high risk of cancer recurrence. This concern may also allow the selection of therapeutic tactics to prevent metastasis. We must fight these invisible enemies simultaneously with surgery. In recent years, drugs that inhibit cancer cell infiltration and vascularization of the primary lesion have been used clinically as antimetastatic agents [48–50]. It is advantageous that these agents cause only slight side effects and may be useful for preventing cancer metastasis perioperatively. The antitumor effects of these agents, in combination with gene diagnosis, should be evaluated by randomized controlled studies in the near future.

References

1. Maehara Y, Emi Y, Baba H, et al (1996) Recurrences and related characteristics of gastric cancer. Br J Cancer 74:975–979
2. Guadagni S, Catarci M, Kinoshit T, et al (1997) Causes of death and recurrence after surgery for early gastric cancer. World J Surg 21:434–439

3. Suzuki S, Kosugi S, Kuwabara S, et al (1998) Tumor recurrence in patients with early gastric cancer: a clinicopathologic evaluation. J Exp Clin Cancer Res 17:187–191
4. Mori M, Mimori M, Ueo H, et al (1998) Clinical significance of molecular detection of carcinoma cells in lymph nodes and peripheral blood by reverse transcription-polymerase chain reaction in patients with gastrointestinal or breast carcinomas. J Clin Oncol 16: 128–132
5. Natsugoe S, Muellr J, Stein HJ, et al (1998) Micrometastasis and tumor cell microinvolvement of lymph nodes from esophageal squamous cell carcinoma. Cancer (Phila) 83:858–866
6. Natsugoe S, Aikou T, Shimada M, et al (1994) Occult lymph node metastasis in gastric cancer with submucosal invasion. Surg Today 24:870–875
7. Isozaki H, Okajima K, Fujii K (1997) Histological evaluation of lymph node metastasis on serial sectioning in gastric cancer with radical lymphadenectomy. Hepatogastroenterology 44:1133–1136
8. Sobin LH, Wittekind CH (2002) TNM classification of malignant tumors, 6th edn. International Union Against Cancer (UICC). Wiley-Liss, New York, pp 10–12
9. Nakajo A, Natsugoe S, Ishigami S, et al (2001) Detection and prediction of micrometastasis in the lymph nodes of patients with pN0 gastric cancer. Ann Surg Oncol 8:158–162
10. Siewert JR, Kestlmeier R, Busch R, et al (1996) Benefit of D2 lymph node dissection for patients with gastric cancer and pN0 and pN1 lymph node metastases. Br J Surg 83: 1144–1147
11. Ishida K, Katsuyama T, Sugiyama A, et al (1997) Immunohistochemical evaluation of lymph node micrometastases from gastric carcinomas. Cancer (Phila) 79:1069–1076
12. Harrison LE, Choe JK, Goldstein M, et al (2000) Prognostic significance of immunohistochemical micrometastases in node negative gastric cancer patients. Surg Oncol 73:153–157
13. Yasuda K, Adachi Y, Shiraishi N, et al (2002) Prognostic effect of lymph node micrometastasis in patients with histologically node-negative gastric cancer. Ann Surg Oncol 9:771–774
14. Lee E, Chae Y, Kim I, et al (2002) Prognostic relevance of immunohistochemically detected lymph node micrometastasis in patients with gastric carcinoma. Cancer (Phila) 94: 2867–2873
15. Stachura J, Zembala M, Heitzman J, et al (1998) Lymph node micrometastases in early gastric carcinoma alone inadequately reflect the new model of metastatic development. Pol J Pathol 49:155–157
16. Kikuchi Y, Tsuchiya A, Ando Y, et al (1999) Immunohistochemical detection of lymph node microinvolvement in node-negative gastric cancer. Gastric Cancer 2:173–178
17. Saragoni L, Gaudio M, Morgagni P, et al (2000) Identification of occult micrometastases in patients with early gastric cancer using anti-cytokeratin monoclonal antibodies. Oncol Rep 7:535–539
18. Fukagawa T, Sasako M, Mann GB, et al (2001) Immunohistochemically detected micrometastases of the lymph nodes in patients with gastric carcinoma. Cancer (Phila) 92:753–760
19. Choi HJ, Kim YK, Kim YH, et al (2002) Occurrence and prognostic implications of micrometastases in lymph nodes from patients with submucosal gastric carcinoma. Ann Surg Oncol 9:13–19
20. Matsumoto M, Natsugoe S, Ishigami S, et al (2003) Rapid immunohistochemical detection of lymph node micrometastasis during operation for upper gastrointestinal carcinoma. Br J Surg 90:563–566
21. Matsumoto M, Natsugoe S, Ishigami S, et al (2002) Lymph node micrometastasis and lymphatic mapping determined by reverse transcriptase-polymerase chain reaction in pN0 gastric carcinoma. Surgery (St. Louis) 131:630–635
22. Noguchi S, Hiratsuka M, Furukawa H, et al (1996) Detection of gastric cancer micrometastases in lymph nodes by amplification of keratin 19 mRNA with reverse transcriptase-polymerase chain reaction. Jpn J Cancer Res 87:650–654
23. Mori M, Mimori K, Inoue H, et al (1995) Detection of cancer micrometastases in lymph nodes by reverse transcriptase-polymerase chain reaction. Cancer Res 55:3417–3420

24. Okada Y, Fujiwara Y, Yamamoto H, et al (2001) Genetic detection of lymph node micrometastases in patients with gastric carcinoma by multiple-marker reverse transcriptase-polymerase chain reaction assay. Cancer (Phila) 92:2056–2064
25. Scheunemann P, Izbicki JR, Pantel K (1999) Tumorigenic potential of apparently tumor-free lymph nodes. N Engl J Med 340:1687
26. Hosch S, Kraus J, Scheunemann P, et al (2000) Malignant potential and cytogenetic characteristics of occult disseminated tumor cells in esophageal cancer. Cancer Res 60:6836–6840
27. Miyazono F, Natsugoe S, Takao S, et al (2001) Surgical maneuvers enhance molecular detection of circulating tumor cells during gastric cancer surgery. Ann Surg 233:189–194
28. Yeh KH, Chen YC, Yeh SH, et al (1998) Detection of circulating cancer cells by nested reverse transcription-polymerase chain reaction of cytokeratin-19 (K19): possible clinical significance in advanced gastric cancer. Anticancer Res 18:1283–1286
29. Majima T, Ichikura T, Takayama E, et al (2000) Detecting circulating cancer cells using reverse transcriptase-polymerase chain reaction for cytokeratin mRNA in peripheral blood from patients with gastric cancer. Jpn J Clin Oncol 30:499–503
30. Nishida S, Kitamura K, Ichikawa D, et al (2000) Molecular detection of disseminated cancer cells in the peripheral blood of patients with gastric cancer. Anticancer Res 20:2155–2159
31. Piva MG, Navaglia F, Basso D, et al (2000) CEA mRNA identification in peripheral blood is feasible for colorectal, but not for gastric or pancreatic cancer staging. Oncology 59:323–328
32. Ikeguchi M, Ohro S, Maeda Y, et al (2003) Detection of cancer cells in the peripheral blood of gastric cancer patients. Int J Mol Med 11:217–221
33. Akimoto T, Kawabe S, Grothey A, et al (1999) Low E-cadherin and beta-catenin expression correlates with increased spontaneous and artificial lung metastases of murine carcinomas. Clin Exp Metastasis 17:171–176
34. Grossniklaus HE (1998) Tumor vascularity and hematogenous metastasis in experimental murine intraocular melanoma. Trans Am Ophthalmol Soc 96:721–752
35. Morris VL, MacDonald IC, Koop S, et al (1993) Early interactions of cancer cells with the microvasculature in mouse liver and muscle during hematogenous metastasis: videomicroscopic analysis. Clin Exp Metastasis 11:377–390
36. Deryugina EI, Soroceanu L, Strongin AY (2002) Up-regulation of vascular endothelial growth factor by membrane-type 1 matrix metalloproteinase stimulates human glioma xenograft growth and angiogenesis. Cancer Res 62:580–588
37. Kim KJ, Li B, Winer J, et al (1993) Inhibition of vascular endothelial growth factor-induced angiogenesis suppresses tumour growth in vivo. Nature (Lond) 362:841–844
38. Baba H, Korenaga D, Okamura T, et al (1989) Prognostic factors in gastric cancer with serosal invasion. Arch Surg 124:1061–1064
39. Koga S, Kaibara N, Iituka Y, et al (1984) Prognostic significance of intraperitoneal free cancer cells in gastric cancer patients. J Cancer Res Clin Oncol 108:236–238
40. Boku T, Nakane Y, Minoura T, et al (1990) Prognostic significance of serosal invasion and free intraperitoneal cancer cells in gastric cancer. Br J Surg 77:436–439
41. Bonenkamp JJ, Songun I, Hermans J, et al (1996) Prognostic value of positive cytology findings from abdominal washings in patients with gastric cancer. Br J Surg 83:672–674
42. Tokuda K, Natsugoe S, Nakajo A, et al (2003) Clinical significance of CEA-mRNA expression in peritoneal lavage fluid from patients with gastric cancer. Int J Mol Med 11:79–84
43. Benevolo M, Mottolese M, Cosimelli M, et al (1998) Diagnostic and prognostic value of peritoneal immunocytology in gastric cancer. J Clin Oncol 16:3406–3411
44. Vogel P, Ruschoff J, Kummel S, et al (1999) Immunocytology improves prognostic impact of peritoneal tumour cell detection compared to conventional cytology in gastric cancer. Eur J Surg Oncol 25:515–519
45. Yonemura Y, Endou Y, Fujimura T, et al (2001) Diagnostic value of preoperative RT-PCR-based screening method to detect carcinoembryonic antigen-expressing free cancer cells in the peritoneal cavity from patients with gastric cancer. ANZ J Surg 71:521–528

46. Yonemura Y, Fujimura T, Ninomiya I, et al (2001) Prediction of peritoneal micrometastasis by peritoneal lavaged cytology and reverse transcriptase-polymerase chain reaction for matrix metalloproteinase-7 mRNA. Clin Cancer Res 7:1647–1653
47. Kodera Y, Nakanishi H, Yamamura Y, et al (1998) Prognostic value and clinical implications of disseminated cancer cells in the peritoneal cavity detected by reverse transcriptase-polymerase chain reaction and cytology. Int J Cancer 79:429–433
48. Boehm T, Folkman J, Browder T, et al (1997) Antiangiogenic therapy of experimental cancer does not induce acquired drug resistance. Nature (Lond) 390:404–407
49. Takao S, Akiyama SI, Nakajo A, et al (2000) Suppression of metastasis by thymidine phosphorylase inhibitor. Cancer Res 60:5345–5348
50. Yi M, Ruoslahti E (2001) A fibronectin fragment inhibits tumor growth, angiogenesis, and metastasis. Proc Natl Acad Sci U S A 98:620–624

Sentinel Node Navigation Surgery: Application to Minimally Invasive and Function-Preserving Surgery for Early Gastric Cancer

Yoshihide Otani[1], Yuko Kitagawa[1], Toshiharu Furukawa[1], Masashi Yoshida[1], Yoshiro Saikawa[1], Tetsuro Kubota[1], Makio Mukai[2], Kaori Kameyama[2], Hirofumi Fujii[3], Atsushi Kubo[3], Koichiro Kumai[4], and Masaki Kitajima[1]

Introduction

Lymphadenectomy in radical gastrectomy for gastric cancer has been generally accepted as a standard technique in many countries. Although gastrectomy with prophylactic lymph node dissection is the standard surgical procedure, the survival benefit of gastrectomy with D2 lymphadenectomy remains controversial [1,2]. Determination of the extent of lymph node dissection required in patients with gastric cancer on the basis of actual node involvement is important because minimalization of dissection may be associated with reduced postoperative morbidity and mortality rates and increased postoperative quality of life (QOL). The development of novel diagnostic procedures for lymph node involvement is therefore crucial to accurate lymph node staging.

The recent increase in the detection rate of T1 gastric cancers in Japan and other countries has highlighted the importance of patients' postoperative QOL. The accurate diagnostic exclusion of cases with lymph node involvement is an essential precondition to the acceptance and use of modified lymphadenectomy such as D0 or D1 for T1 cancers.

What Is the Sentinel Node?

The word "sentinel" is an old military word used to describe a soldier standing as a guard at the entrance of a castle or military base (Fig. 1). The sentinel node (SN) is the first lymph node (LN) encountered by the lymphatic flow as it drains from the primary lesion. SNs are detectable intraoperatively by the injection of a suitable dye or radioactive tracer (Fig. 2). A negative result for metastasis in the SN predicts the absence of the metastases in the other regional lymph nodes. The validity of the SN hypothesis

[1] Department of Surgery, [2] Department of Pathology, and [3] Department of Radiology, [4] Center for Diagnostic and Therapeutic Endoscopy, Keio University School of Medicine, 35 Shinanomachi, Shinjuku-ku, Tokyo 160-8582, Japan
e-mail: otaniy@sc.itc.keio.ac.jp

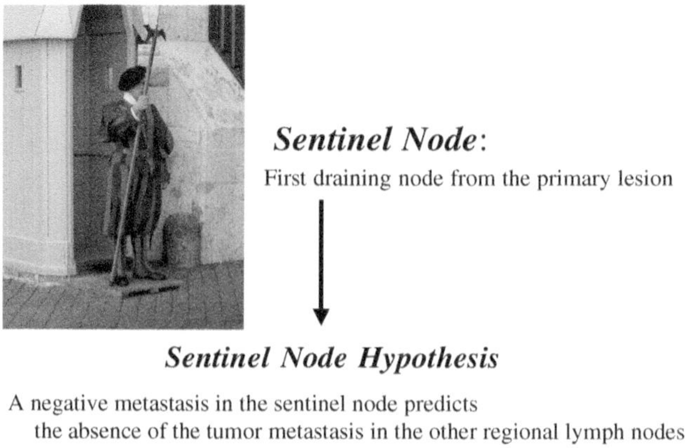

Fig. 1. Definition of sentinel node and sentinel node hypothesis

has been demonstrated in various solid tumors including breast cancers [3,4], malignant melanoma [5], penile cancers [6], and gastrointestinal (GI) cancers [7,8].

Feasibility of Sentinel Node Navigation in Gastric Cancer Surgery

Despite the fact that lymphatic drainage from the GI tract is multidirectional and variable, recent reports from our group and other groups indicate that SN mapping and the detection of metastasis is feasible (Tables 1, 2) [8–32]. Here we introduce the actual methodology of SN navigation surgery and its possible application not only to minimally invasive but also to function-preserving surgery for early gastric cancer.

Endoscopic and Laparoscopic Surgery as a Minimally Invasive Procedure

From the standpoint of minimizing both the invasiveness of the procedure itself and posttreatment loss of gastric volume, endoscopic treatment is superior to other gastric cancer surgeries. Recent progress in endoscopic techniques has enabled the en bloc resection of larger mucosal areas than before, a procedure termed endoscopic submucosal dissection (ESD) (see chapter by M. Fujishiro). The benefit of endoscopic mucosal resection (EMR) can be fully achieved through precise histological examination using resected specimens, so an en bloc resection is always preferable.

Laparoscopic surgery was first introduced into gastric surgery more than a decade ago [33–36] (see chapter by S. Kitano). Since then, the minimal invasiveness of this method has been evidenced in many studies, using a variety of parameters such as postoperative pain, length of postoperative hospital stay, and so on [37,38].

TABLE 1. Summary of sentinel node studies in gastric cancer

Author	No. of patients	Study	Year	Journal	Ref. No.
Kitagawa et al.	36	R	2000	Surg Clin N Am	8
Tsioulias et al.	6	D	2000	Arch Surg	9
Hiratsuka et al.	74	D	2001	Surgery	10
Aikou et al.	18	R, D	2001	Ann Surg Oncol	11
Kitagawa et al.	106	R	2001	Ann Surg Oncol	12
Ichikura et al.	62	D	2002	World J Surg	13
Kitagawa et al.	145	R	2002	Br J Surg	14
Hundley et al.	14	D	2002	Am Surg	15
Carlini et al.	40	D	2002	J Exp Clin Cancer Res	16
Hayashi et al.	31	R, D	2003	J Am Col Surg	17
Yasuda et al.	21	R	2003	Jpn J Clin Oncol	18
Gretschel et al.	15	R	2003	Chirurg	19
Miwa et al.	211	D	2003	Br J Surg	20
Tonouchi et al.	17	R, D	2003	Dig Surg	21
Levine et al.	12	D	2003	J Gastrointest Surg	22
Simsa et al.	22	D	2003	Acta Chir Belg	23
Ajisaka and Miwa	35	D	2003	Br J Surg	24
Ishigami et al.	27	R	2003	J Gastrointest Surg	25
Uenosono et al.	36	R	2003	Cancer Lett	26
Shiozawa et al.	22	D	2003	Hepatogastroenterology	27
Ryu et al.	71	D	2003	Eur J Surg Oncol	28
Song et al.	27	D	2004	Am J Surg	29
Karube et al.	41	R, D	2004	J Surg Oncol	30
Nimura et al.	84	D	2004	Br J Surg	31
Kim et al.	46	R	2004	Ann Surg	32

R, radioactive tracer labeling; D, dye labeling

TABLE 2. Results of sentinel node (SN) biopsy for gastric cancer in Keio University Hospital

Detection rate	97% (262/270)
Number of SN	4.1
Sensitivity	92% (34/37)
Accuracy	99% (259/262)

Source: Keio University Hospital (Jan. 1999–Feb. 2004)

Function-Preserving Gastric Surgery and Its Expected Benefit

Postgastrectomy disturbances such as dumping syndrome, alkaline reflux esophagogastritis, cholecystolithiasis, and reduced food intake from a small gastric volume are unpleasant sequelae in patients undergoing gastrectomy. These conditions lead to body weight loss and malnutrition and may be associated with carcinogenesis in the remnant stomach. A number of methods are now available to minimize or prevent

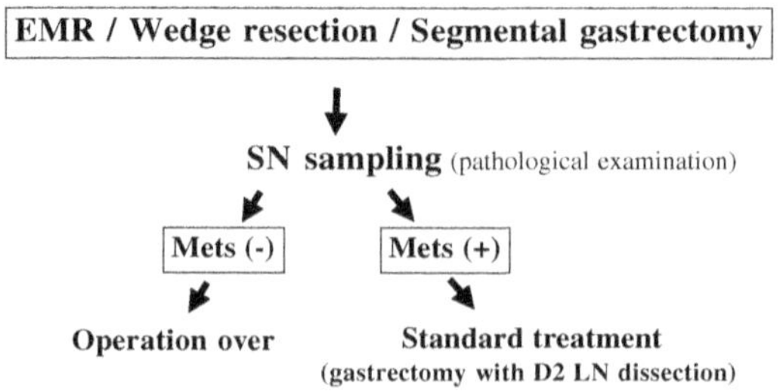

FIG. 3. Strategy for the treatment of early gastric cancer under sentinel node navigation. *EMR*, endoscopic mucosae resection; *LN*, lymph node

these problems. The reduction of resection volume provided by the recently introduced segmental gastrectomy with lymphadenectomy preserves gastric volume and improves QOL in patients with early gastric cancer. Preservation of pylorus function, as a means of avoiding dumping syndrome and duodenal fluid regurgitation, is a current topic of interest among gastric surgeons [39–45]. Further, vagus-sparing gastrectomy involves preservation of the hepatic and celiac branches of the vagus nerve, with the expectation that this will be beneficial in reducing postgastrectomy disturbances as compared with conventional distal gastrectomy.

Treatment Strategy for Early Gastric Carcinoma with Intraoperative Sentinel Node Biopsy

If the SN can be intraoperatively confirmed as negative for metastasis, resection of the cancer lesion with modified LN dissection such as D0, D1 + α, and D1 + β is acceptable. Our treatment protocol under these conditions is shown in Fig. 3. Indications for laparoscopy-assisted segmental gastrectomy for gastric cancer in our institute include the following: (a) T1 (M, SM1), N0, (b) lack of indications for regular EMR, and (c) cancer located in the middle or lower third of the stomach, more than 4 cm from the pyloric ring [46].

Laparoscopy-Assisted Vagus-Sparing Segmental Gastrectomy (LAVSSG) under SN Navigation

We have introduced a novel method of laparoscopy-assisted surgery for early gastric cancer [46] (Fig. 4). For intraoperative SN detection, radiolabeled particles (technetium-99m-radiolabeled tin colloid) are endoscopically injected into the submucosal layer of the lesion 6 h before surgery.

The laparoscopic procedure is done with the patient in the modified lithotomy position. After laparoscopic survey of the abdomen, the gastrocolic ligament is divided 4 cm distal to the epiploic arcade toward the lower pole of the spleen using Ligasure (Valleylab, Boulder, CO, USA). The roots of the left gastroepiploic vessels are exposed and divided using double clips at their origin. The lymph nodes (no. 4sb) along with the left gastroepiploic vessels are dissected from the greater curvature using Ligasure. After division of LN station no. 4d, the root of the right gastroepiploic vein is exposed and secured with double clips and the right gastroepiploic artery is divided at its origin, preserving the infrapyloric artery (Fig. 5).

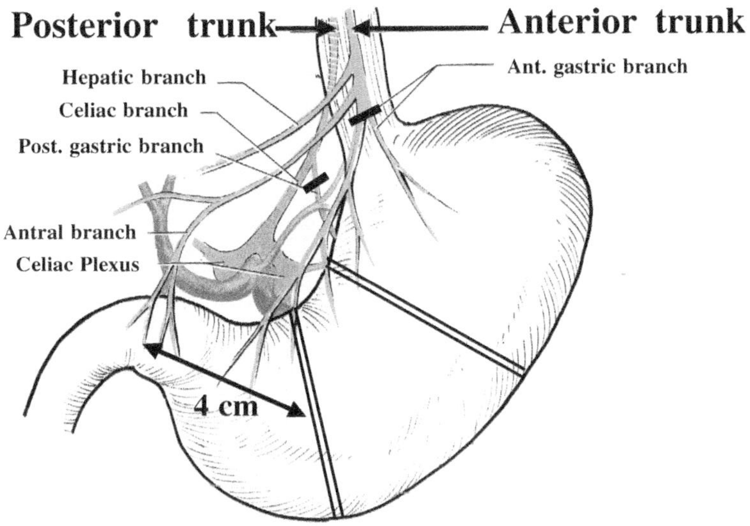

FIG. 4. Surgical anatomy of vagus-sparing segmental gastrectomy (VSSG)

The innervations to the liver (hepatic branch), pylorus (pyloric branch), and small intestine (celiac branch) are preserved (see Fig. 4). The suprapyloric lymph nodes, no. 5, located only on the left side of the vessels, are sampled using the LCS. To preserve vagal nerve innervation of the pylorus, the hepatoduodenal ligament should be kept intact. The gastrohepatic ligament is divided toward the abdominal esophagus to remove the lymph nodes along the lesser curvature. With exposure of the right crus and anterodorsal side of the abdominal esophagus, the white wirelike vagus nerve can be identified under laparoscopic magnified view. The posterior trunk is then isolated with a right-angle clamp and retracted with a vessel loop toward the right side. The stomach is then transected 4 cm proximal to the pylorus using an endoscopic stapling device (60 mm, Endo GIA-II; US Surgical, Norwalk, CT, USA). The lymph nodes along the common hepatic artery, no. 8a, are dissected toward the celiac axis using LCS. Lymph nodes no. 9 and 11p along the common hepatic artery and splenic artery are removed by LCS, exposing the left gastric artery and celiac axis. The celiac branch of the vagus nerve runs down along the lesser curvature to the celiac ganglion together with a branch of the left gastric artery. Retraction of the celiac branch using a vessel loop toward the right side facilitates this procedure (see Fig. 5). Finally, the celiac branch of the posterior vagal trunk is divided from the root of the left gastric artery, which is divided with double clips, thereby keeping the celiac branch and celiac ganglion intact. An en bloc vagus nerve-sparing LN dissection is then completed.

The stomach with perigastric lymph nodes is exteriosed through a midline incisison measuring 5 cm and divided with an ILA 100 stapler (US Surgical). The small abdominal wound is covered with Lap Disc (Ethicon, Cincinnati, OH, USA) and the pneumoperitoneum is established again, confirming the absence of radiolabeled sentinel nodes among residual lymph nodes in the upper abdominal cavity. On a back table, the resected specimen is carefully investigated, and radiolabeled lymph nodes identified with a handheld gamma probe are taken for intraoperative pathological examination (Fig. 6). The gastrogastric anastomosis is created manually with an interrupted layer-to-layer suture. A tube drain is inserted from the right lower trocar wound and placed through the foramen of Winslow, and the abdominal wound is closed. In the case illustrated here, the patient was discharged uneventfully 10 days postoperatively. Postoperative pathological examination revealed that the lesion was mucosal cancer with a negative surgical margin, and no positive lymph nodes were detected including sentinel nodes. On gastroscopy and barium meal 1 year after surgery, gastritis was less obvious than is seen with regular Billroth I anastomosis. Occasionally, peristalsis was observed in the remnant stomach from the oral side to the pyloric ring (Fig. 7).

Unanswered Questions in SN Navigation in Gastric Cancer Surgery

Before SN navigation surgery in gastric cancer treatment can be broadly applied, the following issues require elucidation:

1. Should the tracer be radioactive particles or dye?
2. Should the SN be sampled by pinpoint pickup of the lymph node or lymphatic basin dissection?
3. Should the detection of cancer cells be done using hematoxilin and eosin, immunohistochemistry, or the polymerase chain reaction?

Two nation-wide prospective studies are now examining these issues, one by the Japanese Society of Sentinel Node Navigation Surgery (http://web.sc.itc.keio.ac.jp/surgery/snns/) and the second by the Japan Clinical Oncology Group (http://www.jcog.jp/).

Conclusion

The SN concept in gastric cancer treatment appears ready to assume several important roles in the individualization of treatment in patients with gastric cancer, especially early gastric cancer. The coming decade is likely to see broad general acceptance of minimally invasive and function-preserving surgery based on the sensitive prediction of LN metastasis by SN biopsy.

References

1. Bonenkamp JJ, Hermans J, Sasako M, van de Velde CJ (1999) Extended lymph-node dissection for gastric cancer. N Engl J Med 340:908–914
2. Cuschieri A, Weeden S, Field J, et al. (1999) Patient survival after D1 and D2 resections for gastric cancer: long-term results of the MRC randomized surgical trial. Br J Cancer 340: 1522–1530

3. Giuliano AE, Kirgan DM, Guenther JM, et al. (1994) Lymphatic mapping and sentinel lymphadenectomy for breast cancer. Ann Surg 220:391–401
4. Veronesi U, Paganelli G, Galimberti V, et al. (1997) Sentinel-node biopsy to avoid axillary dissection in breast cancer with clinically negative lymph-nodes. Lancet 349:1864–1867
5. Morton DL, Wen DR, Wong JH, et al. (1992) Technical details of intraoperative lymphatic mapping for early stage melanoma. Arch Surg 127:392–399
6. Cabanas RM (1977) An approach for the treatment of penile carcinoma. Cancer (Phila) 39: 456–466
7. Joosten JJA, Strobbe LJA, Wauters CAP, et al. (1999) Intraoperative lymphatic mapping and sentinel node concept in colorectal carcinoma. Br J Cancer 86:482–486
8. Kitagawa Y, Fujii H, Mukai M, et al. (2000) The role of the sentinel lymph node in gastrointestinal cancer. Surg Clin N Am 80:1799–1809
9. Tsioulias GJ, Wood TF, Morton DL, et al. (2000) Lymphatic mapping and focused analysis of sentinel nodes upstage gastrointestinal neoplasms. Arch Surg 135:926–932
10. Hiratsuka M, Miyashiro I, Ishikawa O, et al. (2001) Application of sentinel node biopsy to gastric cancer surgery. Surgery (St. Louis) 129:335–340
11. Aikou T, Higashi H, Natsugoe S, et al. (2001) Can sentinel node navigation surgery reduce the extent of lymph node dissection in gastric cancer? Ann Surg Oncol 8:90S–93S
12. Kitagawa Y, Ohgami M, Fujii H, et al. (2001) Laparoscopic detection of sentinel lymph nodes in gastrointestinal cancer: a novel and minimally invasive approach. Ann Surg Oncol 8: 86S–89S
13. Ichikura T, Morita D, Uchida T, et al. (2002) Sentinel node concept in gastric carcinoma. World J Surg 26:318–322
14. Kitagawa Y, Fujii H, Mukai M, et al. (2002) Radio-guided sentinel node detection for gastric cancer. Br J Surg 89:604–608
15. Hundley JC, Shen P, Shiver SA, et al. (2002) Lymphatic mapping for gastric adenocarcinoma. Am Surg 68:931–935
16. Carlini M, Carboni F, Petric M, et al. (2002) Sentinel node in gastric cancer surgery. J Exp Clin Cancer Res 21:469–473
17. Hayashi H, Ochiai T, Mori M, et al. (2003) Sentinel node mapping for gastric cancer using a dual procedure with dye- and gamma probe-guided techniques. J Am Coll Surg 196:68–74
18. Yasuda S, Shimada H, Chino O, et al. (2003) Sentinel lymph node detection with Tc-99m tin colloids in patients with esophagogastric cancer. Jpn J Clin Oncol 33:68–72
19. Gretschel S, Bembenek A, Ulmer C, et al. (2003) Lymphatic mapping and sentinel lymph node biopsy in gastric cancer. Chirurg 74:132–138
20. Miwa K, Kinami S, Taniguchi K, et al. (2003) Mapping sentinel nodes in patients with early-stage gastric carcinoma. Br J Surg 90:178–182
21. Tonouchi H, Mohri Y, Tanaka K, et al. (2003) Lymphatic mapping and sentinel node biopsy during laparoscopic gastrectomy for early cancer. Dig Surg 20:421–427
22. Levine EA, Shen P, Shiver SA, et al. (2003) Intraoperative imprint cytology for evaluation of sentinel lymph nodes from visceral malignancies. J Gastrointest Surg 7:687–691
23. Simsa J, Hoch J, Leffler J, et al. (2003) Sentinel node biopsy in gastric cancer: preliminary results. Acta Chir Belg 103:270–273
24. Ajisaka H, Miwa K (2003) Micrometastases in sentinel nodes of gastric cancer. Br J Cancer 18:676–680
25. Ishigami S, Natsugoe S, Uenosono Y, et al. (2003) Infiltration of antitumor immunocytes into the sentinel node in gastric cancer. J Gastrointest Surg 7:735–739
26. Uenosono Y, Natsugoe S, Higashi H, et al. (2003) Evaluation of colloid size for sentinel nodes detection using radioisotope in early gastric cancer. Cancer Lett 200:19–24
27. Shiozawa M, Kawamoto M, Ishiwa, et al. (2003) Clinical usefulness of intraoperative sentinel-node biopsy in gastric cancer. Hepatogastroenterology 50:1187–1189
28. Ryu KW, Lee JH, Kim HS, et al. (2003) Prediction of lymph nodes metastasis by sentinel node biopsy in gastric cancer. Eur J Surg Oncol 29:895–899

29. Song X, Wang L, Chen W, et al. (2004) Lymphatic mapping and sentinel node biopsy in gastric cancer. Am J Surg 187:270–273
30. Karube T, Ochiai T, Shimada H, et al. (2004) Detection of sentinel lymph nodes in gastric cancers based on immunohistochemical analysis of micrometastases. J Surg Oncol 87:32–38
31. Nimura H, Narimiya N, Mitsumori N, et al. (2004) Infrared ray electronic endoscopy combined with indocyanine green injection for detection of sentinel nodes of patients with gastric cancer. Br J Surg 91:575–579
32. Kim MC, Kim HH, Jung GJ, et al. (2004) Lymphatic mapping and sentinel node biopsy using 99mTc tin colloid in gastric cancer. Ann Surg 239:383–387
33. Kitano S, Iso Y, Moriyama M, et al. (1994) Laparoscopy-assisted Billroth I gastrectomy. Surg Laparosc Endosc 4:146–148
34. Uyama I, Ogiwara H, Takahara T, et al. (1994) Laparoscopic and minilaparotomy Billroth I gastrectomy for gastric ulcer using an abdominal wall-lifting method. J Laparoendosc Surg 4:441–445
35. Ohashi S (1995) Laparoscopic intraluminal (intragastric) surgery for early gastric cancer; a new concept in laparoscopic surgery. Surg Endosc 9:169–171
36. Ohgami M, Otani M, Kumai K, et al. (1999) Curative laparoscopic surgery for early gastric cancer: five years experience. World J Surg 23:187–193
37. Yano H, Monden T, Kinuta M, et al. (2001) The usefulness of laparoscopy-assisted distal gastrectomy for early gastric cancer. Gastric Cancer 4:93–97
38. Kitano S, Shiraishi N, Fujii K, et al. (2002) A randomized control trial comparing open vs. laparoscopy-assisted distal gastrectomy for the treatment of early gastric cancer; an interim report. Surgery (St. Louis) 131:S306–S311
39. Isozaki H, Okajima K, Momura E, et al. (1996) Postoperative evaluation of pylorus-preserving gastrectomy for early gastric cancer. Br J Surg 83:266–269
40. Zhang D, Shimoyama S, Kaminishi M (1998) Feasibility of pylorus-preserving gastrectomy with a wider scope of lymphadenectomy Arch Surg 133:993–997
41. Ohwada S, Nakamura S, Ogawa T, et al. (1999) Segmental gastrectomy for early cancer in the mid-stomach. Hepatogastroenterology 46:1229–1233
42. Furukawa H, Hiratsuka M, Imaoka S, et al. (1999) Phase II study of limited surgery for early gastric cancer: segmental gastric resection. Ann Surg Oncol 6:166–170
43. Kodera Y, Yamamura Y, Kanemitsu Y, et al. (2001) Lymph node metastasis in cancer of the middle-third stomach: criteria for treatment with a pylorus-preserving gastrectomy. Surg Today 31:196–203
44. Iseki J, Takagi M, Touyama K, et al. (2003) Editorial comment: feasibility of central gastrectomy for gastric cancer. Surgery (St. Louis) 133:68–73
45. Urushihara T, Sumimoto K, Shimokado K, et al. (2004) Gastric motility after laparoscopically assited distal gastrectomy, with or without preservation of pylorus, for early gastric cancer, as assessed by digital dynamic x-ray imaging. Surg Endosc 18:964–968
46. Otani Y, Furukawa T, Kitagawa Y, et al. (2004) New method of laparoscopy-assisted function-preserving surgery for early gastric cancer: vagus-sparing segmental gastrectomy under sentinel node navigation. J Am Coll Surg 198:1026–1031

Color Plates

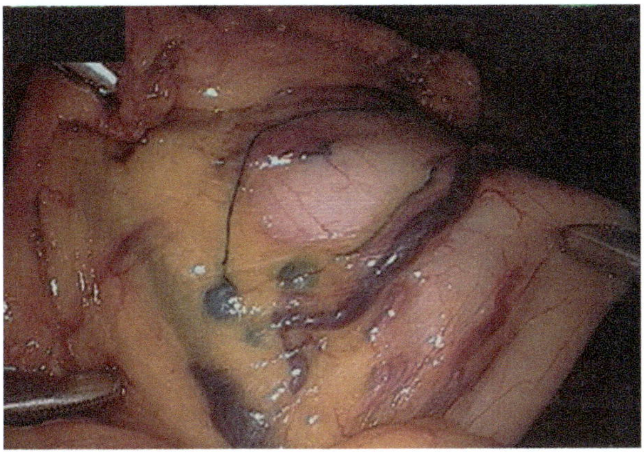

Fig. 2. Laparoscopic detection of sentinel nodes in gastric cancer. Sentinel nodes (lymph node station of no. 4d) are visible after intraoperative injection of blue dye into the submucosal layer under the mucosal cancer lesion

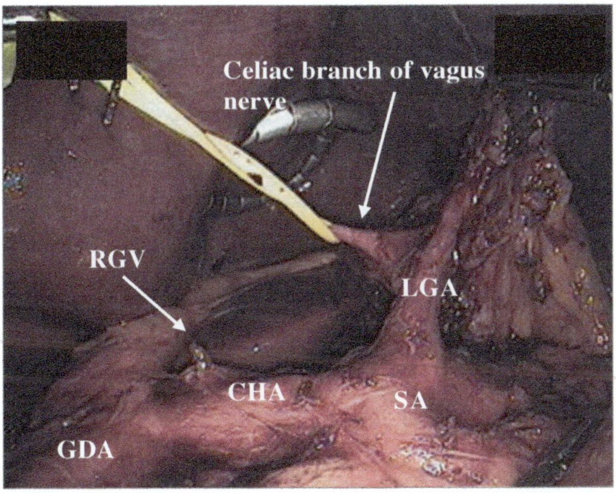

Fig. 5. Preservation of the celiac branch of the vagus nerve. The celiac branch of the posterior trunk is separated from the left gastric artery. Retraction of the celiac branch using a vessel loop toward the right side facilitates this procedure. *CHA*, common hepatic artery; *LGA*, left gastric artery; *SA*, splenic artery; *GDA*, gastroduodenal artery; *RGV*, stump of right gastric vein

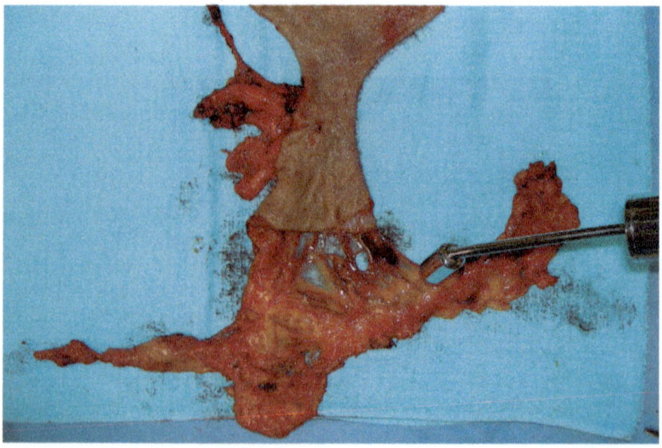

Fig. 6. Detection of radioactive lymph node in the resected specimen on the back table using handheld gamma probe

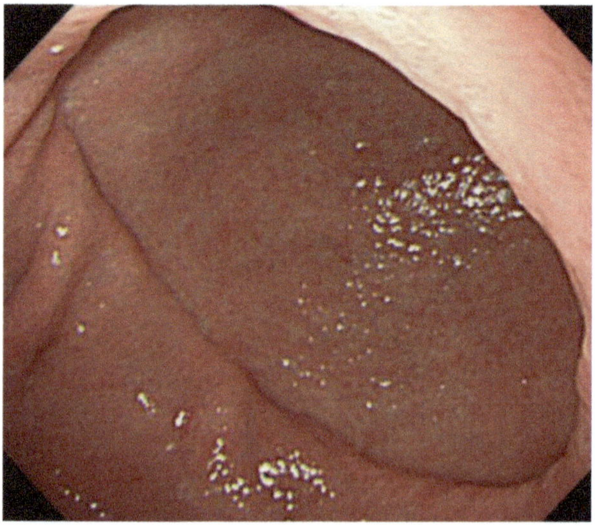

Fig. 7. Findings of endoscopy 1 year after laparoscopic-assisted VSSG (LAVSSG). Mucosal inflammation, which is commonly observed in the residual stomach of Billroth I anastomosis, is not obvious after pylorus preserving (segmental) gastrectomy. Also, peristalsis can be observed in the residual stomach

Index

GPSR Compliance

The European Union's (EU) General Product Safety Regulation (GPSR) is a set of rules that requires consumer products to be safe and our obligations to ensure this.

If you have any concerns about our products, you can contact us on ProductSafety@springernature.com

In case Publisher is established outside the EU, the EU authorized representative is:

Springer Nature Customer Service Center GmbH
Europaplatz 3
69115 Heidelberg, Germany

Batch number: 10755466

Printed by Printforce, the Netherlands